BIOPSY INTERPRETATION SERIES

BIOPSY INTERPRETATION
OF THE PROSTATE

5th Edition

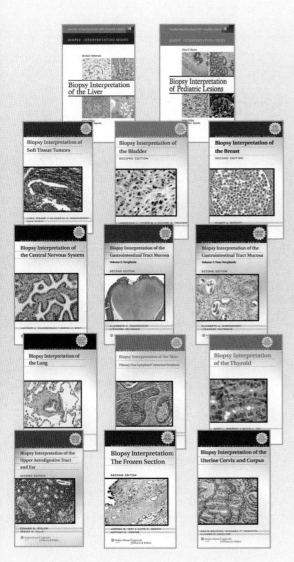

BIOPSY INTERPRETATION SERIES:

BIOPSY INTERPRETATION

OF THE PROSTATE

5th Edition

Jonathan I. Epstein, MD

Professor of Pathology, Urology, and Oncology
The Reinhard Professor of Urological Pathology
Director of Surgical Pathology
The Johns Hopkins Medical Institutions
Baltimore, Maryland

George J. Netto, MD

Professor of Pathology, Urology, and Oncology
Director of Surgical Pathology Molecular Diagnostics
Johns Hopkins Medical Institutions
Baltimore, Maryland

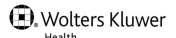

Health

Philadelphia • Baltimore • New York • London
Buenos Aires • Hong Kong • Sydney • Tokyo

Acquisitions Editor: Ryan Shaw
Product Manager: Kate Marshall
Production Product Manager: David Saltzberg
Senior Manufacturing Coordinator: Beth Welsh
Marketing Manager: Dan Dressler
Designer: Doug Smock
Production Service: Absolute Service, Inc.

© 2015 by WOLTERS KLUWER HEALTH
Two Commerce Square
2001 Market Street
Philadelphia, PA 19103 USA
LWW.com

Fourth edition, © 2008 Lippincott Williams & Wilkins
Third edition, © 2002 Lippincott Williams & Wilkins
Second Edition, © 1995 Lippincott-Raven Publishers
First Edition, © 1989 Raven Press

Printed in China

Library of Congress Cataloging-in-Publication Data

Epstein, Jonathan I., author.
  Biopsy interpretation of the prostate / Jonathan I. Epstein, George J. Netto. — Fifth edition.
    p. ; cm. — (Biopsy interpretation series)
  Includes bibliographical references and index.
    ISBN 978-1-4511-8674-1
  I. Netto, George J., author. II. Title. III. Series: Biopsy interpretation series.
  [DNLM: 1. Prostatic Neoplasms—diagnosis. 2. Biopsy, Needle. 3. Prostatic Diseases— diagnosis. WJ 762]
  RC280.P7
  616.99'463—dc23
                                                            2014015250

Care has been taken to confirm the accuracy of the information presented and to describe generally accepted practices. However, the authors, editors, and publisher are not responsible for errors or omissions or for any consequences from application of the information in this book and make no warranty, expressed or implied, with respect to the currency, completeness, or accuracy of the contents of the publication. Application of the information in a particular situation remains the professional responsibility of the practitioner.

The authors, editors, and publisher have exerted every effort to ensure that drug selection and dosage set forth in this text are in accordance with current recommendations and practice at the time of publication. However, in view of ongoing research, changes in government regulations, and the constant flow of information relating to drug therapy and drug reactions, the reader is urged to check the package insert for each drug for any change in indications and dosage and for added warnings and precautions. This is particularly important when the recommended agent is a new or infrequently employed drug.

Some drugs and medical devices presented in the publication have Food and Drug Administration (FDA) clearance for limited use in restricted research settings. It is the responsibility of the health care provider to ascertain the FDA status of each drug or device planned for use in their clinical practice.

To purchase additional copies of this book, call our customer service department at (800) 638-3030 or fax orders to (301) 223-2320. International customers should call (301) 223-2300.

Visit Lippincott Williams & Wilkins on the Internet: at LWW.com. Lippincott Williams & Wilkins customer service representatives are available from 8:30 am to 6 pm, EST.

10 9 8 7 6 5 4 3 2 1

RRS1406

DEDICATION

In 1989, for my first edition of *Prostate Biopsy Interpretation*, I wrote ". . . to my two precious children, David and Jeremy, who make each day a new and wondrous experience full of joy and inspiration." They were 4 and 2 years old, respectively, at the time. It is amazing to think that as I once again dedicate this fifth edition to my sons, they are now residents in internal medicine: David in his final year at UCLA and Jeremy an intern at Hopkins. I could not be more proud of them for being such caring individuals to their friends, family, and patients. I am even more proud that their sensitivity extends beyond their immediate sphere to animal welfare, the environment, and the disadvantaged. Other pathologists often ask if I am disappointed that they are not going into pathology. Quite the opposite, I am just thrilled that they have found their passion and will be great physicians helping people in whatever specialty they have chosen.

—Jonathan Epstein

To my parents Faez and Juliette for their unlimited love and support.

—George Netto

PREFACE

The fifth edition of the *Biopsy Interpretation of the Prostate* brings the field of prostate pathology up to date since the last edition published in 2008. The new edition covers new immunohistochemical markers used for the diagnosis of prostate cancer and its distinction from mimickers. Expanded sections cover common and rare pitfalls of immunohistochemistry in the diagnosis of adenocarcinoma of the prostate. New entities such as fibromyxoid nephrogenic adenoma, high-grade foamy gland carcinoma, new variants of ductal adenocarcinoma and high-grade prostatic intraepithelial neoplasia (PIN), and prostate cancer with aberrant p63 expression are covered. Lesions that were just being introduced in the fourth edition, such as intraductal carcinoma, PIN-like ductal carcinoma, and variants of stromal tumors of the prostate, are now discussed more thoroughly. The fifth edition updates the correlation of needle biopsy carcinoma grade and extent, atypical findings suspicious for carcinoma, and PIN with results at radical prostatectomy. Since the fourth edition, there have been further significant modifications to the Gleason grading system. The current edition covers these changes in detail along with an increased discussion as to how grade impacts clinical decisions. The chapter on neuroendocrine differentiation in the prostate has been totally reworked to reflect the recent consensus conference on this topic. Finally, the fifth edition updates the molecular findings of prostate cancer and how it may affect therapy and predicting prognosis.

Jonathan I. Epstein, MD
George J. Netto, MD

PREFACE TO THE FIRST EDITION

Within the last few years, there has been much change in both our knowledge and our concepts concerning many prostatic entities. The advances in surgical and radiological techniques have led to an increased number of prostate biopsies being performed, and recent pathological techniques have facilitated our evaluation of prostate biopsy material.

New surgical techniques have been developed to enable radical prostatectomy to be performed with minimal morbidity, leading to more aggressive diagnosis and treatment of prostatic carcinoma. Even small, low-grade, incidentally discovered adenocarcinomas of the prostate found in relatively young men may now be treated aggressively because of the lower morbidity and the recently recognized increased risk of long-term progression. The increasing use of transrectal ultrasound and the recent development of biopsy guns that generate thin-core biopsy material with minimal morbidity have resulted in, and will continue to result in, increased numbers of core needle biopsy specimens to evaluate.

Currently, there are only a few general urologic pathology books, and they tend to summarize previous data, often without critically analyzing controversial topics. Furthermore, because of the general nature of these books, only a few photographs are present, and they do not provide the practicing pathologist sufficient help when confronted with diagnostically difficult lesions.

I am very fortunate to practice in an institution at which a wealth of prostate specimens is available for study. More than 600 biopsies (needle and transurethral resection specimens) and almost 200 radical prostatectomies are performed at our institution each year. This book contains an extensive number of photographs culled from these procedures, which will help pathologists in their day-to-day practice with difficult and unusual lesions, as well as common problems encountered in prostate pathology. These include:

1. The distinction between allergic, infectious, posttransurethral resection, and nonspecific granulomatous prostatitis;
2. Differentiation of low-grade adenocarcinoma from adenosis and basal cell hyperplasia;
3. A practical approach to the Gleason grading system on biopsy material correlation with radical prostatectomy findings, and the influence of grade on therapeutic decisions;
4. Use of immunohistochemical techniques, such as a prostate-specific antigen, prostate-specific acid phosphatase, and basal-cell-specific antibodies, in the diagnosis of prostate cancer, along with their limitations and potential pitfalls;
5. diagnosis of limited cancer on needle biopsy specimens; and

6. illustrations of rare and recently described entities, such as post-operative spindle cell nodules involving the prostate, cystosarcoma phyllodes of the prostate, adenoid cystic carcinoma of the prostate, and clear cell cribiforming hyperplasia of the prostate.

Commonly encountered problems such as cautery artifact on transure-thral resection material, crush artifact on needle biopsy specimens, and the distinction between high-grade transitional cell carcinoma and poorly differentiated adenocarcinoma are all dealt with from the experience of a practicing pathologist who deals with these issues on a day-to-day basis. Furthermore, difficult cases have been selected to include those cases in which the patient underwent radical surgery based on the diagnosis, such that the diagnosis of carcinoma was verified.

In addition to thoroughly illustrating diagnostically difficult and unusual lesions, as well as addressing practical problems in the interpretation of prostate biopsies, the text discusses controversial and confusing topics encountered in prostate pathology. These topics include:

1. Classification and prognosis of stage A (incidentally discovered) prostatic carcinoma;
2. Intraductal dysplasia of the prostate, its association with cancer, its distinction from other entities not significantly linked with carcinoma, and the significance of finding dysplasia alone on biopsy material;
3. Current thoughts on unusual variants of prostate cancer, such as prostatic duct carcinoma (endometrioid carcinoma), colloid carcinoma of the prostate, and carcinomas with neuroendocrine differentiation (small cell carcinoma, carcinoid); and
4. Transitional cell carcinoma involving the prostate as it relates to conservative therapy for early bladder cancer, significance of in-situ transitional cell carcinoma involving the prostate, and significance in identification of prostatic stromal invasion by transitional cell carcinoma.

This book will be of interest to all pathologists who evaluate biopsy material from the prostate. In addition, the discussion of the various clinicopathological features concerning each lesion will be a useful reference to pathologists in general.

Jonathan I. Epstein
1989

CONTENTS

Preface vi
Preface to the First Edition vii

1   Clinical Correlates with Biopsy: Serum Prostate-Specific
Antigen, Digital Rectal Examination, and Imaging Techniques 1

2   Needle Biopsy Technique, Tissue Sampling, and
Processing of Needle Biopsy and Transurethral
Resection Specimens 8

3   Gross Anatomy and Normal Histology 16

4   Inflammatory Conditions 25

5   Preneoplastic Lesions in the Prostate:
Prostatic Intraepithelial Neoplasia and
Intraductal Carcinoma of the Prostate 38

6   Diagnosis of Limited Adenocarcinoma
of the Prostate 83

7   Mimickers of Adenocarcinoma of the Prostate 130

8   Reporting Cancer: Influence on Prognosis
and Treatment 185

9   Grading of Prostatic Adenocarcinomas 202

10   Findings of Atypical Glands Suspicious for Cancer 235

11   Prostatic Duct Adenocarcinoma 254

12   Neuroendocrine Differentiation in the Benign
and Malignant Prostate 268

13   Mucinous Differentiation in the Benign and
Malignant Prostate 291

14   Benign and Malignant Prostate following Treatment 298

15   Urothelial Carcinoma 314

16   Mesenchymal Tumors and Tumor-like Conditions 333

17   Miscellaneous Benign and Malignant Lesions 355

18   Prostatic Urethral Lesions 377

19   Emerging Biomarkers for Detection and
Management of Prostate Carcinoma 392

Appendix: Macros 411
Index 418

1

CLINICAL CORRELATES WITH BIOPSY: SERUM PROSTATE-SPECIFIC ANTIGEN, DIGITAL RECTAL EXAMINATION, AND IMAGING TECHNIQUES

Needle biopsies of the prostate are typically performed either because of an abnormal rectal exam or elevated serum prostate-specific antigen (PSA) level; some men are screened because of a strong family history of prostate cancer.

DIGITAL RECTAL EXAMINATION

Asymmetry, induration, and discrete hard nodules are findings on digital rectal examination (DRE) that are suspicious for cancer. The positive predictive value of core needle biopsy of the prostate varies depending on the degree of the palpable abnormality of the prostate, with marked induration or a nodule more likely representing carcinoma than mild firmness.

The positive predictive value of an abnormal DRE is only 22% to 36%.[1] A more serious limitation of DRE is its low sensitivity (i.e., missing cancer). Currently, the majority of cancers clinically detected by needle biopsy are nonpalpable (stage T1c). Although some of these tumors are small, 51% are more than 0.5 cc and located in the peripheral zone, so that one would have expected them to be palpable. Another 15% to 25% of stage T1c prostate cancers are located in the transition zone (anteriorly) where they are not palpable due to their location.[2,3]

There is poor interobserver reproducibility even among urologists as to what is an abnormal DRE.[4]

IMAGING TECHNIQUES

The most commonly used imaging modality for prostate cancer remains transrectal ultrasound (TRUS). The majority of prostate cancers appear

1

on TRUS as hypoechoic relative to the normal peripheral zone, although tumors may also be hyperechoic or isoechoic. Despite initial studies claiming a great value of this test for the detection of prostate cancer, subsequent reports have noted poor sensitivity and specificity limiting its usefulness.[5,6]

Cancer is as likely to be found in areas that are normal by TRUS as they are to be detected in radiographically abnormal areas. Currently, the major role of TRUS is to direct the needle biopsies of the prostate in either a sextant or alternative (see Chapter 2) distribution. Another function of TRUS is to estimate the size of the prostate that can be used to calculate PSA density (see the following text). Even this role of TRUS is limited because there is not a great correlation between prostate volume estimated by TRUS and actual prostate volume.[7]

In part, limitations of TRUS relate to differences in the equipment used and that the exam is heavily operator dependent. Enhanced TRUS modalities include the use of ultrasound contrast agents and color and power Doppler ultrasound, which have only demonstrated incremental improvements over standard gray-scale ultrasonography.

Over the last decade, endorectal magnetic resonance imaging (MRI) and, more recently, multiparametric MRI (mpMRI) have increasingly been used in clinical staging of localized prostate cancer patients. mpMRI adds other modalities beyond the morphology provided by standard T2-weighted images. Some of the more common techniques in mpMRI include diffusion-weighted images (DWI) where the denser packing of prostate cancer relative to benign tissue restricts water diffusion. Another often performed function is dynamic contrast-enhanced (DCE) images where following injection of intravenous contrast, neoangiogenesis can be seen. Less commonly used, mpMRI spectroscopy can quantify the ratio of choline/citrate. Although mpMRI has shown the potential to improve the accuracy of clinical staging and the positive yield (sensitivity) of prostate biopsy,[8–10] its use has yet to become a standard of care given its relatively modest sensitivity and specificity (76% and 82%, respectively) and the need for larger prospective trials. mpMRI role in prostate cancer patients eligible for active surveillance is under intense investigation.[11–13]

Several positron emission tomography (PET) tracers are active in early-stage and late-stage prostate cancer. F18-fluorodeoxyglucose (FDG), C11/F18-choline, and sodium F18-fluoride have been studied most extensively. There is growing evidence supporting the use of choline in early-stage prostate cancer. FDG and sodium F18-fluoride are more valuable in advanced disease, especially for assessing bone metastases. Prostate-specific membrane antigen (PSMA) PET tracers are in the early stages of clinical development. Prospective clinical imaging trials are needed to establish the optimal role of PET in prostate cancer.[14]

PROSTATE-SPECIFIC ANTIGEN

PSA is synthesized in the ductal epithelium and prostatic acini. It is found in normal, hyperplastic, and malignant prostate tissue.[15]

PSA is secreted into the lumina of the prostatic ducts to become a component of the seminal plasma. It reaches the serum by diffusion from the luminal cells through the epithelial basement membrane and stroma where it can pass through the capillary basement membranes. PSA is a serine protease of the human glandular kallikrein family. In the seminal fluid are gel-forming proteins that function to trap spermatozoa at ejaculation. PSA functions to liquefy the coagulum and break down the seminal clot through proteolysis of the gel-forming proteins into smaller, more soluble fragments, thus releasing the spermatozoa.

Total Serum Prostate-Specific Antigen

Numerous studies have shown that patients with prostate cancer have, in general, elevated serum PSA levels relative to men without prostate cancer. The most commonly used cutoff for PSA is 4 ng/mL. When serum PSA concentrations are 4 to 10 ng/mL, the incidence of cancer detection on prostate biopsy in men with a normal DRE is approximately 25%. With serum PSA levels over 10 ng/mL, the incidence of prostate cancer on a biopsy increases to approximately 67%. However, the risk of cancer is proportional to the serum PSA level even at values below 4 ng/mL. With a serum PSA of less than 2 ng/mL, the probability of cancer is less than 2%, rising to about 18% for PSA values of 2.5 to 4.0 ng/mL. As large screening trials have demonstrated clinically significant cancers in men with serum PSA levels of 2.5 to 4.0 ng/mL, some experts have proposed lowering the PSA cutoff to 2.5 ng/mL to improve the early detection of cancer in younger men.[15]

The reason why serum PSA levels are not diagnostic of prostate cancer is that benign prostate tissue also produces serum PSA. Other factors such as prostatitis, infarct, instrumentation of the prostate, and ejaculation also increase serum PSA levels. Routine DRE does not appear to elevate serum PSA levels, although vigorous prostatic massages and prostate needle biopsies do. Following an inciting event, it is recommended that one waits 4 to 6 weeks before using PSA levels to guide clinical decision making. Finasteride, used to treat benign prostatic hyperplasia and hair loss, lowers serum PSA levels on average by approximately 50%. In an attempt to improve the utility of serum PSA tests to detect prostate cancer, while minimizing biopsies performed on men who do not have prostate cancer, variations of the PSA test have been developed.

Prostate-Specific Antigen Density

As noted earlier, benign prostate tissue also contributes to serum PSA levels, although not to the same extent as does cancer. Men with enlarged hyperplastic prostate glands will have higher total serum PSA levels than men with small glands. The measurement of serum PSA density factors out the contribution of benign prostatic tissue to serum PSA levels. Serum PSA density reflects the PSA produced per gram of prostate tissue. It is calculated by dividing the total serum PSA level by the estimated gland volume (usually determined by TRUS measurements) with an upper normal value of approximately 0.15. There are conflicting studies as to the advantage of PSA density over that of total serum PSA to detect prostate cancer. Furthermore, the measurement of prostatic volume by TRUS does not correlate particularly well with actual prostatic volume.

Age-Specific Prostate-Specific Antigen Reference Ranges

As men age, their prostates tend to enlarge with benign prostatic hyperplasia. One would then anticipate that, overall, older men would have higher serum PSA levels than younger men. Derived from measurements of serum PSA levels in a large group of men of varying ages without prostate cancer, the recommended age-specific upper reference ranges for serum PSA are 2.5 ng/mL for men 40 to 49 years of age, 3.5 ng/mL for men 50 to 59 years, 4.5 ng/mL for men 60 to 69 years, and 6.5 ng/mL for men 70 to 79 years. The net effect of using such age-specific PSA reference ranges is that there will be a greater number of biopsies performed in younger men with relatively low serum PSA levels and less biopsies performed in older men with serum PSA levels slightly above the "normal cutoff" of 4.0 ng/mL.

Prostate-Specific Antigen Velocity (Rate of Change of Prostate-Specific Antigen)

PSA velocity is based on data from the Baltimore Longitudinal Study of Aging. This is a long-term prospective aging study by the National Institute of Aging where a large group of male subjects return every 2 years for several days of evaluation, including serum PSA tests. Those men who eventually were diagnosed as having prostate cancer had an increased rate of rise in PSA as compared to men who did not have prostate cancer. The rate of change in PSA that best distinguished between men with and without prostate cancer was 0.75 ng/mL per year. Whereas 72% of men with prostate cancer had a PSA velocity of 0.75 ng/mL per year or more, only 5% of men without prostate cancer had a PSA velocity above this cutoff. In order for this test to be valid, it requires that there be at least three PSA measurements available over a period of 1.5 to 2 years. That is because there is substantial short-term variability (up to 20%) between repeat PSA measurements. In a man who has a significant rise in serum PSA levels even though the latest serum PSA test may be less than 4 ng/mL, this finding is abnormal and should prompt a workup.

Molecular Forms of Prostate-Specific Antigen

In the early 1990s, it was discovered that there are several different molecular forms of PSA in the serum. Once PSA is leaked into the circulation, most is bound to serine protease inhibitors. The three most recognizable inhibitors are α-1 antichymotrypsin (ACT), α-2 macroglobulin, and α-1 protein inhibitor. PSA bound to ACT is the most immunoreactive and is the one clinically most useful in diagnosing prostate cancer. A smaller fraction (5% to 40%) of the measurable serum PSA is free (noncomplexed) PSA. The total serum PSA measured, therefore, reflects both free and complexed PSA.

It has been demonstrated that the percent of free PSA can improve the specificity of PSA testing for prostate cancer. In general, men with a higher percent of free PSA levels in the serum are less likely to have cancer. For men with PSA values of 2.5 to 10 ng/mL, a percent free PSA cutoff of 25% or more is associated with only a 5% risk of prostate cancer and may reduce 20% to 30% unnecessary biopsies. A percent free PSA value of less than 10% is worrisome for cancer. The most common use of this test is for men with a normal DRE and serum PSA values of between 4 and 10 ng/mL in deciding whether to perform a repeat biopsy following an initial negative biopsy.

More recently, additional isoforms of free PSA have been discovered.[15] When PSA is first secreted, it is in the form of a precursor form of PSA termed *pro-PSA*. This inactive PSA form constitutes the majority of free PSA in serum in men with prostate cancer, and a relative increase in pro-PSA is seen in men with prostate cancer. BPSA ("benign PSA") refers to a cleaved form of PSA from BPH tissue. The ratio of pro-PSA/BPSA has been proposed as a means of improving the accuracy of diagnosing cancer in men with very low percent free PSA levels who are at relatively high risk of cancer.[16]

Initially, technical problems with assay development prevented the direct measurement of complexed PSA. Rather, complexed PSA was estimated by subtracting free PSA from total PSA. Complexed PSA can now be directly assayed and in some studies have shown minimal enhancement over other PSA tests. However, in current practice, only percent free-to-total PSA is in routine clinical use among the various molecular forms of PSA.

Prostate-Specific Antigen Relation to Post-therapy Follow-up Biopsies

Serum PSA tests may also be used to monitor various treatments of prostate cancer in deciding whether post-therapy biopsies are needed. Following radical prostatectomy, the serum PSA should drop to undetectable levels. Elevated serum PSA levels following radical prostatectomy (>0.2 ng/mL) indicate recurrent or persistent disease. Ultrasensitive PSA assays allow a lower limit of detection than standard PSA assays and are used by a minority of clinicians to predict earlier biochemical relapse following radical prostatectomy.[17] Following radiotherapy for prostate cancer, serum PSA values will decrease to a nadir although not to the same extent as those following radical prostatectomy. A PSA value that is ≥2 ng/ml than the nadir level after radiation indicates treatment failure.

Finally, the continuous debate on whether current serum PSA–based screening strategies are warranted and whether they are potentially leading to "overtreatment" of a subset of prostate cancer patients has fueled a strong interest in pursuing clinicopathologic and molecular parameters that may help identify patients with biologically "significant" prostate cancers (see Chapter 19).

A large multi-institutional trial (Prostate, Lung, Colorectal, and Ovarian [PLCO] Cancer Screening Trial) was undertaken to determine whether there is a reduction in prostate cancer mortality from screening using serum PSA testing and DRE. Surprisingly, the study found an almost identical cumulative mortality rates (3.7 and 3.4 deaths per 10,000 person-years) from prostate cancer in patients who were annually screened and those who were not showing no statistically significant survival advantage.[18,19]

However, there are major criticisms of the PLCO Trial in that there was significant contamination of the control arm with men who had prior PSA testing. The findings are in contrast to those of the "European Randomized Study of Screening for Prostate Cancer" that pointed to a relative reduction in the risk of death from prostate cancer in the serum PSA screening group of 29%. The absolute reduction in mortality from prostate cancer in the screening group was 1.07 deaths per 1,000 men who underwent randomization. The fact remained, however, that there was no significant difference between the two groups in all-cause mortality, and in order to prevent one death from prostate cancer at 11 years of follow-up, 1,055 men would need to be invited for screening and 37 cancers would need to be detected and treated.[20–22]

A recently introduced American Urological Association (AUA) guideline on detection of prostate cancer suggests that the strongest evidence that benefits of serum PSA screening may outweigh harms is in men aged 55 to 69 years undergoing PSA-based screening. This led the AUA panel to recommend shared decision making for these men at average risk but recommend against routine screening for other age groups at below average risk.[23,24]

REFERENCES

1. Scardino PT, Weaver R, Hudson MA. Early detection of prostate cancer. *Hum Pathol.* 1992;23:211–222.
2. Epstein JI, Walsh PC, Carmichael M, et al. Pathologic and clinical findings to predict tumor extent of nonpalpable (stage T1c) prostate cancer. *JAMA.* 1994;271:368–374.
3. Carter HB, Sauvageot J, Walsh PC, et al. Prospective evaluation of men with stage T1C adenocarcinoma of the prostate. *J Urol.* 1997;157:2206–2209.
4. Angulo JC, Montie JE, Bukowsky T. Interobserver consistency of digital rectal examination in clinical setting of localized prostatic carcinoma. *Urol Oncol.* 1995;1:199–205.

5. Carter HB, Hamper UM, Sheth S, et al. Evaluation of transrectal ultrasound in the early detection of prostate cancer. *J Urol*. 1989;142:1008–1010.

6. Coffield KS, Speights VO, Brawn PN, et al. Ultrasound detection of prostate cancer in postmortem specimens with histological correlation. *J Urol*. 1992;147:822–826.

7. Matthews GJ, Motta J, Fracehia JA. The accuracy of transrectal ultrasound prostate volume estimation: clinical correlations. *J Clin Ultrasound*. 1996;24:501–505.

8. Trabulsi EJ, Merriam WG, Gomella LG. New imaging techniques in prostate cancer. *Curr Urol Rep*. 2006;7:175–180.

9. Wu LM, Xu JR, Ye YQ, et al. The clinical value of diffusion-weighted imaging in combination with T2-weighted imaging in diagnosing prostate carcinoma: a systematic review and meta-analysis. *AJR Am J Roentgenol*. 2012;199:103–110.

10. Delongchamps NB, Rouanne M, Flam T, et al. Multiparametric magnetic resonance imaging for the detection and localization of prostate cancer: combination of T2-weighted, dynamic contrast-enhanced and diffusion-weighted imaging. *BJU Int*. 2011;107:1411–1418.

11. Robertson NL, Emberton M, Moore CM. MRI-targeted prostate biopsy: a review of technique and results. *Nat Rev Urol*. 2013;10:589–597.

12. Park BH, Jeon HG, Choo SH, et al. Role of multiparametric 3.0 tesla magnetic resonance imaging in prostate cancer patients eligible for active surveillance [published online ahead of print August 23, 2013]. *BJU Int*. doi:10.1111/bju.12423.

13. Mullins JK, Bonekamp D, Landis P, et al. Multiparametric magnetic resonance imaging findings in men with low-risk prostate cancer followed using active surveillance. *BJU Int*. 2013;111:1037–1045.

14. Fox JJ, Schoder H, Larson SM. Molecular imaging of prostate cancer. *Curr Opin Urol*. 2012;22:320–327.

15. Gretzer MB, Partin AW. PSA markers in prostate cancer detection. *Urol Clin North Am*. 2003;30:677–686.

16. Khan MA, Sokoll LJ, Chan DW, et al. Clinical utility of proPSA and "benign" PSA when percent free PSA is less than 15%. *Urology*. 2004;64:1160–1164.

17. Shen S, Lepor H, Yaffee R, et al. Ultrasensitive serum prostate specific antigen nadir accurately predicts the risk of early relapse after radical prostatectomy. *J Urol*. 2005;173:777–780.

18. Andriole GL, Crawford ED, Grubb RL III, et al. Prostate cancer screening in the randomized Prostate, Lung, Colorectal, and Ovarian Cancer Screening Trial: mortality results after 13 years of follow-up. *J Natl Cancer Inst*. 2012;104:125–132.

19. Andriole GL, Crawford ED, Grubb RL III, et al. Mortality results from a randomized prostate-cancer screening trial. *N Engl J Med*. 2009;360:1310–1319.

20. Schroder FH, Hugosson J, Roobol MJ, et al. Screening and prostate-cancer mortality in a randomized European study. *N Engl J Med*. 2009;360:1320–1328.

21. Schroder FH, Hugosson J, Roobol MJ, et al. Prostate-cancer mortality at 11 years of follow-up. *N Engl J Med*. 2012;366:981–990.

22. Bokhorst LP, Bangma CH, van Leenders GJ, et al. Prostate-specific antigen-based prostate cancer screening: reduction of prostate cancer mortality after correction for nonattendance and contamination in the Rotterdam Section of the European Randomized Study of Screening for Prostate Cancer. *Eur Urol*. 2014;65:329–336.

23. Carter HB. American Urological Association (AUA) guideline on prostate cancer detection: process and rationale. *BJU Int*. 2013;112:543–547.

24. Carter HB, Albertsen PC, Barry MJ, et al. Early detection of prostate cancer: AUA guideline. *J Urol*. 2013;190:419–426.

2

NEEDLE BIOPSY TECHNIQUE, TISSUE SAMPLING, AND PROCESSING OF NEEDLE BIOPSY AND TRANSURETHRAL RESECTION SPECIMENS

NEEDLE BIOPSY TECHNIQUE

In the past, the standard method used to diagnose prostate cancer was that of ultrasound-guided systematic sextant biopsy.[1] Routine sextant biopsies sample the parasagittal midlobe region of the prostate despite the recognition that many prostate cancers arise posterolaterally.[2] In recent years, studies have suggested alternative needle biopsy sampling techniques to increase prostate cancer detection. Three general modifications of the sextant biopsy technique have been proposed: (a) addition of transition zone biopsies, (b) addition of biopsies for enlarged prostates, and (c) modifying the location of the nontransition zone biopsies. Investigations of nonpalpable (stage T1c) prostate cancer note that 15% to 22% of tumors are located anteriorly within the transition zone.[3,4]

However, most studies demonstrate a low incidence of cancer found solely in the transition zone biopsy.[5,6] A recognized use of transition zone biopsies is when findings are very suspicious for cancer, yet the initial biopsy is benign.[7] Modifications of routine sextant biopsies have also been proposed based on the size of the prostate gland. Several studies have shown that with larger prostates, there is decreased detection of prostate cancer.[8–12]

More recently, emphasis on transition zone sampling have been placed in the setting of active surveillance protocols based on the findings by our group and others from radical prostatectomy specimens in patients who were converted from active surveillance to surgical resection. The greatest concern for adopting active surveillance in very low–risk patients remains the risk of missing a high-risk cancer due to undersampling on prostate biopsy. This is particularly worrisome in men with a life expectancy of greater than 15 years. To reduce the risk of undersampling, our group has added transition zone sampling to surveillance biopsy protocol since 2009. Similarly, other programs have added repeat diagnostic biopsy or saturation biopsy to their protocol.[13]

The recommendation for adding two cores from the transition zone was based on data obtained from reviewing 48 radical prostatectomy specimens from our cohort of active surveillance patients who underwent surgery due to needle biopsy evidence of higher grade or more extensive disease. All 10 tumors with a dominant nodule size greater than 1 cm^3 were located predominantly anteriorly.[13–16] A subsequent study from our group involving African American patients also revealed that Black men with very low–risk prostate cancer at diagnosis have a significantly higher prevalence of anterior cancer foci that are of higher grade and larger volume.[17] The use of transition zone biopsies in providing evidence of disease progression in active surveillance has been called into questions by others.[18] An alternative to transition zone biopsies to evaluate the transition zone may be multiparametric magnetic resonance imaging (MRI) (see Chapter 1).

Several studies have demonstrated that extra biopsies enhance the detection of prostate cancer in larger prostates.[19] Another issue that has recently been brought forward is that tumors detected in large prostate glands have a better outcome than those found in smaller prostates.[20] It remains to be studied whether increased sampling to detect tumors in large prostates may result in a relative increase in the detection of more indolent tumors.

The addition of midline peripheral zone needle biopsies is not supported by most studies.[21–23] Most studies, however, have concentrated on the utility of more posterolaterally guided biopsies.[21–25] If one were to only perform six needle biopsies of the prostate, then these biopsies should be aimed more toward the posterolateral aspect of the gland. However, combining both routine sextant and posterolateral needle biopsies maximizes the detection of cancer and results in more accurate prediction of pathologic stage and whole prostate Gleason score.[21–32] The importance of posterolateral biopsies is even more dramatized by the preponderance of significant cancers that would be missed by not sampling the posterolateral region.[21] In men with multiple negative prior biopsies and increasingly worrisome prostate-specific antigen (PSA) parameters, other options that are rarely used include saturation biopsy (extensive prostate biopsy, often >20 cores) to rule out a peripheral zone cancer and diagnostic transurethral resection to rule out a transition zone malignancy.[33,34] At our institution, urologists currently perform routine sampling of both the sextant and posterolateral aspects of the gland with 12 cores sampled per patient. As indicated earlier, in patients under consideration for or managed by active surveillance, 2 additional cores from the transition zones are obtained, for a total of 14 cores sampled per patient.

Several types of local anesthesia are now available for use to alleviate the pain associated with the biopsy procedures. Periprostatic nerve block has proved to be the most effective method to reduce pain during biopsy. It remains controversial whether other medications should be added to periprostatic nerve block.[35] In an attempt to increase accuracy of prostatic biopsy and reduce unnecessary prostate biopsy, color and power Doppler imaging, with or without contrast enhancement, and elastography have been proposed, but their routine use is still controversial.[35]

NEEDLE BIOPSY PROCESSING—FIXATIVE

Although the most common fixative used for prostate needle biopsy is formalin, other fixatives, such as Bouin or Hollande solutions, are also used to provide enhanced nuclear detail. The disadvantage of these fixatives is that one can see visible nucleoli even in benign glands, such that the significance of finding nucleoli in atypical glands suspicious for carcinoma is not as powerful as when more prominent nucleoli are seen in formalin-fixed tissue. When using fixatives such as Bouin, one must judge what are prominent nucleoli relative to the nucleoli seen in adjacent benign glands. If one does not see nucleoli in the majority of prostate cancers sampled on needle biopsy, it is not necessary to switch from formalin to these other alternative fixatives. Rather, careful attention to microtomy and staining can improve the situation; sections that are too thick or overstained result in hyperchromatic nuclei without visible nucleoli.

NEEDLE BIOPSY PROCESSING—NUMBER OF LEVELS

It is recommended that three levels be prepared from each prostate biopsy paraffin block so that adequate visualization of the needle biopsy cores is possible, because fewer levels may miss atypical foci or cancer.[36,37] In a survey of urologic pathologists, three levels of needle biopsies were used routinely by the majority.[38] It is better to have three levels on different slides as opposed to doing all the three levels on a single slide. In a difficult case, it is useful to have multiple profiles of the area in question rather than just three if the levels are all done on one slide.

NEEDLE BIOPSY PROCESSING—INTERVENING UNSTAINED SLIDES

Immunohistochemistry stains for high molecular weight cytokeratin may demonstrate the presence or absence of basal cells in a small focus of atypical glands, helping to establish a benign or malignant diagnosis, receptively. From January 1994 to present, we have generated intervening unstained slides on all prostate needle biopsies for potential immunohistochemistry stains for high molecular weight cytokeratin, because lesions may not survive deeper sectioning into the block. Of 1,105 prostate needle biopsy cases seen at Johns Hopkins from January 1994 to December 1996, immunohistochemistry staining for high molecular weight cytokeratin was initially done on 94 (8.5%). To see if lesions would still have been present for evaluation if we did not have intervening slides, we repeated the immunohistochemistry stains for high molecular weight cytokeratin off of the paraffin blocks in 81 cases where material was available for study.[39] Care was taken to not trim the blocks. In 52 cases, the original high molecular weight cytokeratin helped to establish a diagnosis: In 31 of these cases, the lesion was not present on repeat immunohistochemistry stains from the block. Of these 31 cases, the original high molecular weight cytokeratin from intervening unstained slides helped to establish a cancer ($n = 23$) or benign ($n = 8$) diagnosis. The use of intervening unstained slides was critical to establish a diagnosis in 31/1,105 (2.8%) of prostate needle biopsies. Each laboratory must decide whether these data justify the cost of preparing extra unstained slides. Approximately one-half of urologic pathologists keep unstained intervening sections for immunohistochemistry.[38]

NEEDLE BIOPSY PROCESSING—NUMBER OF TISSUE CORES PER BLOCK/SLIDE

A major concern with placing multiple cores into one jar is that the urologist loses information as to where these cores are coming from. In 5% to 10% of prostate needle biopsies, the pathologist will render an "atypical, suspicious for carcinoma" diagnosis, necessitating a repeat biopsy. We have demonstrated that the cancer is often near or adjacent to these atypical sites.[40] Consequently, if one knows the sextant region where the initial atypical site has come from, one can focus the repeat biopsy by doing more repeat biopsies in this region and in the adjacent regions. It makes no sense to know where the cores are coming from and have the specific information, only to lose it by throwing all the cores, for example, from the left side into one jar.

There is another reason why it is important to know the location of each core. Within the central zone toward the base of the prostate around the ejaculatory duct, there is a close mimicker of high-grade prostatic intraepithelial neoplasia (PIN).[41] If pathologists know that the biopsy that they are looking at comes from the base of the prostate, it is easier for the pathologist to recognize this central zone histology as a mimicker of high-grade PIN rather than overdiagnose these lesions as high-grade PIN. Recognizing mimickers of high-grade PIN can prevent false-positive biopsies and obviate the need for unnecessary repeat needle biopsy.

The final reason why it is important to separate cores into six distinct jars depending on the sextant location is to help the pathologist identify tumor in the radical prostatectomy specimen when the tumor is extremely focal. In approximately 5% of radical prostatectomy specimens, it may be extremely difficult to identify prostate cancer.[42] These cases represent very small tumors that have been incidentally hit by needle biopsy. If the pathologist knows the approximate location (i.e., sextant region) of the cancer on needle biopsy, the pathologist can then focus his or her hunt in the radical prostatectomy for prostate cancer in these regions by performing cutdowns and flipping paraffin blocks. We are aware of at least one case where the urologist has been sued when no cancer was found in the radical prostatectomy, despite an accurate diagnosis of minute cancer of the prostate on needle biopsy. Patients are naturally suspicious when they undergo a major surgical operation and no cancer is found. Knowing the site of origin of the cancer on needle biopsy within the prostate can minimize the likelihood that prostates will be signed out showing no evidence of residual carcinoma.

Pathologists should ideally place two and at most three cores in a single cassette. The first problem is that when there are multiple cores in a given jar, the histotechnologist in processing these needle biopsy specimens cannot guarantee that the cores will all remain in the same plane of section within the paraffin. This results in histologic slides where they may be missing gaps of prostate tissue that the pathologist will not see.[43] This can be critical, because the key focus within a prostate needle biopsy showing the only malignancy may be present in one of these gaps of tissue. It has also been demonstrated that specimens submitted in 1 to 2 containers have a higher incidence of "atypical" diagnoses as compared to specimens submitted individually in 6 to 12 containers.[44] Pre-embedded specimens where cores are stretched and oriented between meshes in tissue cassettes before being placed in formalin also decrease atypical foci and increase the yield of cancer.[45] It is difficult to section cases with multiple tissue cores, such that atypical foci tend to be lost on deeper sectioning for both hematoxylin and eosin (H&E) and immunohistochemical stains. It is also more difficult to match up the H&E-stained sections with the immunohistochemical stains for basal cells when there are multiple tangled fragmented cores.

SAMPLING OF TRANSURETHRAL RESECTION SPECIMENS

In order to minimize undersampling of a high-grade cancer component, tissue should be evenly placed within cassettes, such that there is no overlapping of transurethral resection of the prostate (TURP) chips.[46]

1. Initially, submit eight cassettes of tissue in a random fashion. Submission of eight cassettes will identify almost all stage T1b cancers (see Chapter 8) and approximately 90% of stage T1a tumors (see Chapter 8).[28-31] Submit the specimen in its entirety if it requires nine cassettes or less.
2. In younger men (<65 years of age), submission of all the tissue may be justified to identify all stage T1a lesions, because studies have shown these men are at increased risk of progression with long-term follow-up and they may be given the option of definitive therapy at some institutions.

3. When stage T1b carcinoma is found on the initial eight slides, it is not necessary to submit additional tissue. We have demonstrated that a review of additional material, beyond that of the initial eight cassettes, will not change the stage based on the percent of tumor involvement.[46] Although the percent of tumor changed in some cases, the magnitude of the change was never sufficient to change a lesion from less than 5% (T1a) to greater than 5% (T1b) or vice versa. This finding is expected because the tissue is randomly submitted, and examination of eight cassettes should be representative of the percent of tumor involvement for the entire specimen.

4. When stage T1a carcinoma is found on the initial eight slides reviewed, the remaining tissue should be submitted for review.[46] The rationale for submitting the remaining tissue for stage T1a lesions is as follows. There is a small potential of upstaging based on finding high-grade cancer in the additionally submitted tissue. The decision to submit the remaining tissue should not be burdensome because it occurs in only approximately 1.5% of TURP specimens: Approximately 10% to 15% of TURPs have cancer and only 15% of these cases are stage T1a lesions requiring more than nine cassettes for complete submission. In the few cases with excessive amounts of tissue, it is not unreasonable to submit a maximum total of 16 cassettes, because the potential for upstaging based on grade is relatively small.

REFERENCES

1. Hodge KK, McNeal JE, Terris MK, et al. Random systematic versus directed ultrasound guided transrectal core biopsies of the prostate. *J Urol*. 1989;142:71–74; discussion 74–75.

2. Stamey TA, McNeal JE, Freiha FS, et al. Morphometric and clinical studies on 68 consecutive radical prostatectomies. *J Urol*. 1988;139:1235–1241.

3. Carter HB, Sauvageot J, Walsh PC, et al. Prospective evaluation of men with stage T1C adenocarcinoma of the prostate. *J Urol*. 1997;157:2206–2209.

4. Epstein JI, Walsh PC, Carmichael M, et al. Pathologic and clinical findings to predict tumor extent of nonpalpable (stage T1c) prostate cancer. *JAMA*. 1994;271:368–374.

5. Bazinet M, Karakiewicz PI, Aprikian AG, et al. Value of systematic transition zone biopsies in the early detection of prostate cancer. *J Urol*. 1996;155:605–606.

6. Fleshner NE, Fair WR. Indications for transition zone biopsy in the detection of prostatic carcinoma. *J Urol*. 1997;157:556–558.

7. Liu IJ, Macy M, Lai YH, et al. Critical evaluation of the current indications for transition zone biopsies. *Urology*. 2001;57:1117–1120.

8. Epstein JI, Walsh PC, Sauvageot J, et al. Use of repeat sextant and transition zone biopsies for assessing extent of prostate cancer. *J Urol*. 1997;158:1886–1890.

9. Karakiewicz PI, Bazinet M, Aprikian AG, et al. Outcome of sextant biopsy according to gland volume. *Urology*. 1997;49:55–59.

10. Epstein JI, Walsh PC, Akingba G, et al. The significance of prior benign needle biopsies in men subsequently diagnosed with prostate cancer. *J Urol*. 1999;162:1649–1652.

11. Naughton CK, Smith DS, Humphrey PA, et al. Clinical and pathologic tumor characteristics of prostate cancer as a function of the number of biopsy cores: a retrospective study. *Urology*. 1998;52:808–813.

12. Uzzo RG, Wei JT, Waldbaum RS, et al. The influence of prostate size on cancer detection. *Urology*. 1995;46:831–836.

13. Tosoian JJ, JohnBull E, Trock BJ, et al. Pathological outcomes in men with low risk and very low risk prostate cancer: implications on the practice of active surveillance. *J Urol*. 2013;190:1218–1222.

14. Duffield AS, Lee TK, Miyamoto H, et al. Radical prostatectomy findings in patients in whom active surveillance of prostate cancer fails. *J Urol*. 2009;182:2274–2278.

15. Lee S, Walsh S, Woods CG, et al. Reliable identification of transition zone prostatic adenocarcinoma in preoperative needle core biopsy. *Hum Pathol*. 2013;44:2331–2337.

16. Ploussard G, de la Taille A, Terry S, et al. Detailed biopsy pathologic features as predictive factors for initial reclassification in prostate cancer patients eligible for active surveillance. *Urol Oncol*. 2013;31:1060–1066.

17. Sundi D, Kryvenko ON, Carter HB, et al. Pathological examination of radical prostatectomy specimens in men with very low risk disease at biopsy reveals distinct zonal distribution of cancer in black American men. *J Urol*. 2014;191:60–67.

18. RiChard JL, Motamedinia P, McKiernan JM, et al. Routine transition zone biopsy during active surveillance for prostate cancer rarely provides unique evidence of disease progression. *J Urol*. 2012;188:2177–2180.

19. Eskicorapci SY, Guliyev F, Akdogan B, et al. Individualization of the biopsy protocol according to the prostate gland volume for prostate cancer detection. *J Urol*. 2005;173:1536–1540.

20. D'Amico AV, Whittington R, Malkowicz SB, et al. A prostate gland volume of more than 75 cm3 predicts for a favorable outcome after radical prostatectomy for localized prostate cancer. *Urology*. 1998;52:631–636.

21. Epstein JI, Walsh PC, Carter HB. Importance of posterolateral needle biopsies in the detection of prostate cancer. *Urology*. 2001;57:1112–1116.

22. Terris MK, Wallen EM, Stamey TA. Comparison of mid-lobe versus lateral systematic sextant biopsies in the detection of prostate cancer. *Urol Int*. 1997;59:239–242.

23. Eskew LA, Woodruff RD, Bare RL, et al. Prostate cancer diagnosed by the 5 region biopsy method is significant disease. *J Urol*. 1998;160:794–796.

24. Norberg M, Egevad L, Holmberg L, et al. The sextant protocol for ultrasound-guided core biopsies of the prostate underestimates the presence of cancer. *Urology*. 1997;50:562–566.

25. Chang JJ, Shinohara K, Bhargava V, et al. Prospective evaluation of lateral biopsies of the peripheral zone for prostate cancer detection. *J Urol*. 1998;160:2111–2114.

26. Singh H, Canto EI, Shariat SF, et al. Six additional systematic lateral cores enhance sextant biopsy prediction of pathological features at radical prostatectomy. *J Urol*. 2004;171:204–209.

27. Naya Y, Ochiai A, Troncoso P, et al. A comparison of extended biopsy and sextant biopsy schemes for predicting the pathological stage of prostate cancer. *J Urol*. 2004;171:2203–2208.

28. Elabbady AA, Khedr MM. Extended 12-core prostate biopsy increases both the detection of prostate cancer and the accuracy of Gleason score. *Eur Urol*. 2006;49:49–53; discussion 53.

29. Eichler K, Hempel S, Wilby J, et al. Diagnostic value of systematic biopsy methods in the investigation of prostate cancer: a systematic review. *J Urol*. 2006;175:1605–1612.

30. Emiliozzi P, Maymone S, Paterno A, et al. Increased accuracy of biopsy Gleason score obtained by extended needle biopsy. *J Urol*. 2004;172:2224–2226.

31. King CR, McNeal JE, Gill H, et al. Extended prostate biopsy scheme improves reliability of Gleason grading: implications for radiotherapy patients. *Int J Radiat Oncol Biol Phys*. 2004;59:386–391.

32. Mian BM, Lehr DJ, Moore CK, et al. Role of prostate biopsy schemes in accurate prediction of Gleason scores. *Urology*. 2006;67:379–383.

33. Fleshner N, Klotz L. Role of "saturation biopsy" in the detection of prostate cancer among difficult diagnostic cases. *Urology*. 2002;60:93–97.

34. Bratt O. The difficult case in prostate cancer diagnosis—when is a "diagnostic TURP" indicated? *Eur Urol*. 2006;49:769–771.

35. Scattoni V, Zlotta A, Montironi R, et al. Extended and saturation prostatic biopsy in the diagnosis and characterisation of prostate cancer: a critical analysis of the literature. *Eur Urol*. 2007;52:1309–1322.

36. Brat DJ, Wills ML, Lecksell KL, et al. How often are diagnostic features missed with less extensive histologic sampling of prostate needle biopsy specimens? *Am J Surg Pathol*. 1999;23:257–262.

37. Renshaw AA. Adequate tissue sampling of prostate core needle biopsies. *Am J Clin Pathol*. 1997;107:26–29.

38. Egevad L, Allsbrook WC, Epstein JI. Current practice of diagnosis and reporting of prostatic intraepithelial neoplasia and glandular atypia among genitourinary pathologists. *Mod Pathol*. 2006;19:180–185.

39. Green R, Epstein JI. Use of intervening unstained slides for immunohistochemical stains for high molecular weight cytokeratin on prostate needle biopsies. *Am J Surg Pathol*. 1999;23:567–570.

40. Allen EA, Kahane H, Epstein JI. Repeat biopsy strategies for men with atypical diagnoses on initial prostate needle biopsy. *Urology*. 1998;52:803–807.

41. Srodon M, Epstein JI. Central zone histology of the prostate: a mimicker of high-grade prostatic intraepithelial neoplasia. *Hum Pathol*. 2002;33:518–523.

42. DiGiuseppe JA, Sauvageot J, Epstein JI. Increasing incidence of minimal residual cancer in radical prostatectomy specimens. *Am J Surg Pathol*. 1997;21:174–178.

43. Kao J, Upton M, Zhang P, et al. Individual prostate biopsy core embedding facilitates maximal tissue representation. *J Urol*. 2002;168:496–499.

44. Gupta C, Ren JZ, Wojno KJ. Individual submission and embedding of prostate biopsies decreases rates of equivocal pathology reports. *Urology*. 2004;63:83–86.

45. Rogatsch H, Moser P, Volgger H, et al. Diagnostic effect of an improved preembedding method of prostate needle biopsy specimens. *Hum Pathol*. 2000;31:1102–1107.

46. McDowell PR, Fox WM, Epstein JI. Is submission of remaining tissue necessary when incidental carcinoma of the prostate is found on transurethral resection? *Hum Pathol*. 1994;25:493–497.

3

GROSS ANATOMY AND NORMAL HISTOLOGY

GROSS ANATOMY

The prostate weighs approximately 30 to 40 g in adult men without prominent benign prostatic hyperplasia (BPH). It has the shape of an inverted cone with the base located proximally at the bladder neck and the apex distally at the urogenital diaphragm. The prostatic urethra runs through the center of the gland with a 35-degree anterior bend at the verumontanum.[1] Posteriorly, a thin, filmy layer of connective tissue known as Denonvilliers fascia separates the prostate and seminal vesicles from the rectum.

Initially, the prostate was thought to be composed of distinct anatomic lobes. Today's anatomic theories divide the prostate into inner and outer regions, although right and left lobes are still referred to based on palpation of a midline furrow. The inner zone is affected predominantly by BPH, and the outer zone has a predilection for carcinoma, although some carcinomas occur centrally and BPH nodules may be seen peripherally.[2] The prostate is divided into four zones: (a) anterior fibromuscular stroma; (b) central zone; (c) peripheral zone; and (d) preprostatic region, which encompasses the periurethral ducts and the larger transition zone[1] (Fig. 3.1).

The anterior fibromuscular stroma, which occupies approximately one-third of the prostate, contains very few glands and consists of smooth muscle tissue and dense fibrous tissue. The central zone forms a cone-shaped volume surrounding the ejaculatory ducts with its apex at the verumontanum and its base at the bladder neck. The peripheral zone is the largest zone and contains 75% of the glandular tissue of the prostate. The peripheral zone is distal to the central zone and corresponds to a horseshoe-shaped structure extending posteriorly, posterolaterally, and laterally around the inner aspect of the prostate. The most critical area of the preprostatic region is the transition zone, which is most affected by hyperplasia. The rationale for separating the outer aspect of the prostate into central and peripheral zones is in part based on both histologic differences and differences in the diseases affecting these two areas. From a diagnostic standpoint, central zone histology may mimic high-grade

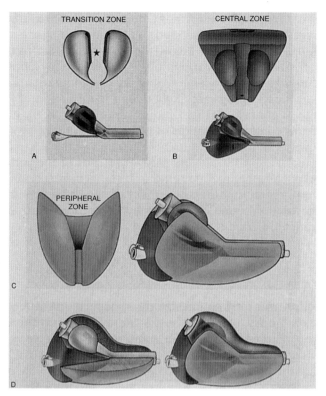

FIGURE 3.1 Zonal anatomy of the prostate. (From Epstein JI, Wojno KJ. The prostate and seminal vesicles. In: Sternberg SS, ed. *Diagnostic Surgical Pathology*. 3rd ed. Philadelphia, Pa: Lippincott William & Wilkins, 1999, with permission.)

prostatic intraepithelial neoplasia (PIN) (see Chapter 5). The peripheral zone is much more frequently affected by carcinoma. The central zone is an uncommon site for origin of carcinoma, although it may be secondarily invaded by large peripheral zone tumors. Despite these differences, experts in the field still find difficulties in distinguishing between the central and peripheral zones and often will combine them into one zone when investigating various aspects of prostatic disease. From this standpoint, McNeal's[1] more complicated scheme is often simplified into a two-zone concept, corresponding to the inner (transition zone) and outer (peripheral and central zones) sections of the prostate.

According to the previously mentioned widely accepted McNeal's[1] anatomic model, the transition zone and central zone do not extend below the verumontanum. Recent use of magnetic resonance imaging (MRI) of the prostate gland has pointed to the difficulty in reliably differentiating the transition zone from the central zone. The term *central gland* is coined and used by radiologists to refer to the area encompassing both transition and central zones. A recent study analyzing anatomic findings in 63 patients undergoing multiparametric endorectal MRI[3] seems to suggest that the central gland (combination of the central zone and transition zone) extended below the verumontanum in the majority (95%) of patients. Positive correlation was found between age and the amount of central gland extension below the verumontanum. The authors suggested that their findings are likely due to deformation of the gland by BPH with age. If confirmed, their findings should be taken into consideration for accurate characterization of the zonal origin of prostate cancer below the level of the verumontanum. Based on McNeal's[1] model, nearly all of the anterior prostate cancers below the level of the verumontanum are classified as peripheral zone tumors. If the central gland does extend below the verumontanum, the adjustment of the transition zone and peripheral zone tumoral zone of origin may have prognostic implications, given that transition zone cancers may have a more favorable outcome.[3-5]

HISTOLOGY

Rather than provide a complete description of the histology of the prostate, this section will only emphasize those aspects that affect interpretation of prostate biopsy material. The discussion of some topics of prostate histology (i.e., neuroendocrine differentiation) will be deferred to sections of the book dealing with pathology related to these topics. The prostate consists of epithelial and stromal cells. The epithelial cells are arranged in glands consisting of ducts, which branch out from the urethra and terminate into acini. Distinction between a prostatic duct and acinus primarily is based on its architecture as determined on low magnification. Ducts consist of elongated tubular structures with branching as opposed to acini, which are more rounded structures grouped in lobular units. Smaller ducts cut on cross section are indistinguishable from acini.

Epithelial cells in the prostate are (a) urothelial (transitional) cells, (b) secretory cells, (c) basal cells, and (d) neuroendocrine cells. The proximal portions of the prostatic ducts are lined by urothelium similar to the urethra. In distal portions of the prostatic ducts as well as in scattered prostatic acini, there may be alternating areas of cuboidal and columnar epithelium admixed with urothelium. When urothelium is seen within the more peripheral prostatic ducts and acini, it is referred to as urothelial metaplasia (Fig. 3.2, eFigs. 3.1 to 3.3). Urothelial metaplasia may be a misnomer in that there is no evidence that this process results from metaplasia of a different epithelial cell type. It may be seen in infants and neonates throughout the prostate (author's personal observations). The urothelium is composed of spindle-shaped epithelial cells with occasional nuclear grooves, which are often oriented with their long axes parallel to the basement membrane. Urothelium may undermine the cuboidal pale-staining prostatic glandular epithelium.

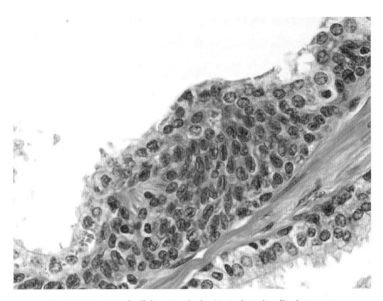

FIGURE 3.2   Urothelial metaplasia. Note longitudinal grooves.

Columnar secretory epithelial cells are tall with pale to clear cyto-plasm (eFigs. 3.4 and 3.5). These cells are terminally differentiated and stain positively with prostate-specific antigen (PSA), and prostate-specific acid phosphatase (PSAP). Secretory cells lack immunoreactivity with antibodies to high molecular weight cytokeratin.[6] Corpora amylacea are seen in approximately 25% of prostate glands in men aged 20 to 40 years, whereas they are rare in carcinomas.[7,8] Corpora amylacea are round lami-nated hyaline eosinophilic structures that may become calcified (eFig. 3.6). Although lipofuscin was initially thought to be diagnostic of seminal ves-icle epithelium, it may be seen in approximately 50% of cases of benign prostate glands in hematoxylin and eosin (H&E)–stained sections and in almost all cases when studied by special stains such as Fontana-Masson.[9] On H&E-stained sections, these granules may be either yellow-brown or pale gray-brown with a dark blue rim (Fig. 3.3, eFigs. 3.7 to 3.12).

Basal cells lie beneath the secretory cells (eFig. 3.5). Basal cell nuclei are cigar-shaped or resemble those of fibroblasts and are oriented paral-lel to the basement membrane (Fig. 3.4). The cells may be inconspicuous in benign glands and may be difficult to distinguish from surrounding fibroblasts. It is important to recognize basal cells and differentiate them from fibroblasts or an artifactual two-cell layer in cancer, because basal cells are absent in adenocarcinoma of the prostate and may be identified in conditions that mimic prostate cancer.[10,11] Whereas fibroblasts have extremely hyperchromatic and pointed nuclei, basal cells may be recogniz-able by their more ovoid nuclei with lighter chromatin resembling those of smooth muscle cells. In some institutions' material, basal cell nuclei are

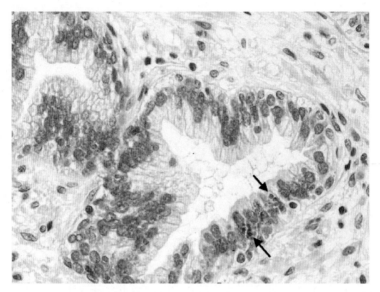

FIGURE 3.3 Lipofuscin in benign prostate glands. In addition to red-orange lipofuscin, lipofuscin may have a brown-purple appearance *(arrows)*.

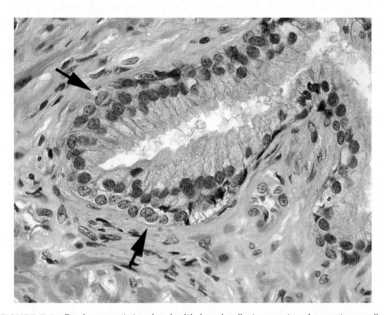

FIGURE 3.4 Benign prostate gland with basal cells *(arrows)* and secretory cells.

more blue-gray and may be surrounded by a halo, whereas secretory cell nuclei appear reddish violet (Fig. 3.4). Basal cells may show prominent nucleoli, mimicking high-grade PIN (see Chapter 5). Basal cells also may be identified by their immunohistochemical reaction with antibodies to high molecular weight cytokeratin (eFig. 3.13).[6] Basal cells in hyperplastic glands usually are uniformly labeled with these antibodies, although an occasional gland stains discontinuously or even not at all. Basal cells are less differentiated than secretory cells and are almost devoid of secretory products, such as PSA and PSAP.[12] Basal cells are not myoepithelial cells and do not react with antibodies to muscle-specific actin or S-100, and ultrastructural studies reveal a lack of contractile elements.[13,14] It is thought that the basal cells are the stem cell population of the secretory cells; the largest proportion of proliferating cells in the prostate is basal cells.[15]

The fourth group of prostatic epithelial cells is those with neuro-endocrine differentiation. The prostate contains the largest number of endocrine-paracrine cells of any genitourinary organ (see Chapter 12).

Stromal cells are skeletal and smooth muscle cells, fibroblasts, nerves, and endothelial cells. In the most distal (apical) portion of the prostate gland, skeletal muscle of the urogenital diaphragm extends into the prostate.[16,17] Although mostly exterior to the gland, skeletal muscle fibers do not uncommonly extend into the peripheral portion of the prostate gland, especially apically and anteriorly (Fig. 3.5, eFig. 3.14). The finding of skeletal muscle fibers on transurethral resection does not result in an increase in incontinence.[18] In the normal prostate, one can also find small nerve bundles. Occasionally, ganglion cells and paraganglia may be

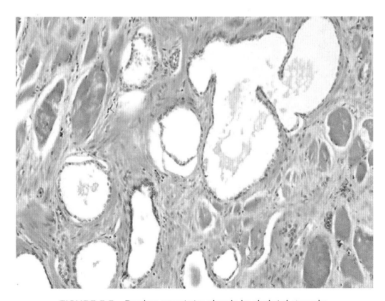

FIGURE 3.5 Benign prostate glands in skeletal muscle.

seen in the prostate, although they are more commonly identified exterior to the gland (see Chapter 7). Cowper gland may also occasionally be seen on needle biopsy (see Chapter 7).

BENIGN PROSTATIC HYPERPLASIA

BPH, also referred to as nodular hyperplasia, is the most common urologic disease to affect men. Clinically, hyperplasia is classified into lateral enlargement, middle lobe enlargement, and posterior lobe hyperplasia. Typical hyperplasia of tissue lateral to the urethra is designated as lateral lobe enlargement. Middle lobe enlargement refers to a nodule arising at the bladder neck, which may then project into the bladder, creating a ball-valve obstruction. In posterior lobe hyperplasia, there is a bar of tissue, termed the *median bar*, which arises in the posterior aspect of the urethra. Because of the strategic location of middle or posterior lobe enlargement, relatively small prostates may be associated with marked urinary obstructive symptoms.[19]

Franks described five histologic subtypes of prostatic hyperplasia based on their differing epithelial and stromal components.[20] The smallest nodules are predominantly stromal, often composed of loose mesenchyma containing prominent small round vessels (eFig. 3.15 to 3.19). In a needle biopsy specimen, these vessels help differentiate between a mesenchymal tumor and a stromal nodule (Fig. 3.6). These nodules are located in the periurethral submucosa and seldom reach large size except near the bladder neck, where they may protrude into the bladder lumen as a solitary midline mass.

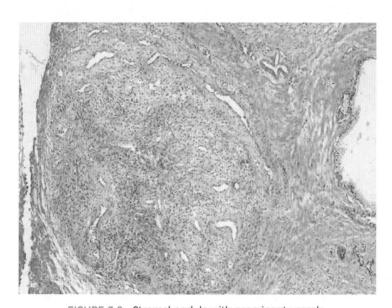

FIGURE 3.6 Stromal nodule with prominent vessels.

Occasionally, there are small pure stromal nodules composed almost entirely of smooth muscle.[21] Some of these lesions have been reported as leiomyomas of the prostate (eFigs. 3.20 to 3.23). However, the diagnosis of prostatic leiomyoma should be restricted to only large symptomatic masses of smooth muscle. The issue of distinguishing atypical stromal hyperplasia from stromal neoplasms of the prostate is discussed in Chapter 16.

The largest and most numerous hyperplastic nodules are almost always laterally situated and tend to occur in the periurethral zone near the proximal end of the verumontanum.[1] The glandular component is made up of small and large acini, some showing papillary infoldings and projections containing central fibrovascular cores. The stroma consists of smooth muscle and fibrous tissue, which can occasionally display nuclear palisading mimicking a neural tumor (eFig. 3.24). Within hyperplastic areas, there often is an infiltrate of lymphocytes and plasma cells around the glands. Usually, these are not associated with any infection nor with symptoms of prostatitis.[22,23] In more limited hyperplasia, tissue removed by transurethral resection of the prostate (TURP) contains a higher percentage component of bladder neck and anterior fibromuscular tissue.[24] In larger specimens, usually obtained by enucleation, glandular-stromal nodules become a more dominant feature.

In many cases, the histologic diagnosis of nodular hyperplasia does not relate to specific histologic findings but rather to the clinical findings of an enlarged prostate resulting in obstructive symptoms. The presence of papillary infoldings, although more prominent in hyperplasia, is not specific. Only the histologic identification of nodules is diagnostic for hyperplasia. By definition, TURP specimens may be diagnosed as hyperplasia, because surgery has been performed for urinary obstructive symptoms. Needle biopsy specimens should not be diagnosed as showing hyperplasia. First, many needle biopsy specimens do not even sample the transition zone. Second, histologic findings on needle biopsy, with the exception of stromal nodules, do not correlate with size of the prostate or urinary obstructive symptoms.[25]

Finally, signing out a specimen as "BPH" may falsely reassure the urologist that he has sampled the palpable or hypoechoic lesion of concern. Benign needle biopsy specimens of the prostate should be diagnosed as "benign prostate tissue" not as BPH.

REFERENCES

1. McNeal JE. Normal and pathologic anatomy of prostate. *Urology.* 1981;17:11–16.
2. Oyen RH, Van de Voorde WM, Van Poppel HP, et al. Benign hyperplastic nodules that originate in the peripheral zone of the prostate gland. *Radiology.* 1993;189:707–711.
3. Hansford BG, Peng Y, Jiang Y, et al. Revisiting the central gland anatomy via MRI: does the central gland extend below the level of verumontanum? *J Magn Reson Imaging.* 2014;39:167–171.
4. Al-Ahmadie HA, Tickoo SK, Olgac S, et al. Anterior-predominant prostatic tumors: zone of origin and pathologic outcomes at radical prostatectomy. *Am J Surg Pathol.* 2008;32:229–235.

5. Fine SW, Al-Ahmadie HA, Gopalan A, et al. Anatomy of the anterior prostate and extraprostatic space: a contemporary surgical pathology analysis. *Adv Anat Pathol.* 2007;14:401–407.

6. Hedrick L, Epstein JI. Use of keratin 903 as an adjunct in the diagnosis of prostate carcinoma. *Am J Surg Pathol.* 1989;13:389–396.

7. Andrews GS. The histology of the human foetal and prepubertal prostates. *J Anat.* 1951;85:44–54.

8. Humphrey PA, Vollmer RT. Corpora amylacea in adenocarcinoma of the prostate: prevalence in 100 prostatectomies and clinicopathologic correlations. *Surg Pathol.* 1990;3:389–396.

9. Brennick JB, O'Connell JX, Dickersin GR, et al. Lipofuscin pigmentation (so-called "melanosis") of the prostate. *Am J Surg Pathol.* 1994;18:446–454.

10. Totten RS, Heinemann MW, Hudson PB, et al. Microscopic differential diagnosis of latent carcinoma of prostate. *AMA Arch Pathol.* 1953;55:131–141.

11. Brandes D, Kircheim D, Scott WW. Ultrastructure of the human prostate: normal and neoplastic. *Lab Invest.* 1964;13:1541–1560.

12. Warhol MJ, Longtine JA. The ultrastructural localization of prostatic specific antigen and prostatic acid phosphatase in hyperplastic and neoplastic human prostates. *J Urol.* 1985;134:607–613.

13. Srigley JR, Dardick I, Hartwick RW, et al. Basal epithelial cells of human prostate gland are not myoepithelial cells. A comparative immunohistochemical and ultrastructural study with the human salivary gland. *Am J Pathol.* 1990;136:957–966.

14. Howat AJ, Mills PM, Lyons TJ, et al. Absence of S-100 protein in prostatic glands. *Histopathology.* 1988;13:468–470.

15. Bonkhoff H, Stein U, Remberger K. The proliferative function of basal cells in the normal and hyperplastic human prostate. *Prostate.* 1994;24:114–118.

16. Kost LV, Evans GW. Occurrence and significance of striated muscle within the prostate. *J Urol.* 1964;92:703–704.

17. Manley CB Jr. The striated muscle of the prostate. *J Urol.* 1966;95:234–240.

18. Graversen PH, England DM, Madsen PO, et al. Significance of striated muscle in curettings of the prostate. *J Urol.* 1988;139:751–753.

19. Bartsch G, Muller HR, Oberholzer M, et al. Light microscopic stereological analysis of the normal human prostate and of benign prostatic hyperplasia. *J Urol.* 1979;122:487–491.

20. Franks LM. Benign nodular hyperplasia of the prostate: a review. *Ann R Coll Surg Engl.* 1953;14:92–106.

21. Moore R. Benign hypertrophy of the prostate: a morphologic study. *J Urol.* 1943;50:680–710.

22. Kohnen PW, Drach GW. Patterns of inflammation in prostatic hyperplasia: a histologic and bacteriologic study. *J Urol.* 1979;121:755–760.

23. Nielsen ML, Asnaes S, Hattel T. Inflammatory changes in the noninfected prostate gland. A clinical, microbiological and histological investigation. *J Urol.* 1973;110:423–426.

24. McNeal J. Pathology of benign prostatic hyperplasia. Insight into etiology. *Urol Clin North Am.* 1990;17:477–486.

25. Viglione M, Epstein JI. Should benign prostatic hypertrophy be diagnosed on needle biopsy? *Mod Pathol.* 2002;33:796–800.

4

INFLAMMATORY CONDITIONS

ACUTE AND CHRONIC PROSTATIC INFLAMMATION

Although acute and chronic prostatitis are common diseases in urologic practice, they are usually diagnosed clinically and treated with antibiotics such that the histologic examination of specimens removed for symptomatic prostatitis is uncommon. Acute bacterial prostatitis consists of sheets of neutrophils within and around acini, intraductal desquamated cellular debris, stromal edema, and hyperemia, in contrast to the focal nonspecific acute inflammation that is much frequently seen (eFigs. 4.1 to 4.3). With the onset of effective antibiotics, symptomatic prostatic abscess formation is now infrequently seen.[1-4] Prostatic abscesses most commonly arise in individuals with preexisting bladder outlet obstruction secondary to a lower urinary tract infection, usually due to coliform organisms. Much less frequently, prostatic abscesses result by dissemination from an extraurinary source of infection, the most common being staphylococcal infections of the skin. Prostatic abscess may also arise as a complication of biopsy or instrumentation. Other risk factors include immunosuppression, diabetes, internal prosthesis, chronic renal failure, indwelling catheters, and chronic prostatitis.

Histologically, symptomatic chronic prostatitis cannot be distinguished from the chronic inflammation that is commonly seen in specimens removed for benign prostatic hyperplasia. Chronic inflammation typically involves the prostate in a periglandular distribution and contains an admixture of plasma cells (Fig. 4.1, eFig. 4.4). Several studies have shown that in many prostatic specimens with prominent chronic inflammation, organisms cannot be cultured.[5,6] Also, in prostatic specimens with positive cultures, there is frequently an absence of prominent inflammation within the tissue.[7] It is preferable to diagnose inflamed prostate specimens as showing "acute or chronic inflammation" as opposed to "acute or chronic prostatitis."

Clinical prostatitis may give rise to elevated serum prostate-specific antigen (PSA) elevations.[8] There are conflicting studies as to whether histologic evidence of either acute or chronic inflammation on biopsy correlates with an increase in total serum PSA levels.[9-13] We comment on the histologic presence of chronic inflammation only when it is prominent, as it is fairly ubiquitous. The presence of acute inflammation, except if

25

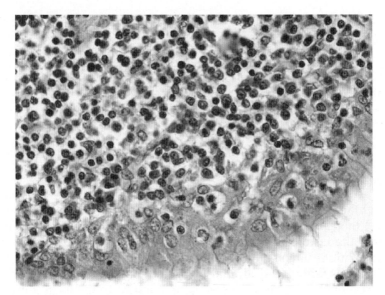

FIGURE 4.1   Benign prostate gland surrounded by lymphocytes admixed with plasma cells.

only very focal, is noted in the report. Acute and chronic inflammation may result in both architectural and cytologic abnormalities that may be confused with carcinoma (see Chapter 10).

MALAKOPLAKIA

As in the bladder, the majority of men with prostatic malakoplakia have urinary tract infections, most frequently with *Escherichia coli*.[14–16] Malako-plakia may clinically mimic cancer, resulting in prostatic induration and a hypoechoic lesion seen on transrectal ultrasound. Histologically, the lesions are indistinguishable from those occurring in other sites (Fig. 4.2, eFig. 4.5).

SARCOIDOSIS

Sarcoidosis of the prostate is an extremely rare occurrence. Only four cases have been reported in the literature where clinically documented sarcoidosis was associated with sarcoidal lesions on prostate biopsy. Like nonprostatic sites, ruling out an infectious etiology is a prerequisite for the diagnosis.[17]

GRANULOMATOUS PROSTATITIS

Granulomatous prostatitis is subclassified into infectious granulomas, non-specific granulomatous prostatitis, postbiopsy resection granulomas, and sys-temic granulomatous prostatitis.[18,19] In a series of 200 cases of granulomatous prostatitis, nonspecific granulomatous prostatitis (138 cases) and postbiopsy granulomas (49 cases) were the most common. Infectious granulomatous

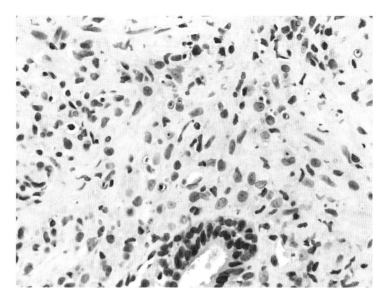

FIGURE 4.2   Malakoplakia with numerous Michaelis-Gutmann bodies.

prostatitis occurred in only 7 cases, with the remaining 6 due to systemic granulomatous disorders.[18]

MYCOTIC PROSTATITIS

Fungal infections of the prostate usually occur in immunocompromised hosts with disseminated mycoses.[20] Blastomycosis, coccidiomycosis, paracoccidioidomycosis, and cryptococcosis are the most common diseases (eFigs. 4.6 to 4.9). Cases have also been reported of histoplasmosis, paracoccidiomycosis, aspergillosis, and candidiasis of the prostate. The histology in these cases is identical to that seen in nonprostatic sites.[21–25]

MYCOBACTERIAL PROSTATITIS

Mycobacterial prostatitis may occur in patients with systemic tuberculosis, but today it is more commonly seen as a complication of bacillus Calmette-Guérin (BCG) immunotherapy for superficial bladder carcinoma.

The incidence of prostatic involvement in systemic tuberculosis ranges from 3% to 12%; in over 90% of these cases, there is coexisting pulmonary tuberculosis. In patients with urogenital tuberculosis, the prostate is involved in 75% to 95% of the cases.[26,27] However, in only 7% to 13% of cases of urogenital tuberculosis is the prostate the sole organ involved. Most cases of tuberculous prostatitis appear to arise from hematogenous dissemination rather than contact with infected urine. Atypical mycobacterial infections of the prostate are exceedingly rare.[28,29]

Chuang et al.[30] recently reported the rare occurrence of granulomatous prostatitis due to *Mycobacterium abscessus* in five patients who experienced poor wound healing following radical prostatectomy for prostate cancer. *M. abscessus* was cultured from the debridement specimens, and acid-fast–positive bacilli were identified histologically within the prostates. The authors further identified seven additional radical prostatectomy specimens with *M. abscessus* granulomatous prostatitis. Morphologically, suppurative necrotizing granulomatous inflammation extensively involved the prostate and frequently the extraprostatic soft tissue, seminal vesicles, and vas deferens. In addition to prolonged wound healing, urethrorectal fistula formation and pelvic abscess were encountered.[30]

Following BCG immunotherapy for superficial bladder carcinoma, patients may have fever, mild hematuria, and urinary frequency. Approximately 40% of these men have an abnormal digital rectal exam and 55% have ultrasonographic abnormalities of the prostate.[31-33] These lesions may further mimic carcinoma on magnetic resonance imaging (MRI) and positron emission tomography–computed tomography (PET-CT) imaging[34-36] and by elevating serum PSA levels. Following BCG, biopsies show caseating or noncaseating granulomas in 22% of cases and acid-fast stains are positive in approximately 50% of these cases. Histologically, the findings in BCG prostatitis are indistinguishable from those of tuberculous prostatitis occurring as a result of systemic infection. Small noncaseating granulomas are found in the periglandular stroma, as seen in early hematogenous dissemination of systemic tuberculosis (Fig. 4.3, eFig. 4.10). As these granulomas enlarge, they may eventually destroy glands (eFig. 4.11). There also

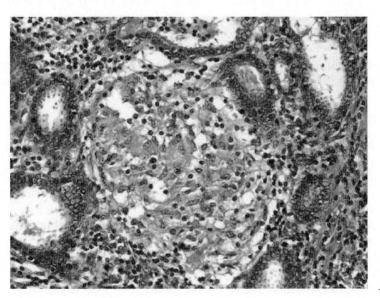

FIGURE 4.3   Periglandular BCG granulomas.

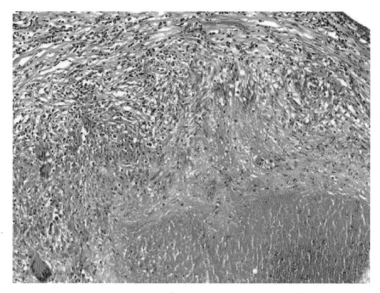

FIGURE 4.4 Caseation seen in BCG granulomas.

may be large granulomas with caseous necrosis, consisting of grumous fine granular debris, as opposed to coagulative necrosis seen in postbiopsy resection granulomas (eFigs. 4.12 and 4.13). Large caseating granulomas predominate within the peripheral zone of the prostate, although the transition zone or central zone may also be involved (Fig. 4.4). In addition to the more peripherally located caseating and noncaseating granulomas, there are almost always small suburethral granulomas. In some instances, the suburethral granulomas are well-formed and discrete, and in other cases, more ill-defined granulomatous inflammation is seen. Regardless of the histologic pattern of BCG-related granulomatous prostatitis or the presence of acid-fast bacilli on special stains, patients are usually asymptomatic and require no specific therapy.[31,32] It is not necessary in a man with a history of BCG therapy to perform stains for acid-fast organisms to evaluate prostatic granulomas; it is debatable whether stains for fungi should be done for completeness. Rarely, patients develop disseminated infection with BCG, accompanied by systemic signs and symptoms.

NONSPECIFIC GRANULOMATOUS PROSTATITIS

The most commonly diagnosed granulomatous process within the prostate is nonspecific granulomatous prostatitis. In a study of 25,387 benign prostate specimens, the incidence of nonspecific granulomatous prostatitis was 0.5%.[18] Lesions occurred over broad ages ranging from 18 to 86 years of age with a mean and median age of 62 years. Common symptoms included irritative voiding symptoms (50%), fever (46%), chills (44%), and obstructive voiding symptoms (32%). In 82% of men, there was pyuria, and in 46% there was hematuria. Seventy-one percent of men experienced a urinary tract infection at an average of 4 weeks prior to diagnosis. In 59% of the men, the rectal exam revealed an indurated prostate suspicious for adenocarcinoma. The etiology of this lesion is thought to be a reaction to bacterial toxins, cell debris, and secretions spilling into the stroma from blocked ducts.

Nonspecific granulomatous prostatitis mimics prostate carcinoma on rectal exam ultrasound and MRI exams[34,37] and can result in an elevated serum PSA level. At the same time, the pathologist could be confronted with a biopsy where the histology may closely mimic carcinoma[38,39] (see Chapter 7).

The earliest lesion in nonspecific granulomatous prostatitis consists of dilated ducts and acini filled with neutrophils, debris, foamy histiocytes, and desquamated epithelial cells (Fig. 4.5, eFigs. 4.14 and 4.15). Rupture of these ducts and acini results in a localized granulomatous and chronic inflammatory reaction (eFig. 4.16). Extension of the infiltrate into surrounding ductal and acinar units gives rise to the characteristic lobular dense infiltrate of lymphocytes, plasma cells, and histiocytes typical of more advanced nonspecific granulomatous prostatitis (Fig. 4.6, eFigs. 4.17 to 4.19). Many of the histiocytes have foamy cytoplasm and some are multinucleated. Neutrophils and eosinophils make up a smaller component of the inflammatory infiltrate. Often within the center of these large inflammatory nodules are dilated and partially effaced acini. Older lesions of nonspecific granulomatous prostatitis show a more prominent fibrous component.

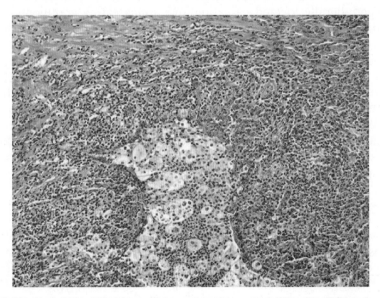

FIGURE 4.5 Early lesion of nonspecific granulomatous prostatitis with dilated gland containing foamy histiocytes and inflammation.

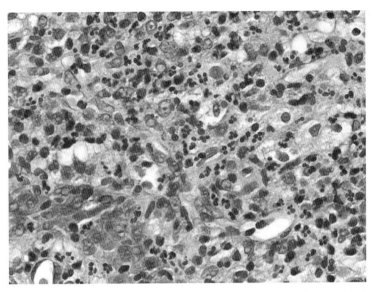

FIGURE 4.6 Nonspecific granulomatous prostatitis with numerous acute and chronic inflammatory cells, histiocytes, and eosinophils.

In most cases, there is little histologic similarity between nonspecific granulomatous prostatitis and infectious granulomatous inflammation of the prostate, and special stains for organisms need not be performed. In general, the lesions of nonspecific granulomatous prostatitis are not as granulomatous as those due to infection and are composed of a more mixed inflammatory infiltrate. Though discrete small granulomas can be seen in nonspecific granulomatous prostatitis, they are invariably seen with the early lesion surrounding a ruptured dilated duct or acinus. In contrast, early infectious noncaseating granulomas surround intact acini. Although small abscesses may be present at the center of nodules of nonspecific granulomatous prostatitis, caseous necrosis is absent. In some instances, nonspecific granulomatous prostatitis may resemble an infectious granulomatous process, justifying the performance of special stains for organisms (Fig. 4.7).

Recognition that nonspecific granulomatous prostatitis may contain abundant eosinophils should prevent a misdiagnosis of allergic granulomatous prostatitis. The eosinophils reflect a subacute inflammatory reaction rather than an allergic disorder. Allergic symptoms are absent and only rarely do these men have hypereosinophilia.

Nonspecific granulomatous prostatitis is treated with warm sitz baths, fluids, and antibiotics if a urinary tract infection is documented. Most patients' symptoms resolve within a few months although slightly over 50% of men have a persistent abnormal rectal exam 2 to 8 years following diagnosis.

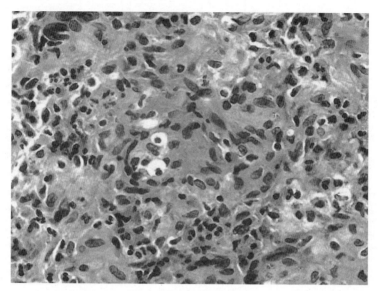

FIGURE 4.7   Nonspecific granulomatous prostatitis resembling infectious granulomas.

POSTBIOPSY GRANULOMAS

Prostatic granulomas are frequent sequelae after transurethral resection.[19,40] The post-transurethral resection interval with which these granulomas may be identified ranges from 9 days to 52 months. Although it is much more common to have a granulomatous reaction following transurethral resection, similar linear granulomas may rarely develop following needle biopsy (eFig. 4.20).

Postbiopsy granulomas are composed of a central region of fibrinoid necrosis surrounded by palisading epithelioid histiocytes (Fig. 4.8, eFig. 4.21). In contrast to infectious granulomas, the necrosis in postbiopsy granulomas often contains ghostlike structures of vessels, acini, and stroma (Fig. 4.8). Though these lesions can assume a multitude of shapes, some of the more common shapes observed are those of wedge-shaped granulomas, ovoid granulomas, and long tortuous granulomas dissecting through the tissue (Fig. 4.9). The irregularity of their shapes also distinguishes these granulomas from infectious granulomas. Following transurethral resection of the prostate (TURP), nonspecific foreign body giant cell granulomas are frequently seen in addition to the characteristic necrobiotic granulomas (eFig. 4.22). Postbiopsy granulomas also rarely occur following a needle biopsy.

In cases where the prior transurethral resection occurred within the last month, abundant eosinophils may be identified. Prior to the recognition of this disorder, postbiopsy granulomas with numerous eosinophils had been reported in the literature as allergic granulomatous prostatitis. In contrast to allergic granulomatous prostatitis, the eosinophils are

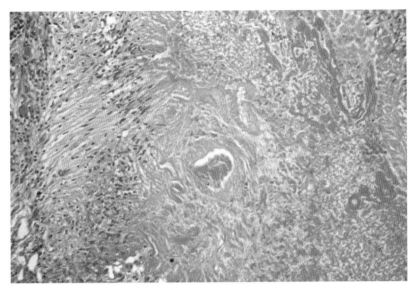

FIGURE 4.8 Post-TUR granuloma with coagulative necrosis showing residual outlines of vessels and connective tissue with peripheral palisading of histiocytes.

localized around postbiopsy granulomas rather than diffusely infiltrating the stroma. Inflammation surrounding postbiopsy granulomas where there is a longer interval from the prior transurethral resection is usually minimal consisting predominantly of lymphocytes and plasma cells with scattered eosinophils.

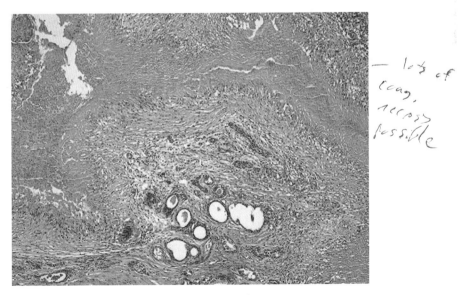

— lots of coag, necrosy possible

FIGURE 4.9 Post-TUR granulomas.

The postbiopsy granuloma appears to be a reaction to altered epithelium and stroma from the trauma of previous cautery. The recognition of similar postbiopsy granulomas in other sites following cautery argues against the process resulting solely from altered epithelium or secretions unique to the prostate. The lesion is so characteristic and distinct from infectious granulomas, so that stains for organisms are usually not necessary. Postbiopsy granulomas are asymptomatic, incidental findings requiring no treatment.

SYSTEMIC GRANULOMATOUS PROSTATITIS

This category encompasses cases with tissue eosinophilia such as allergic granulomatous prostatitis and Churg-Strauss syndrome, as well as those without eosinophilia, such as Wegener granulomatous prostatitis.[18,41] Allergic granulomatous prostatitis as part of a more generalized allergic reaction is an exceedingly rare condition.[18,19,42] Of the 12 patients with allergic granulomatous prostatitis reported in the literature, all have had either asthma or evidence of systemic allergic reaction at the time of diagnosis of their prostatic lesions. Furthermore, the majority of the effected individuals had increased blood eosinophil counts. In some instances, the severity of the asthmatic symptoms fluctuated synchronously with the severity of the urinary obstructive symptoms. In a few cases, the condition was systemic with granulomas found in other organs, and in one instance, the systemic granulomatous process contributed to a patient's death. Because allergic granulomatous prostatitis may be systemic in nature requiring prompt aggressive treatment with steroids, it is important to distinguish the rare allergic granulomatous prostatitis from the more common postbiopsy granulomas with eosinophils.

Histologically, allergic granulomatous prostatitis consists of multiple small, ovoid granulomas surrounded by numerous eosinophils (Fig. 4.10, eFigs. 4.23 to 4.25). The regularity of the size and shape of these granulomas, the eosinophilic necrosis within the granulomas, and the extensive infiltration of eosinophils throughout the stroma, not just surrounding the granulomas, separate this entity from that of postbiopsy granulomas with eosinophils. Rarely following a recent prior transurethral resection, the granulomas may resemble those seen in allergic granulomatous prostatitis. In these instances, the history of a recent prior-transurethral resection as well as the localization of eosinophils around the granulomas, rather than diffusely infiltrating the stroma, distinguish postbiopsy granulomas from allergic granulomatous prostatitis. Nonspecific granulomatous prostatitis with numerous eosinophils must also be distinguished from allergic granulomatous prostatitis.

MISCELLANEOUS INFECTIONS

Rare cases of cytomegalovirus and herpes zoster involving the prostate have been reported.[43,44] Other prostatic infections, some of which are

FIGURE 4.10   Allergic granulomatous prostatitis. (Courtesy of Dr. B. Bhagavan, Baltimore, MD.)

more commonly seen in developing countries, are exceedingly rare in North America and Europe. These include schistosomiasis, amoebic prostatitis, syphilis, actinomycosis, echinococcosis, and brucellosis.[45–50]

REFERENCES

1. Meares EM Jr. Prostatitis and related disorders. In: Walsh PC, Retik AB, Stamey TA, et al, eds. *Campbell's Urology.* 6th ed. Philadelphia, PA: WB Saunders; 1992:807–822.
2. Granados EA, Riley G, Salvador J, et al. Prostatic abscess: diagnosis and treatment. *J Urol.* 1992;148:80–82.
3. Sohlberg OE, Chetner M, Ploch N, et al. Prostatic abscess after transrectal ultrasound guided biopsy. *J Urol.* 1991;146:420–422.
4. Mamo GJ, Rivero MA, Jacobs SC. Cryptococcal prostatic abscess associated with the acquired immunodeficiency syndrome. *J Urol.* 1992;148:889–890.
5. Gorelick JI, Senterfit LB, Vaughan ED Jr. Quantitative bacterial tissue cultures from 209 prostatectomy specimens: findings and implications. *J Urol.* 1988;139:57–60.
6. Kohnen PW, Drach GW. Patterns of inflammation in prostatic hyperplasia: a histologic and bacteriologic study. *J Urol.* 1979;121:755–760.
7. Nielsen ML, Asnaes S, Hattel T. Inflammatory changes in the non-infected prostate gland. A clinical, microbiological and histological investigation. *J Urol.* 1973;110:423–426.
8. Neal DE Jr, Clejan S, Sarma D, et al. Prostate specific antigen and prostatitis. I. Effect of prostatitis on serum PSA in the human and nonhuman primate. *Prostate.* 1992;20: 105–111.
9. Hasui Y, Marutsuka K, Asada Y, et al. Relationship between serum prostate specific antigen and histological prostatitis in patients with benign prostatic hyperplasia. *Prostate.* 1994;25:91–96.
10. Ornstein DK, Smith DS, Humphrey PA, et al. The effect of prostate volume, age, total prostate specific antigen level and acute inflammation on the percentage of free serum

prostate specific antigen levels in men without clinically detectable prostate cancer. *J Urol.* 1998;159:1234–1237.

11. Jung K, Meyer A, Lein M, et al. Ratio of free-to-total prostate specific antigen in serum cannot distinguish patients with prostate cancer from those with chronic inflammation of the prostate. *J Urol.* 1998;159:1595–1598.

12. Okada K, Kojima M, Naya Y, et al. Correlation of histological inflammation in needle biopsy specimens with serum prostate-specific antigen levels in men with negative biopsy for prostate cancer. *Urology.* 2000;55:892–898.

13. Nadler RB, Humphrey PA, Smith DS, et al. Effect of inflammation and benign prostatic hyperplasia on elevated serum prostate specific antigen levels. *J Urol.* 1995;154:407–413.

14. Koga S, Arakaki Y, Matsuoka M, et al. Malakoplakia of prostate. *Urology.* 1986;27: 160–161.

15. Sujka SK, Malin BT, Asirwatham JE. Prostatic malakoplakia associated with prostatic adenocarcinoma and multiple prostatic abscesses. *Urology.* 1989;34:159–161.

16. Sarma HN, Ramesh K, al Fituri O, et al. Malakoplakia of the prostate gland—report of two cases and review of the literature. *Scand J Urol Nephrol.* 1996;30:155–157.

17. Furusato B, Koff S, McLeod DG, et al. Sarcoidosis of the prostate. *J Clin Pathol.* 2007; 60:325–326.

18. Stillwell TJ, Engen DE, Farrow GM. The clinical spectrum of granulomatous prostatitis: a report of 200 cases. *J Urol.* 1987;138:320–323.

19. Epstein JI, Hutchins GM. Granulomatous prostatitis: distinction among allergic, non-specific, and post-transurethral resection lesions. *Hum Pathol.* 1984;15:818–825.

20. Wise GJ, Silver DA. Fungal infections of the genitourinary system. *J Urol.* 1993;149: 1377–1388.

21. Seo IY, Jeong HJ, Yun KJ, et al. Granulomatous cryptococcal prostatitis diagnosed by transrectal biopsy. *Int J Urol.* 2006;13:638–639.

22. Yurkanin JP, Ahmann F, Dalkin BL. Coccidioidomycosis of the prostate: a determination of incidence, report of 4 cases, and treatment recommendations. *J Infect.* 2006;52: e19–e25.

23. Sohail MR, Andrews PE, Blair JE. Coccidioidomycosis of the male genital tract. *J Urol.* 2005;173:1978–1982.

24. de Arruda PF, Gatti M, de Arruda JG, et al. Prostatic paracoccidioidomycosis with a fatal outcome: a case report. *J Med Case Rep.* 2013;7:126.

25. Wada R, Nakano N, Yajima N, et al. Granulomatous prostatitis due to *Cryptococcus neoformans*: diagnostic usefulness of special stains and molecular analysis of 18S rDNA. *Prostate Cancer Prostatic Dis.* 2008;11:203–206.

26. Auerbach O. Tuberculosis of the genital system. *Q Bull Sea View Hosp.* 1942;7:188–207.

27. Moore RA. Tuberculosis of the prostate gland. *J Urol.* 1937;37:372–384.

28. Mikolich DJ, Mates SM. Granulomatous prostatitis due to Mycobacterium avium complex. *Clin Infect Dis.* 1992;14:589–591.

29. Lee LW, Burgher LW, Price EB Jr, et al. Granulomatous prostatitis. Association with isolation of Mycobacterium kansasii and Mycobacterium fortuitum. *JAMA.* 1977;237: 2408–2409.

30. Chuang AY, Tsou MH, Chang SJ, et al. *Mycobacterium abscessus* granulomatous prostatitis. *Am J Surg Pathol.* 2012;36:418–422.

31. Oates RD, Stilmant MM, Freedlund MC, et al. Granulomatous prostatitis following bacillus Calmette-Guerin immunotherapy of bladder cancer. *J Urol.* 1988;140:751–754.

32. Mukamel E, Konichezky M, Engelstein D, et al. Clinical and pathological findings in prostates following intravesical bacillus Calmette-Guerin instillations. *J Urol.* 1990;144: 1399–1400.

33. Miyashita H, Troncoso P, Babaian RJ. BCG-induced granulomatous prostatitis: a comparative ultrasound and pathologic study. *Urology.* 1992;39:364–367.

34. Bour L, Schull A, Delongchamps NB, et al. Multiparametric MRI features of granulomatous prostatitis and tubercular prostate abscess. *Diagn Interv Imaging.* 2013; 94:84–90.

35. Wilkinson C, Chowdhury F, Scarsbrook A, et al. BCG-induced granulomatous prostatitis—an incidental finding on FDG PET-CT. *Clin Imaging.* 2012;36:413–415.

36. Suzuki T, Takeuchi M, Naiki T, et al. MRI findings of granulomatous prostatitis developing after intravesical Bacillus Calmette-Guerin therapy. *Clin Radiol.* 2013;68:595–599.

37. Lee HY, Kuo YT, Tsai SY, et al. Xanthogranulomatous prostatitis: a rare entity resembling prostate adenocarcinoma with magnetic resonance image picture. *Clin Imaging.* 2012; 36:858–860.

38. Warrick J, Humphrey PA. Nonspecific granulomatous prostatitis. *J Urol.* 2012;187: 2209–2210.

39. Montironi R, Scarpelli M, Mazzucchelli R, et al. The spectrum of morphology in nonneoplastic prostate including cancer mimics. *Histopathology.* 2012;60:41–58.

40. Mies C, Balogh K, Stadecker M. Palisading prostate granulomas following surgery. *Am J Surg Pathol.* 1984;8:217–221.

41. Bray VJ, Hasbargen JA. Prostatic involvement in Wegener's granulomatosis. *Am J Kidney Dis.* 1991;17:578–580.

42. Kelalis PP, Harrison EG Jr, Greene LF. Allergic granulomas of the prostate in asthmatics. *JAMA.* 1964;188:963–967.

43. Benson PJ, Smith CS. Cytomegalovirus prostatitis. *Urology.* 1992;40:165–167.

44. Clason AE, McGeorge A, Garland C, et al. Urinary retention and granulomatous prostatitis following sacral Herpes Zoster infection. A report of 2 cases with a review of the literature. *Br J Urol.* 1982;54:166–169.

45. Zaher MF, el-Deeb AA. Bilharziasis of the prostate: its relation to bladder neck obstruction and its management. *J Urol.* 1971;106:257–261.

46. Goff DA, Davidson RA. Amebic prostatitis. *South Med J.* 1984;77:1053–1054.

47. Thompson L. Syphilis of the prostate. *Am J Syph.* 1920;4:323–341.

48. de Souza E, Katz DA, Dworzack DL, et al. Actinomycosis of the prostate. *J Urol.* 1985;133:290–291.

49. Houston W. Primary hydatid cyst of the prostate gland. *J Urol.* 1975;113:732–733.

50. Kelalis PP, Greene LF, Weed LA. Brucellosis of the urogenital tract: a mimic of tuberculosis. *J Urol.* 1962;88:347–353.

5

PRENEOPLASTIC LESIONS IN THE PROSTATE: PROSTATIC INTRAEPITHELIAL NEOPLASIA AND INTRADUCTAL CARCINOMA OF THE PROSTATE

PROSTATIC INTRAEPITHELIAL NEOPLASIA

This lesion was first described in the 1960s by McNeal and more precisely characterized in 1986 by McNeal and Bostwick at which time the entity was called intraductal dysplasia; currently, it is referred to as prostatic intraepithelial neoplasia (PIN).[1-4] PIN consists of architecturally benign prostatic acini or ducts lined by cytologically atypical cells. PIN is currently subcategorized into two grades, low- and high-grade PIN. The distinction between low- and high-grade PIN is the finding of prominent nucleoli in high-grade PIN (Figs. 5.1 and 5.2). There are no standard criteria defining how prominent or how frequent the nucleoli must be before they are sufficient to warrant a diagnosis of high-grade PIN. The criteria we use for diagnosing high-grade PIN is that nucleoli should be visible using a 20× lens, which has allowed us to achieve greater consistency in its diagnosis and prevent its overdiagnosis. High-grade PIN, defined accordingly, has also correlated with outcome in various studies from our institution.

Low-grade PIN consists of preexisting benign prostate glands with minimal epithelial proliferation in terms of nuclear stratification, where nuclei are minimally enlarged without prominent nucleoli (Figs. 5.3 and 5.4, eFigs. 5.1 to 5.19). If one has to hunt at 40× lens in a gland for a rare cell with prominent nucleoli, then the case should not be diagnosed as high-grade PIN. It may represent low-grade PIN, but for the reasons described in the following case should merely be signed out as benign prostate tissue without mentioning PIN.

Although high-grade PIN is characterized by nuclear atypia, there is often accompanying architectural abnormalities. At low magnification, basophilic glands that are separated by a modest amount of stroma and

38

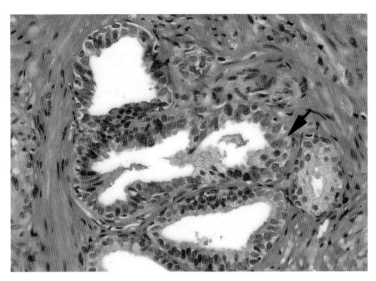

FIGURE 5.1   Flat high-grade PIN with nucleoli *(arrow).*

have a normal overall architectural pattern characterize high-grade PIN (Fig. 5.5). These glands resemble benign glands in that they are large, branch, and typically have papillary and undulating luminal surfaces. (Fig. 5.6, eFigs. 5.20 and 5.21). Their basophilic appearance is due to a combination of features including nuclear enlargement, hyperchromasia, overlapping, and amphophilic cytoplasm (Fig. 5.7, eFig. 5.22). Flat high-grade

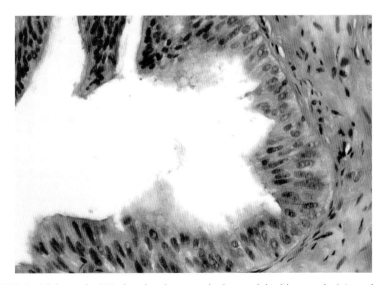

FIGURE 5.2   High-grade PIN showing large vesicular nuclei with prominent nucleoli that have lost their basal orientation and have become crowded and overlapping. Most of the gland has a flat morphology with tufting seen at *top.*

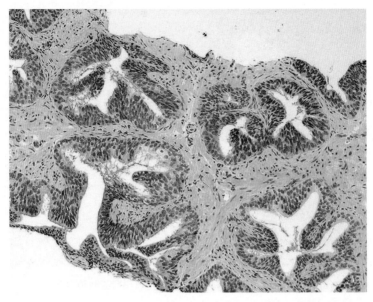

FIGURE 5.3 Low magnification of architecturally benign glands, which appear more baso-philic at low magnification.

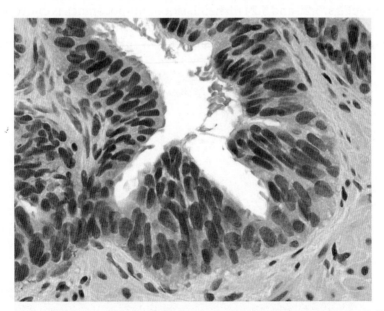

FIGURE 5.4 Same case as Figure 5.3 with tufting proliferation of crowded nuclei. The lack of prominent nucleoli is diagnostic of low-grade PIN.

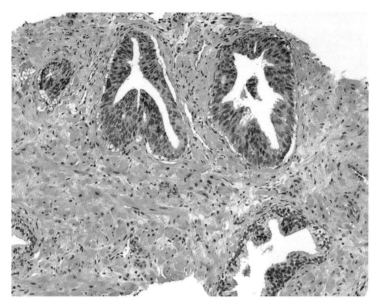

FIGURE 5.5   Low magnification of high-grade PIN with tufting, which appear more baso-philic at low magnification. Note benign gland with lighter appearance *(lower right)*.

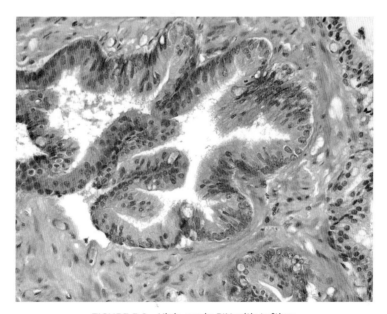

FIGURE 5.6   High-grade PIN with tufting.

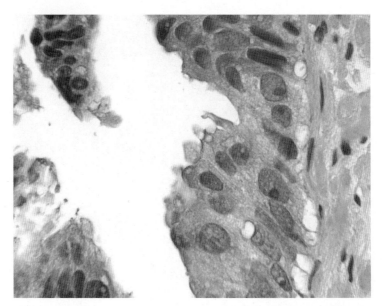

FIGURE 5.7   Higher magnification of high-grade PIN with prominent nucleoli.

PIN is characterized by nuclear atypia without significant epithelial hyperplasia (Fig. 5.8). The basal cell layer may or not be visible and the demarcation between atypical and normal nuclei is frequently abrupt. With more hyperplastic forms of high-grade PIN, nuclei become more piled up into tufts and can develop micropapillary projections (Figs. 5.9 and 5.10).

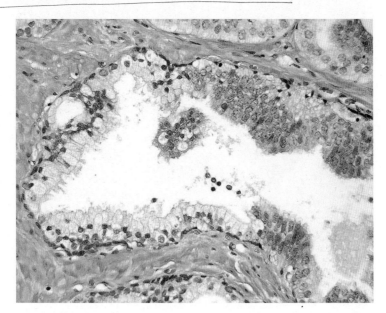

FIGURE 5.8   Abrupt transition between benign epithelium and flat high-grade PIN.

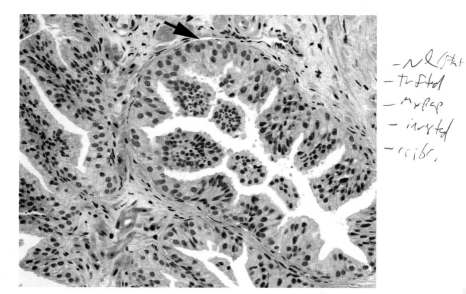

FIGURE 5.9 Micropapillary high-grade PIN. Prominent nucleoli are seen at the edge of the gland against the basement membrane *(arrow)*. Toward the luminal surface, the nuclei appear more benign.

These micropapillary projections are similar to those seen with micropapillary intraductal carcinoma of the breast, in that they are composed of tall epithelial buds, typically lacking fibrovascular cores.

An interesting phenomenon in high-grade PIN is that nuclei toward the center of the gland tend to have more bland cytology, as compared to the nuclei peripherally located up against the basement membrane (Fig. 5.11, eFig. 5.23). Small cell–like change in the center of glands with high-grade PIN is an uncommon finding, which may be a more pronounced manifestation of this phenomenon where there is an abrupt transition between mostly centrally located populations of small cells with bland nuclei and scant cytoplasm and large more typical PIN cells with enlarged nuclei and prominent nucleoli at the periphery.[5] The grade of PIN is assigned based on assessment of the nuclei peripherally located up against the basement membrane (eFigs. 5.24 to 5.82).

With further epithelial hyperplasia, more complex architectural patterns appear such as Roman bridge and cribriform formation (Figs. 5.12 to 5.14). The various patterns of PIN have been designated as flat (eFigs. 5.24 to 5.29), tufting (eFigs. 5.30 to 5.38), micropapillary (eFigs. 5.39 to 5.52, 5.80 to 5.82), and cribriform (eFigs. 5.53 to 5.67).[6] Unusual subtypes of high-grade PIN include PIN with signet-ring features, small cell neuroendocrine PIN, PIN with mucinous features (Fig. 5.15, eFigs. 5.68 to 5.73), foamy PIN (Fig. 5.16, eFigs. 5.20, 5.74 to 5.79), PIN with inverted nuclei (Fig. 5.17, eFig. 5.21), and desquamating apoptotic PIN.[5,7–11]

(text continues on p. 48)

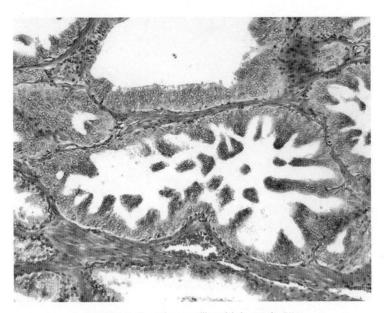

FIGURE 5.10   Micropapillary high-grade PIN.

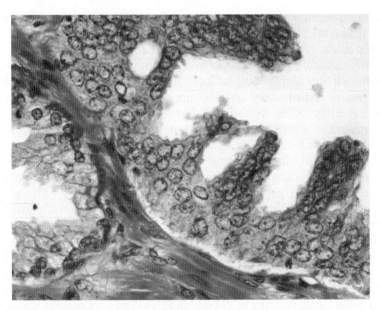

FIGURE 5.11   Higher magnification of Figure 5.10, where more prominent nucleoli are seen at the edge of the gland and nuclei appear more benign toward the luminal surface. Compare atypical cytology to benign gland *(lower left)*.

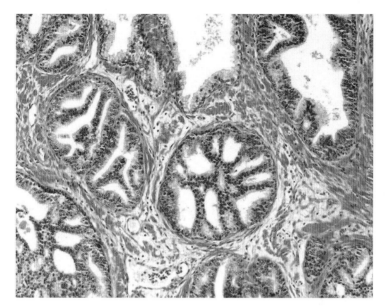

FIGURE 5.12   Cribriform high-grade PIN.

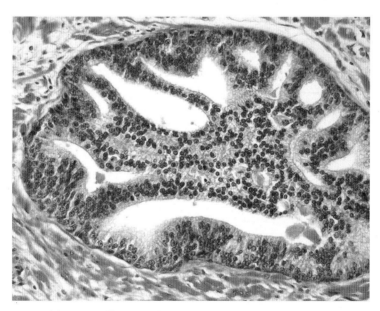

FIGURE 5.13   Higher magnification of Figure 5.12, where more benign–appearing nuclei are toward the center of the gland.

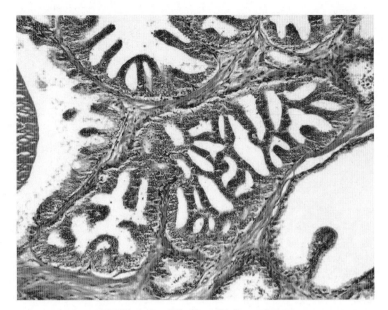

FIGURE 5.14   Cribriform high-grade PIN.

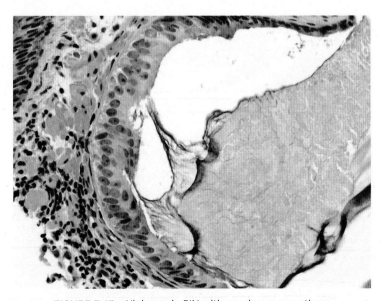

FIGURE 5.15   High-grade PIN with mucinous secretions.

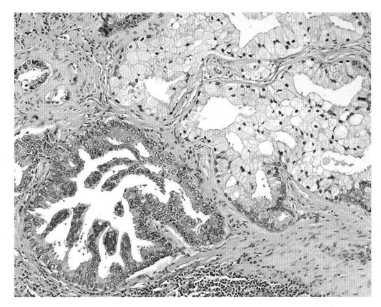

FIGURE 5.16   High-grade PIN of the usual type *(lower left)* and with foamy gland features *(upper right).*

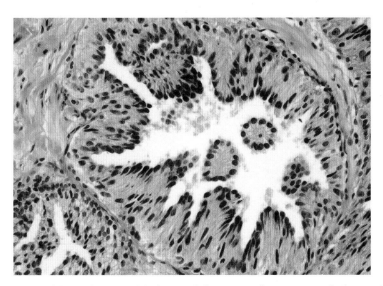

FIGURE 5.17   High-grade PIN with inverted features, where many of the nuclei are oriented to the luminal surface.

PIN attenuated basal cells

EVIDENCE LINKING PROSTATIC INTRAEPITHELIAL NEOPLASIA TO CANCER

Comparing prostates with carcinoma to those without carcinoma, there is an increase in the size and number of high-grade PIN foci, in addition to an increased incidence of high-grade PIN.[12,13] Also, with increasing amounts of high-grade PIN, there are a greater number of multifocal carcinomas. This observation follows if high-grade PIN is a precursor to some carcinomas, since with more precursor lesion, one would expect that there would be more early carcinomas. The finding of zones of high-grade PIN from which there appears to be budding off glands of carcinoma is further histologic evidence that high-grade PIN is a precursor to some prostate carcinomas. McNeal[14] has designated these foci as "transitive glands," although most other investigators prefer the term *high-grade PIN with microinvasive carcinoma*. Several studies have also noted an increase of high-grade PIN in the peripheral zone of the prostate, corresponding to the site of origin for most adenocarcinomas of the prostate.[15] Also, the expression of various biomarkers in high-grade PIN is either (a) the same in high-grade PIN and carcinoma as opposed to benign prostate tissue or (b) intermediate between benign prostate tissue and carcinoma.[12,15,16] All these findings would be expected if high-grade PIN is a precursor lesion to carcinoma of the prostate.

It has been shown that high-grade PIN is more closely related to peripheral, as opposed to transition zone cancers. Intermediate- or high-grade cancers are also more likely to be associated with high-grade PIN, compared to low-grade cancer. This weaker association of high-grade PIN to low-grade transition zone carcinomas is also supported by the histologic differences of high-grade PIN and transition zone carcinomas.[17] Centrally located low-grade adenocarcinomas tend to have bland cytology, often lacking nuclear enlargement or nucleoli in contrast to high-grade PIN. Peripherally located intermediate-grade carcinomas often have identical cytologic features to those of high-grade PIN.

MIMICKERS OF PIN

Central Zone Histology

Glands within the central zone up at the base of the prostate are complex and large with numerous papillary infoldings and often are lined by tall pseudostratified epithelium with eosinophilic cytoplasm (eFigs. 5.83 to 5.90). Occasionally, a prominent basal cell layer surrounds these glands, whereas with high-grade PIN, the basal cell layer is typically indistinct (Fig. 5.18). Central zone glands are frequently overdiagnosed as high-grade PIN because their nuclei are piled up and they may be arranged in Roman bridge and cribriform glandular patterns.[18] However, within these central zone glands, nuclei stream parallel to the glandular bridges, in contrast to the more rigid bridges seen in high-grade PIN (Fig. 5.19). Most important, central zone glands are distinguished from high-grade PIN by their lack of cytologic atypia.

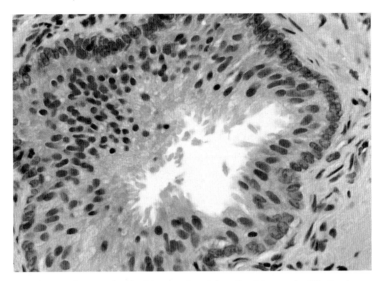

FIGURE 5.18   Central zone gland with prominent basal cell layer, stratified columnar secretory cells, and amphophilic cytoplasm.

Clear Cell Cribriform Hyperplasia   *spectrum of BPH*

Clear cell cribriform hyperplasia consists of crowded cribriform glands, with clear cytoplasm sometimes growing as a nodule and in other instances more diffusely (Figs. 5.20 and 5.21, eFig. 5.91).[19] The key distinguishing feature of clear cell cribriform hyperplasia from high-grade PIN is the lack

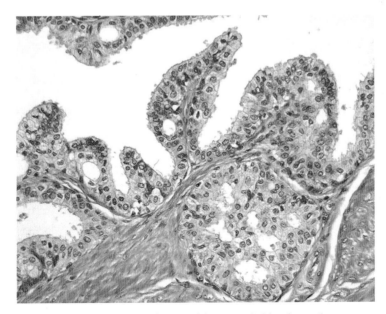

FIGURE 5.19   Central zone with Roman bridge formation.

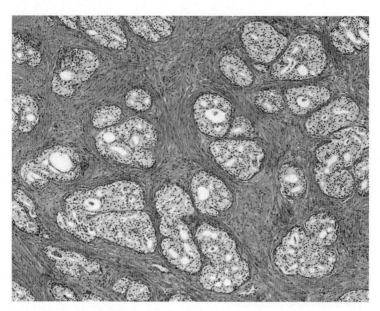

FIGURE 5.20   Clear cell cribriform hyperplasia composed of nests of glands with clear cells growing in a prominent cribriform pattern.

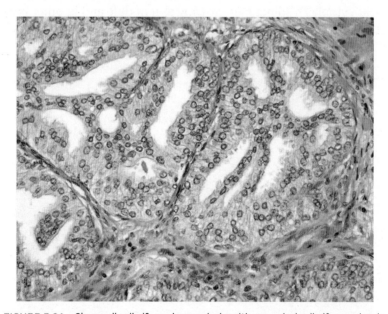

FIGURE 5.21   Clear cell cribriform hyperplasia with crowded cribriform glands.

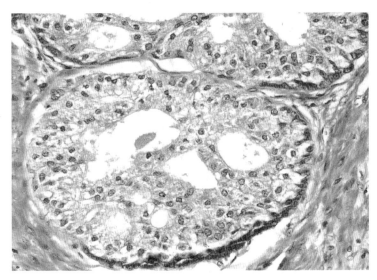

FIGURE 5.22 Higher magnification of clear cell cribriform hyperplasia shows striking basal cell layer and benign cytology in contrast to high-grade PIN.

of nuclear atypia. Furthermore, within a nodule of clear cell cribriform hyperplasia, at least some of the cribriform glands show a strikingly evident basal cell layer, which as noted earlier is not typically seen in high-grade PIN (Fig. 5.22). Immunostaining with antibodies to basal cells cannot distinguish between the two entities, since both have a patchy basal cell layer. Clear cell cribriform hyperplasia is typically located in the transition zone, whereas high-grade PIN predominates in the peripheral zone.

Basal Cell Hyperplasia

Otherwise typical basal cell hyperplasia may show prominent nucleoli along with mitotic activity[20,21] (Fig. 5.23, eFigs. 5.92 to 5.103). Because of the prominent nucleoli, these lesions may be mistaken for high-grade PIN. Although occasionally, the distinction between these two entities may be difficult, usually they are distinct (Table 5.1). There is a proliferation of small round crowded glands in basal cell hyperplasia, whereas in high-grade PIN, the atypical nuclei fill preexisting larger benign glands that are separated from each other by a greater amount of stroma. The nuclei in basal cell hyperplasia tend to be round and at times form small solid basaloid nests. In contrast, the nuclei in high-grade PIN tend to be more pseudostratified and columnar and do not occlude the glandular lumina. Within areas of basal cell hyperplasia, atypical basal cells can be seen undermining overlying benign-appearing secretory cells. The basal cells in these foci tend to have a streaming morphology parallel to the basement membrane. High-grade PIN has full thickness cytologic atypia, with the nuclei oriented perpendicular to the basement membrane. In cases of full thickness basal cell hyperplasia, where an overlying secretory cell layer may

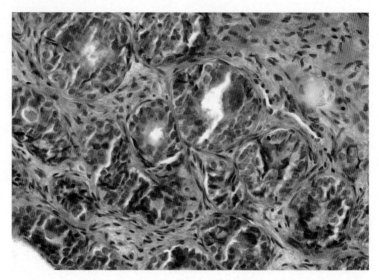

FIGURE 5.23   Crowded tubules of basal cell hyperplasia with prominent nucleoli.

TABLE 5.1 Differential Diagnosis of Basal Cell Hyperplasia with Nucleoli versus High-Grade Prostatic Intraepithelial Neoplasia	
Basal Cell Hyperplasia with Nucleoli	**High-Grade Prostatic Intraepithelial Neoplasia**
More prevalent in transition zone	More common in peripheral zone
Proliferation of small glands	Architecturally benign (large glands without crowding)
Occasional small solid nests	Glands with well-formed lumina
Basal cells with atypical nuclei (blue) undermining benign secretory cells with bland nuclei (red)	No distinct two-cell population
Basal cells stream parallel to basement membrane	Atypical cells perpendicular to basement membrane
Nuclei often round	Nuclei pseudostratified columnar
Pseudocribriform glands	True cribriform glands
Basal cell markers show multilayered positivity	Basal cell markers with flattened single basal cell layer that can be patchy or even negative in occasional glands

not be apparent, the luminal cytoplasm is atrophic, whereas in high-grade PIN, the luminal cells have apical cytoplasm. An additional difference between the two entities is that most cases of basal cell hyperplasia are found in transurethral resection of the prostate (TURP) specimens, indicating growth in the transition zone, in contrast to high-grade PIN's preferential location in the periphery of the prostate. Occasionally, when there are only a few glands to evaluate, such as on needle biopsy, immunohistochemical stains are needed to distinguish the two. Basal cell hyperplasia reveals high molecular weight cytokeratin or p63 positivity in multilayered nuclei, although in some cases, the more centrally located cells are not immunoreactive[22] (Fig. 5.24, eFig. 5.104). In high-grade PIN, high molecular weight cytokeratin or p63 labels only flattened cytologically benign basal cells beneath the negatively stained atypical cells of PIN. Basal cells in benign glands, even when not proliferative, can also have prominent nucleoli and be mistaken for high-grade PIN (Fig. 5.25, eFigs. 5.105 to 5.109). In some institutions' material, basal cell nuclei have a blue-gray appearance, in contrast to the red-violet hue of secretory cell nuclei. Basal cell hyperplasia may also be cribriform, further mimicking high-grade PIN (Fig 5.26, eFigs. 5.110 to 5.113). Whereas cribriform high-grade PIN glands represent a single glandular unit with punched out lumina, many of the glands within a focus of cribriform basal cell hyperplasia appeared as fused individual basal cell hyperplasia glands (pseudocribriform). The use of basal cell immunohistochemistry can help in difficult cases. Cribriform basal cell hyperplasia shows multilayered staining of the basal cells in some of the glands and a continuous layer of immunoreactivity. Cribriform high-grade PIN demonstrates an interrupted immunoreactive single cell layer of basal cells.

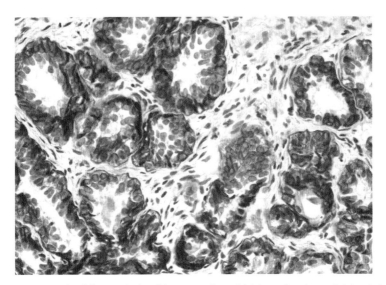

FIGURE 5.24 Basal cell hyperplasia with expression of high molecular weight cytokeratin. Note some of the multilayered cells with prominent nucleoli are positive, although some centrally located cells are negative.

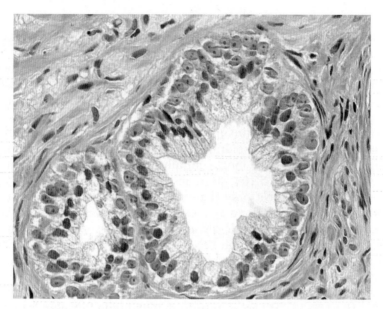

FIGURE 5.25 Benign prostate gland with basal cell nuclei have a lighter gray-purple hue as opposed to more red-purple color of overlying secretory cell nuclei. Note prominent nucleoli in basal cells.

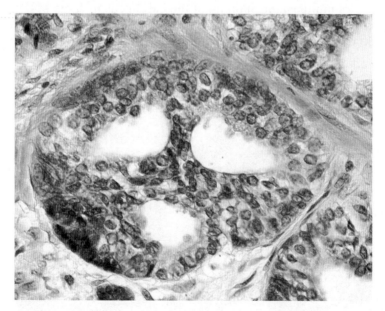

FIGURE 5.26 Pseudocribriform basal cell hyperplasia with fused discrete glands of basal cell hyperplasia.

Acinar (Usual) Adenocarcinoma

In some cases, it is difficult to distinguish cribriform high-grade PIN from cribriform Gleason pattern 3 adenocarcinoma.[23] Although the distinction between cribriform Gleason pattern 3 cancer and cribriform high-grade PIN may be difficult, from a diagnostic standpoint, this is usually not critical. Almost always, when there are atypical cribriform glands, they are accompanied by small atypical infiltrating glands where the diagnosis of infiltrating tumor can be made (Fig. 5.27). Only when cytologically atypical cribriform glands are so large, back-to-back, or outside of the prostate that they are inconsistent with cribriform PIN should infiltrating cribriform carcinoma be diagnosed on hematoxylin and eosin (H&E)–stained sections in the absence of small atypical infiltrating glands (eFigs. 5.15 to 5.23). Immunohistochemistry with antibodies to basal cell markers can be used in difficult cases to differentiate these two entities. In the setting of numerous atypical cribriform glands, a negative reaction in all of the glands is diagnostic of carcinoma; positive staining, even if patchy, verifies the lesion as cribriform PIN. If there are only a few cribriform glands, negative for basal cell markers, it is not diagnostic of carcinoma. This results from the patchy nature with which basal cell markers label high-grade PIN and the recognition that even benign glands may occasionally not be labeled with these antibodies.[22] When there is only one or a few small cribriform glands on needle biopsy without small glands of infiltrating carcinoma, these cases in general are not diagnostic of infiltrating carcinoma. Instead, the diagnosis is "focus of atypical cribriform glands" with a comment that "the distinction

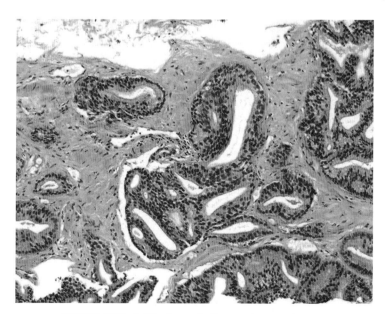

FIGURE 5.27 Infiltrating cribriform acinar carcinoma.

between cribriform high-grade PIN and cribriform carcinoma cannot be made with certainty, and a repeat biopsy is recommended" (eFigs. 5.124 to 5.132). This finding is associated with a higher association of cancer on repeat biopsy (50%) than the finding of high-grade PIN on a biopsy.[24]

The other more common scenario where it is difficult to distinguish acinar adenocarcinoma from high-grade PIN is when there are a few atypical glands immediately adjacent to high-grade PIN.[23] The differential diagnosis is whether these small glands represent tangential sectioning or outpouching off of the high-grade PIN glands or a small focus of carcinoma adjacent to the high-grade PIN (Figs. 5.28 to 5.31, eFigs. 5.133 to 5.149). We refer to these foci at PINATYP. A diagnosis of carcinoma can be rendered only if the small atypical glands are too numerous or too far away from the high-grade PIN glands to represent outpouching or tangential sectioning from the PIN glands (Figs. 5.32 and 5.33, eFigs. 5.150 to 5.159). In cases of PINATYP, the lack of basal cells in the small atypical glands can be construed as evidence that these glands represent infiltrating cancer only if there are more than a few such glands. As high-grade PIN glands can have discontinuous basal cells, one can envision tangential sections off PIN glands in which all cells would appear negative for basal cell markers, such that a few negative small atypical glands adjacent to PIN is not diagnostic of cancer.[25] If the PIN gland has a continuous basal cell later, then one can more confidently diagnose adjacent small focus of carcinoma (Figs. 5.34 and 5.35). Some cases may have the appearance of PINATYP yet will be entirely negative for basal cell markers; these foci may be diagnostic of cancer if there are many glands that are

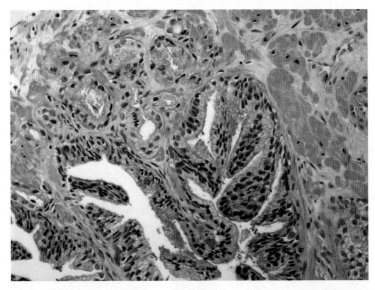

FIGURE 5.28   PINATYP with high-grade PIN with adjacent small atypical glands suspicious for infiltrating carcinoma.

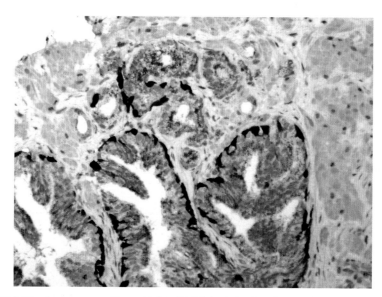

FIGURE 5.29   Same case as Figure 5.28 with triple stain showing both high-grade PIN and many of the small atypical glands with patchy basal cell layer stained with p63 and high molecular weight cytokeratin *(brown)*. Both are also positive for AMACR *(red)*. A definitive diagnosis of infiltrating carcinoma cannot be made.

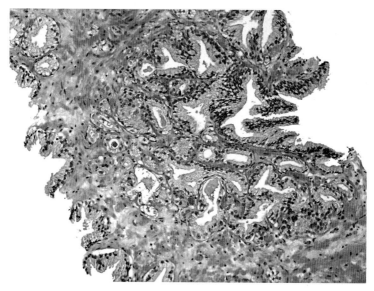

FIGURE 5.30   PINATYP with high-grade PIN with adjacent small atypical glands suspicious for infiltrating carcinoma.

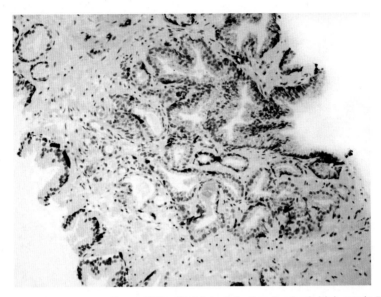

FIGURE 5.31   Same case as Figure 5.30 with triple stain showing both high-grade PIN and many of the small atypical glands with patchy basal cell layer stained with p63 and high molecular weight cytokeratin *(brown)*. Both are also positive for AMACR *(red)*. Due to patchy staining in some of the small glands, a definitive diagnosis of infiltrating carcinoma cannot be made.

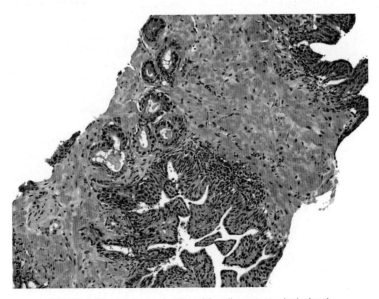

FIGURE 5.32   High-grade PIN with adjacent atypical glands.

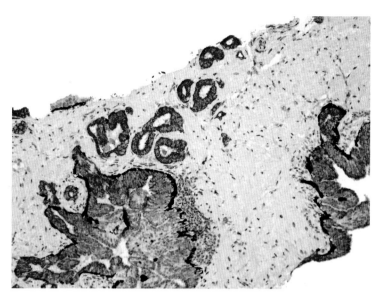

FIGURE 5.33 Same case as Figure 5.32 with small glands lacking a basal cell later *(brown)*. There are a sufficient number of small negative glands that extend far enough away from the high-grade PIN to establish a diagnosis of high-grade PIN with adjacent infiltrating carcinoma.

not immunoreactive. One may also see classic high-grade PIN where some of the glands show the expected patchy basal cell layer and a few identical glands are negative for the basal cell markers; these cases we would still diagnose as high-grade PIN. Racemase does not differentiate between high-grade PIN and cancer because both typically express this antigen.[26,27] Immunohistochemical expression of ERG in high-grade PIN has been

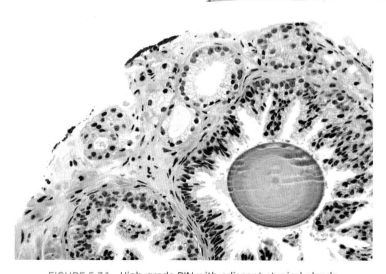

FIGURE 5.34 High-grade PIN with adjacent atypical glands.

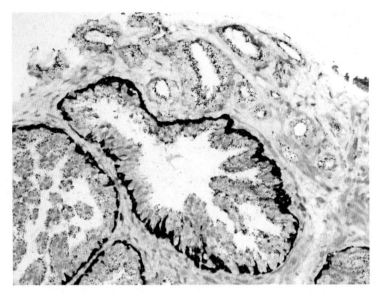

FIGURE 5.35 Same case as Figure 5.44 with small glands negative for basal cell markers *(brown)*. The small glands cannot be outpouching or tangential sectioning of the adjacent high-grade PIN because the latter has an intact basal cell layer.

reported in 5% to 16% of cases, whereas it is seen in approximately 50% of prostate cancers, such that ERG expression cannot be used to discriminate between the two entities.[28,29]

Ductal Adenocarcinoma

A difficult distinction is between high-grade PIN and ductal adenocarcinoma of the prostate (see Chapter 11) (Table 5.2).[30-32] Ductal adenocarcinomas are aggressive tumors, often of advanced pathologic stage, and

TABLE 5.2 Differential Diagnosis of Ductal Adenocarcinoma versus High-Grade Prostatic Intraepithelial Neoplasia

Ductal Adenocarcinoma	High-Grade Prostatic Intraepithelial Neoplasia
More common transition zone	Uncommon in transition zone
True papillary fronds	Micropapillary
May be back-to-back or larger than normal glands	Architecturally benign
May see necrosis	Lacks necrosis
May have detached cancer on needle cores	Lacks detached epithelium on needle core
May have patchy or negative basal cells	May have patchy or negative basal cells

associated with a poor prognosis. Their distinction from cribriform PIN is critical. There are several features that distinguish these two lesions. Ductal adenocarcinomas are often centrally located in the periurethral region and sampled on TURP (eFigs. 5.160 and 5.161). PIN is uncommonly found within the periurethral region and infrequently seen on TURP. Ductal adenocarcinomas often contain true papillary fronds with well-established fibrovascular cores, whereas high-grade PIN more frequently reveals micropapillary fronds with tall columns of epithelium without fibrovascular stalks (eFig. 5.162). Ductal adenocarcinomas frequently contain comedonecrosis, which may be extensive (eFig. 161). High-grade PIN lacks comedonecrosis. Finally, ductal adenocarcinomas may consist of very large and/or back-to-back glands, whereas glands involved by PIN are of the size and distribution of benign glands (eFig. 5.163). The use of basal cell markers in this differential diagnosis may be problematic, as both high-grade PIN and ductal adenocarcinoma may display a patchy basal cell layer. However, absence of a basal cell layer in numerous glands rules out PIN.[33]

Although the most common forms of ductal adenocarcinoma mimic cribriform and micropapillary high-grade PIN, ductal adenocarcinoma may be composed of simple glands lined by stratified columnar epithelium with cytologic and architectural features of flat and tufting high-grade PIN. These PIN-like ductal cancers are distinguished from high-grade PIN either because the atypical glands are too crowded to represent high-grade PIN or there are too many atypical glands that are negative for basal cell markers to be consistent with high-grade PIN.[34,35] Additional differences are in PIN-like ductal adenocarcinoma, many of the glands are lined by flat epithelium (an uncommon pattern in high-grade PIN) and the glands are often cystically dilated (Figs. 5.36 to 5.38, eFigs. 5.164 to 5.169) (see Chapter 11).

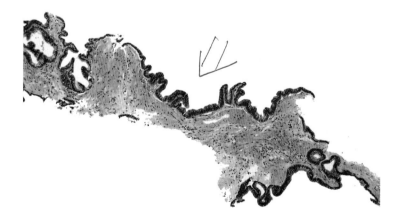

FIGURE 5.36 PIN-like ductal adenocarcinoma with dilated ducts on needle biopsy characterized by long strips of epithelium along the sides of the core.

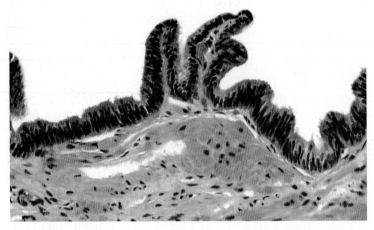

FIGURE 5.37 Same case as Figure 5.36 with ducts lined by pseudostratified columnar epithelium. In contrast, high-grade PIN does not have dilated ducts and would have more prominent nucleoli.

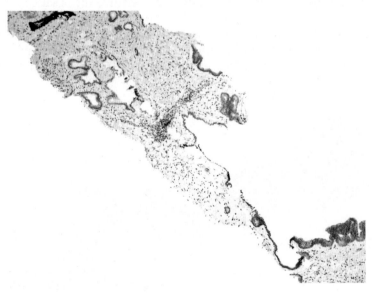

FIGURE 5.38 Same case as Figures 5.36 and 5.37 with lack of basal cells (brown).

LOW-GRADE PROSTATIC INTRAEPITHELIAL NEOPLASIA: RISK OF CANCER ON A REBIOPSY

Low-grade PIN should not be documented as a finding in pathology reports for several reasons. First, there is a lack of reproducibility in its diagnosis even by uropathologists.[23] McNeal's[36] quotation summarizes his consideration of low-grade PIN: "There is not a sharp line of demarcation between grade 1 dysplasia (i.e., low-grade PIN) and mild degrees of deviation from normal histology." More important, there does not appear to be a higher risk of cancer following a diagnosis of low-grade PIN on a biopsy as compared to that following a benign diagnosis on a biopsy.[37] If a diagnosis of low-grade PIN is rendered on a needle biopsy pathology report, it may lead to multiple unnecessary repeat biopsies, which result not only in added costs to the health care system but also to potential patient morbidity and concern.

HIGH-GRADE PROSTATIC INTRAEPITHELIAL NEOPLASIA ON BIOPSY: INCIDENCE, RISK OF CANCER ON A REBIOPSY, AND A REBIOPSY STRATEGY

High-Grade Prostatic Intraepithelial Neoplasia: Incidence on a Biopsy

There is marked variation within the literature on the incidence of high-grade PIN on needle biopsy, ranging from 0% to 24.6%.[37] The mean reported incidence of high-grade PIN on needle biopsy is 7.6%, with a median value of 5.2%. There is no consistent trend in the incidence of high-grade PIN on biopsy as it relates to the type of practice setting (i.e., community hospital, commercial laboratory, academic institution). Although one might expect that greater sampling of the prostate would increase the likelihood of identifying high-grade PIN on needle biopsy, there does not appear to be a relationship between the number of cores sampled and the incidence of high-grade PIN on needle biopsy. There is also no trend for the reported incidence of high-grade PIN over time.

There are several potential explanations for the observed variation in the incidence of high-grade PIN. The hallmark distinguishing low- and high-grade PIN is the presence of prominent nucleoli. Beyond this relatively vague definition, there is much latitude for interpretation. There are no standard criteria defining how prominent or how frequent the nucleoli must be before they are sufficient to warrant a diagnosis of high-grade PIN; as noted at the beginning of this chapter, we use nucleoli visible with the 20× lens as the threshold for diagnosing high-grade PIN. In a survey of urologic pathologists, the majority diagnosed high-grade PIN if any visible nucleoli were present.[38] However, a third of urologic pathologists required nucleoli in at least 10% of the cells in the gland. Allam et al.[39] demonstrated that some general pathologists reviewing a prostate biopsy considered nucleoli were sufficiently prominent to render a diagnosis of high-grade PIN, whereas others looking at the same case felt that the nucleoli were not large enough. Another problem noted by Allam was that while partial involvement of the gland was sufficient for the diagnosis of high-grade PIN for some of the observers, for others it was not. Even within partially involved glands, the number of nucleoli sufficient for the diagnosis of high-grade PIN varied among observers. In another study, 75% of cases diagnosed as high-grade PIN by outside pathologists sent to a genitourinary pathology expert at the request of either the patient or urologist were confirmed as high-grade PIN.[40]

Technical factors relating to the processing of needle biopsy specimens can also contribute to the reported variability in the incidence of high-grade PIN on biopsy. In several studies with higher incidences of high-grade PIN, nonstandard fixatives were used to preserve specimens, which tend to enhance nuclear detail and nucleolar prominence. Technical factors can also potentially explain lower incidences of high-grade PIN reported in the literature. In cases with suboptimal microtomy, sections are thick, resulting in increased uptake of dyes used to stain the tissue that can obscure fine nuclear detail. The resulting difficulty in visualizing nucleoli would lead to a lower reported incidence of high-grade PIN.

Although one study has reported that African American men have a higher incidence of high-grade PIN than Caucasian men, this by itself is unlikely an explanation for the marked variation seen in the literature.[41] An incidence of high-grade PIN between 4% and 8% is a reasonable figure with which a pathologist can benchmark his or her practice. Incidences markedly lower or higher raise the question of either underdiagnosing or overdiagnosing high-grade PIN on needle biopsy.

High-Grade Prostatic Intraepithelial Neoplasia on Biopsy: Overall Risk of Cancer

The most important clinical aspect of high-grade PIN is the risk of cancer for a patient who has been diagnosed with high-grade PIN on needle biopsy. The initial studies evaluating this question in the early 1990s on relatively few cases reported a high percentage of cancer following the diagnosis of high-grade PIN, with most studies citing the risk of cancer to be around 50%.[37] Analyzing more contemporary data published in the year 2000 or later, 23 studies report that the median risk of cancer following a diagnosis of high-grade PIN on biopsy is only 21%.[37]

In order to assess the significance of high-grade PIN on needle biopsy, it is not enough to know the risk of cancer on rebiopsy. However, one must compare the risk of cancer on repeat biopsy following a high-grade PIN diagnosis to the risk of cancer on repeat biopsy following a benign diagnosis. It is widely recognized that even with more extensive sampling of the prostate, a certain percentage of cancers will remain undetected due to sampling error. The median risk of finding cancer in a repeat biopsy following a benign diagnosis is 19%,[37] which is not appreciably different than the risk following a diagnosis of high-grade PIN. Of nine publications that have examined in the same study the risk of cancer on rebiopsy following a needle biopsy diagnosis of high-grade PIN to that following a benign diagnosis, seven showed no statistically significant difference. Subsequent studies have in general shown similar findings, including a study using saturation biopsy.[42,43]

High-Grade Prostatic Intraepithelial Neoplasia on Biopsy: Risk of Cancer Stratified by Clinical Predictors

As several studies have shown that high-grade PIN by itself does not elevate serum prostate-specific antigen (PSA) levels, one might hypothesize that an elevated serum PSA level in a man with high-grade PIN is more likely the result of an associated carcinoma.[44,45] However, most studies have found that serum PSA levels are not predictive of cancer on rebiopsy.[37] Several studies have also examined PSA velocity, free to total PSA, and PSA density with most showing no correlation with risk of cancer on rebiopsy. The results of digital rectal exam, transrectal ultrasound, age, and family history of prostate cancer are also not influential in predicting which men with high-grade PIN on needle biopsy will have carcinoma on rebiopsy.[37] In summary, there does not appear to be any clinical parameter that helps to identify men with high-grade PIN on a needle biopsy who are more likely to have cancer on rebiopsy.

High-Grade Prostatic Intraepithelial Neoplasia on a Biopsy: Risk of Cancer Stratified by Pathologic Predictors

In contemporary studies, the one feature that has correlated with an increased risk of cancer on rebiopsy is the number of cores involved with high-grade PIN. In the largest study by Merrimen et al.,[46,47] there was approximately a 30% chance of cancer on rebiopsy following the diagnosis of high-grade PIN in 2 or more cores. Contemporary smaller studies have also reported an increased risk of cancer on rebiopsy with increased numbers of involved cores. Some of these studies have used a higher cutoff in terms of the number of cores with high-grade PIN (i.e., $\geq$3 or $\geq$4) where 2 or more cores with high-grade PIN may not have been statistically significantly associated with an increased risk of subsequent cancer due to the smaller number of cases.[48–50] Other studies have found an increased risk of cancer with bilateral high-grade PIN or increased proportion of the cores involved by high-grade PIN.[51,52]

Most studies have not found that the morphology of high-grade PIN (flat vs. tufting vs. micropapillary vs. cribriform) can predict which high-grade PIN lesions are at greater risk of being associated with carcinoma on repeat biopsy.[53–56] A caveat to the previous conclusion is that pathologists must use strict criteria to differentiate cribriform high-grade PIN and cribriform carcinoma.

Racemase (alpha-methylacyl coenzyme A racemase [AMACR]) is upregulated both in carcinoma and high-grade PIN and not in benign prostate tissue.[26] In one study utilizing radical prostatectomy specimens, high-grade PIN lesions adjacent to carcinoma had more AMACR overexpression (56%) than high-grade PIN lesions away from cancer (14%).[27]

Further studies are needed to determine whether AMACR expression of high-grade PIN lesions on needle biopsy could help predict which patients are more likely to have cancer.

There are conflicting studies as to the relation of ERG on high-grade PIN biopsies and the subsequent risk of cancer. In the study by He et al.[28] from the Cleveland Clinic, positive ERG immunohistochemical expression was not associated with an increased cancer detection in subsequent repeat biopsies. In the other study to assess this marker, a greater number of patients (56 of 59, 94.9%) with an ERG rearrangements rate of 1.6% or greater on initial biopsy were diagnosed with prostate cancer during repeat biopsy follow-ups as compared with those (5 of 103, 4.9%) with an ERG rearrangements rate of less than 1.6% ($P < 0.001$) using fluorescent in situ hybridization (FISH). Although there was a significant positive correlation between the ERG rearrangement rate by FISH and the ERG protein expression, the authors did not state that using ERG immunohistochemistry was useful to predict which PIN lesions on biopsy were associated with cancer on rebiopsy.[57]

High-Grade Prostatic Intraepithelial Neoplasia on Biopsy: Risk of Cancer Stratified by Number of Cores Sampled

A major contributing factor to the decreased incidence of cancer following a diagnosis of high-grade PIN on needle biopsy in the contemporary era relates to increased needle core biopsy sampling. Relatively poor sampling (i.e., sextant biopsies) on the initial biopsy misses associated cancers resulting in only high-grade PIN on the initial biopsy. With rebiopsy, some of these initially missed cancers are detected, yielding a high risk of cancer following a sextant needle biopsy diagnosis of high-grade PIN. Sampling more extensively on the initial biopsy detects many associated cancers, such that when only high-grade PIN is found, they often truly represent isolated high-grade PIN; therefore, rebiopsy even with good sampling does not detect many additional cancers.[58]

High-Grade Prostatic Intraepithelial Neoplasia on Biopsy: Repeat Biopsy Strategy and Technique

Recommendations for following men with high-grade PIN on biopsy have varied widely. It is the recommendation of these reviewers that men do not need a routine repeat needle biopsy within the first year following the diagnosis of a single core with high-grade PIN in the absence of other clinical indicators of cancer. Unifocal high-grade PIN is not associated with an increased risk of cancer on rebiopsy that is much different than men with a benign diagnosis on the initial biopsy. If there are 2 or more cores with high-grade PIN, the risk of cancer is sufficiently high (30% to 40%), justifying rebiopsy within 6 months.

Studies from New York University Medical Center have raised the question of whether repeat biopsy should be performed several years following a high-grade PIN diagnosis because men with high-grade PIN have a continued risk of developing prostate cancer during long-term follow-up.[59-61] However, these studies did not report the number of cores with high-grade PIN.

Data from Cleveland Clinic reported estimated cancer rates of 3.6%, 12.5%, and 22.4% for patients with a benign diagnosis; 4.4%, 14.7%, and 26.1% for patients with unifocal high-grade PIN; and 9.1%, 29.0%, and 47.8% for patients with multifocal high-grade PIN, at 1, 3, and 5 years, respectively.[52] At 3 and 5 years' follow-up after the initial biopsy, there were no significant differences in the risk of cancer between an initial benign diagnosis and a diagnosis of unifocal high-grade PIN. It is therefore questionable whether men with a single core with high-grade PIN ever need a repeat biopsy.

A limited number of studies have evaluated where cancer is found on rebiopsy. The risk of cancer being found in the contralateral lobe to where high-grade PIN is initially diagnosed ranges in studies from 10% to 40% with an average of 30%. The risk of finding cancer in the same sextant site where high-grade PIN was initially found is reported to be on average 55%.[62–65] In one of these studies, there was a 74% probability of cancer on repeat biopsy being in the same sextant site as the initial high-grade PIN and an 89% risk of cancer being in the same and adjacent sextant sites as the initial high-grade PIN.[64] If cancer was randomly distributed throughout the prostate in men with high-grade PIN on needle biopsy, one would expect the risk of cancer in any given sextant site to be one-sixth (16.7%). Based on these data, it is recommended that if rebiopsy is performed for high-grade PIN, sampling should be proportionally more in the region of the original high-grade PIN site and in adjacent sites, although the entire prostate should be sampled.

High-Grade Prostatic Intraepithelial Neoplasia: Significance on Transurethral Resection of the Prostate Material

The significance of finding high-grade PIN on TURP is more controversial. Whereas two studies have found that high-grade PIN on TURP places an individual at higher risk for the subsequent detection of cancer, a long-term study from Norway demonstrated no association between the presence of high-grade PIN on TURP and the incidence of subsequent cancer.[66–68] In a younger man with high-grade PIN on TURP, we would recommend that needle biopsies be performed to rule out a peripheral zone cancer. In an older man without elevated serum PSA levels, clinical follow-up is probably sufficient. When high-grade PIN is found on TURP, some pathologists recommend sectioning deeper into the corresponding block and most pathologists recommend processing the entire specimen.[67]

High-Grade Prostatic Intraepithelial Neoplasia on Biopsy: Findings at Subsequent Radical Prostatectomy

Men who are found to have high-grade PIN then cancer on repeat biopsy needle who subsequently undergo radical prostatectomy have more favorable pathologic stage than cases where cancer is diagnosed on the first biopsy. Tumor size at radical prostatectomy is also small in cases where the initial diagnosis is high-grade PIN followed by cancer on repeat needle biopsy. These findings likely reflect cancers associated with high-grade PIN, in which the cancers were missed on the initial biopsy as a result of smaller size.[69]

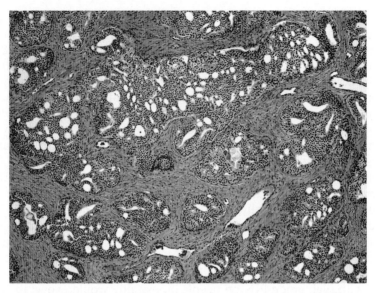

FIGURE 5.39 Intraductal carcinoma with dense cribriform pattern.

INTRADUCTAL CARCINOMA OF THE PROSTATE

Intraductal carcinoma of the prostate (IDC-P) in radical prostatectomy specimens is described as an atypical glandular lesion that spans the entire lumen of prostatic ducts or acini while the normal architecture of ducts or acini is still maintained (Figs. 5.39 and 5.40).[70-74] Rarely, IDC-P may

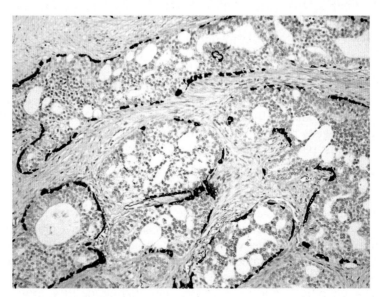

FIGURE 5.40 Same case as Figure 5.39 with intact basal layer (p63 and high molecular weight cytokeratin) around each cribriform glands.

TABLE 5.3	Definition of Intraductal Carcinoma of the Prostate

Malignant epithelium filling large acini or ducts with preservation of basal cells and:

- Solid or dense cribriform pattern

  or

- Loose cribriform or micropapillary pattern with either (a) marked nuclear atypia (nuclei 6× normal) or (b) necrosis

be identified on biopsy material in the absence of infiltrating carcinoma. Our definition of IDC-P on needle biopsy was derived to identify objective morphologic criteria that either architecturally or cytologically clearly exceed those seen in high-grade PIN (Table 5.3) [75] (Figs. 5.41 to 5.49, eFigs. 5.170 to 5.182). A dense cribriform pattern was one where there were overtly more solid than luminal areas (i.e., ratio of solid to luminal areas >70%). IDC-P may also rarely show small cell–like change, which may also be seen in high-grade PIN and infiltrating carcinoma (Fig. 5.50).[5] IDC-P on prostate biopsies is frequently associated with high-grade cancer and poor prognostic parameters at radical prostatectomy. In the largest study, of 21 radical prostatectomies, there was extraprostatic extension without seminal vesicle invasion in 38% and seminal vesicle invasion in 13% of cases. Organ-confined disease was present in 38% of cases and intraductal carcinoma without identifiable invasive cancer was seen in 10%. Average Gleason score was 7.9.[76] These findings support prior

(text continues on p. 74)

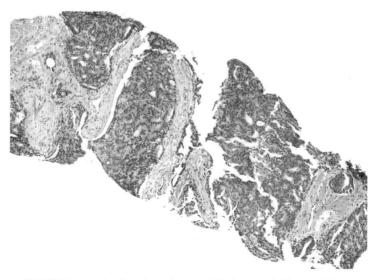

FIGURE 5.41 Intraductal carcinoma with dense cribriform pattern.

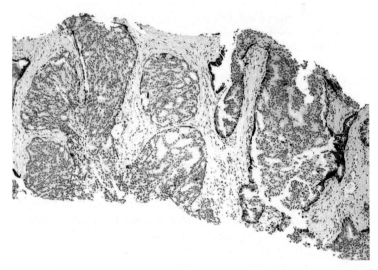

FIGURE 5.42 Same case as Figure 5.41 with intact basal layer (p63 and high molecular weight cytokeratin) around each cribriform glands.

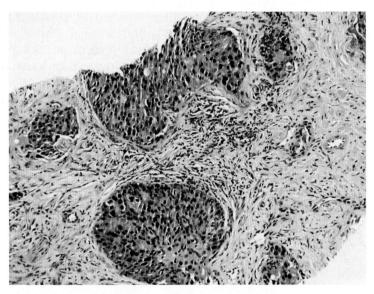

FIGURE 5.43 Intraductal carcinoma with solid nested pattern.

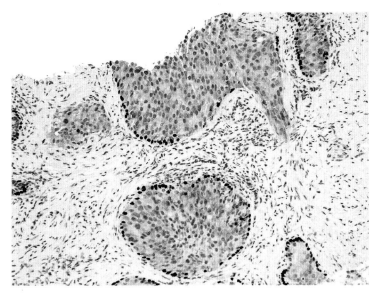

FIGURE 5.44 Same case as Figure 5.43 with intact basal layer (p63) around each nest of cells.

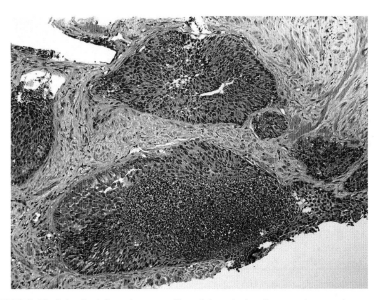

FIGURE 5.45 Intraductal carcinoma with solid nested pattern and comedonecrosis.

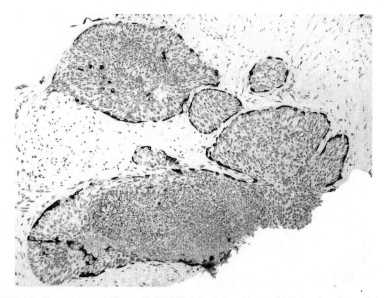

FIGURE 5.46   Same case as Figure 5.45 with intact basal layer (high molecular weight cyto-keratin) around each nest of cells.

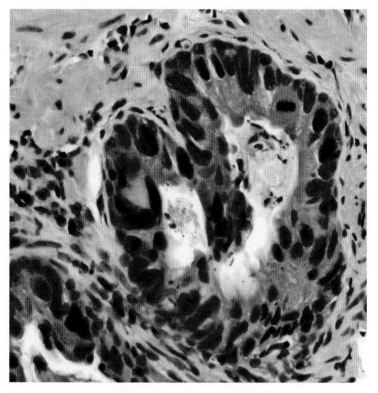

FIGURE 5.47   Intraductal carcinoma with markedly pleomorphic nuclei.

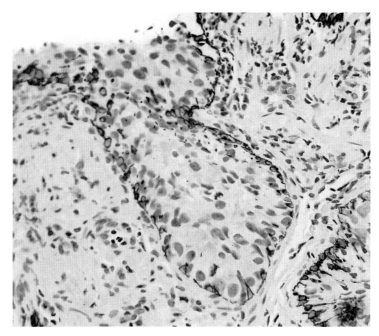

FIGURE 5.48   Same case as Figure 5.47 with intact basal layer (high molecular weight cytokeratin) around each nest of cells.

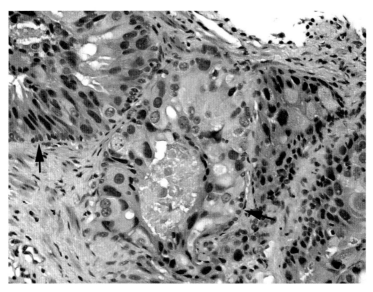

FIGURE 5.49   Intraductal carcinoma with markedly pleomorphic nuclei. A basal cell layer is visible on H&E stain (arrows).

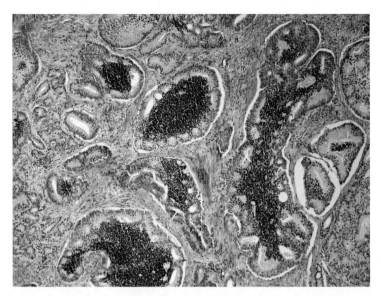

FIGURE 5.50 Intraductal carcinoma with small cell–like change and adjacent small glands of infiltrating carcinoma *(left)*. A basal cell layer was present around all the larger cribriform glands.

studies that IDC-P represents an advanced stage of tumor progression with intraductal spread of tumor in most cases. However, in some cases, IDC-P is precursor distinct and more likely to be associated with aggressive prostate cancer than high-grade PIN.

Infiltrating cribriform acinar adenocarcinoma (Gleason pattern 4 or Gleason pattern 5 with comedonecrosis) closely mimics cribriform IDC-P (Table 5.4). Most cases of IDC-P would be diagnosed as cribriform carcinoma if immunohistochemistry demonstrating basal cells had not been performed (Figs. 5.51 and 5.52). In some cases, the contour and branching pattern of normal duct architecture suggests the diagnosis of IDC-P as opposed to infiltrating carcinoma. As described in the following

TABLE 5.4 Cribriform Acinar Adenocarcinoma versus Cribriform Intraductal Carcinoma of the Prostate

Cribriform Acinar Adenocarcinoma	Cribriform Intraductal Carcinoma of the Prostate
Lacks branching glands	May have branching glands
Much larger than normal glands	Can be larger than normal glands
Irregular, infiltrative borders	Rounded, circumscribed glands
Absence of basal cells	Basal cells present

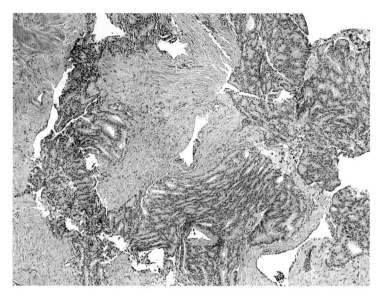

FIGURE 5.51 Cribriform carcinoma, which by H&E stain only could be misdiagnosed as infiltrating cribriform carcinoma.

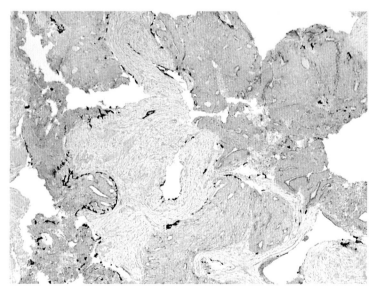

FIGURE 5.52 Same case as Figure 5.51 with intact basal layer (high molecular weight cyto-keratin and p63) around each cribriform gland, diagnostic of intraductal carcinoma.

text, the treatment recommendations for IDC-P and infiltrating high-grade prostate adenocarcinomas are identical, such that the distinction on biopsy is usually not critical. Consequently, some experts have suggested that IDC-P should be diagnosed as Gleason pattern 4 if IDC-P is composed of cribriform glands without necrosis or Gleason pattern 5 if consisting of solid nests or cribriform glands with necrosis. Whereas in most cases following this proposal would be consistent with findings at radical prostatectomy, some cases of IDC-P on biopsy are shown to have only IDC-P at resection without infiltrating carcinoma. For these men, it would be inaccurate to label them as having aggressive disease with a predicted poor prognosis on biopsy, where pure IDC-P at radical prostatectomy would be 100% cured by surgery. From a practical standpoint, if there is obvious infiltrating Gleason pattern 4 or higher grade adenocarcinoma on a biopsy core associated with possible IDC-P, typically, stains for basal cells to prove IDC-P is not recommended. If there is IDC-P identifiable on H&E-stained sections along with infiltrating high-grade carcinoma, then the cores are diagnosed as infiltrating carcinoma with intraductal spread and the measurement of the cancer includes both the infiltrating and IDC-P components. If there is no definitive infiltrating carcinoma on H&E-stained sections and a suggestion of IDC-P in a core, then basal stains are recommended to differentiate IDC-P from infiltrating carcinoma. In cases where there is Gleason pattern 3 infiltrating carcinoma and IDC-P on biopsy, we add a note that IDC-P is typically associated with high-grade adenocarcinoma, which is not present most likely due to sampling error.

There is significant morphologic overlap between ductal adenocarcinoma of the prostate and IDC-P (Table 5.5). Distinguishing features seen in ductal adenocarcinoma include tall pseudostratified columnar epithelium usually with amphophilic cytoplasm, classically arranged in cribriform patterns with slitlike spaces and/or true papillary fronds. In contrast, IDC-P has cuboidal cells, cribriform patterns with rounded lumina, and micropapillary tufts without fibrovascular cores. In addition, basal cells are generally absent in ductal adenocarcinoma, although occasionally, there may be partial retention of basal cells as ductal adenocarcinoma can also spread within prostatic ducts.

TABLE 5.5 Ductal Adenocarcinoma versus Intraductal Carcinoma of the Prostate

Ductal Adenocarcinoma	Intraductal Carcinoma of the Prostate
Cribriform with slitlike spaces	Cribriform with rounded lumina
Pseudostratified columnar cells	Cuboidal cells
Papillary fronds	Micropapillary fronds
Basal cells variably present	Basal cells always present

TABLE 5.6 **Intraductal Urothelial Carcinoma versus Intraductal Carcinoma of the Prostate**

Intraductal Urothelial Carcinoma	Intraductal Carcinoma of the Prostate
Rarely associated with glands	Often glandular or cribriform
Often solid nests	Occasional solid nests
Often marked pleomorphism	Occasional marked pleomorphism
Prostatic markers negative (PSA, P501S, NKX3.1)	Prostate markers positive
Urothelial markers positive (GATA3, thrombomodulin, p63, HMWCK)	Urothelial markers negative

PSA, prostate-specific antigen; HMWCK, high molecular weight cytokeratin.

Solid patterns of IDC-P may mimic intraductal spread of urothelial carcinoma in the prostate, as both demonstrate solid intraductal–acinar involvement (Table 5.6).[77] Other overlapping morphologic features include marked nuclear pleomorphism, frequent mitotic activity, and comedonecrosis. However, solid patterns of IDC-P are often associated with cribriform or glandular patterns. When it is difficult to distinguish IDC-P from urothelial carcinoma, immunohistochemical studies generally resolve the problem, as IDC-P is usually positive for PSA, P501S, and NKX3.1 but negative for high molecular weight cytokeratin, p63, thrombomodulin, and GATA3, opposite to what is typically seen with urothelial carcinoma.

The most critical distinction is between high-grade PIN and IDC-P, as the former is typically not treated with definitive therapy and there is a question whether high-grade PIN on needle biopsy even requires immediate rebiopsy within the first year following its diagnosis. It has been questioned whether reproducible criteria can be developed to distinguish IDC-P from high-grade PIN.[12] Both entities share cytologic features such as nuclear enlargement, hyperchromasia, and enlarged nucleoli. Although the solid and dense cribriform patterns are not architectural patterns associated with high-grade PIN, loose cribriform and micropapillary patterns overlap between the two entities. To establish the diagnosis of IDC-P in the latter two patterns, other cytologic features such as markedly enlarged nuclei (six times larger than those in adjacent nonneoplastic cells) and comedonecrosis are required. Cases that do not satisfy the strict criteria for IDC-P on needle biopsy yet appear more atypical either architecturally or cytologically than usual high-grade PIN can be diagnosed as borderline between IDC-P and high-grade PIN with a strong recommendation for repeat biopsy.

Despite its morphology resembling high-grade PIN, IDC-P in most cases is not likely to be a preinvasive neoplastic condition. Whereas high-grade PIN is often present in prostate glands that have not yet developed invasive carcinoma, IDC-P is almost always associated with invasive cancer. Dawkins et al.[78] studied allelic instability in prostate cancers to define the position of IDC-P in the sequence of prostate cancer progression. They found that 29% of Gleason pattern 4 cancers and 60% of IDC-P demonstrated loss of heterozygosity (LOH) of certain microsatellite markers, while LOH was rarely observed in PIN and Gleason pattern 3 adenocarcinoma. In another study, ERG rearrangement was absent (0 of 16) in isolated cribriform high-grade PIN, whereas it was present in 75% (36 of 48) of IDC-P.[79] Confirming these findings, Lotan et al.[80] from our institution found that ERG immunohistochemical expression was identified in 58% (26 of 45) of intraductal carcinoma compared with 13% (5 of 39) of PIN. More discriminating was that cytoplasmic PTEN loss was identified in 84% (38 of 45) of the intraductal carcinoma yet was never observed in PIN (0 of 39).[80] PTEN genomic and PTEN protein loss in prostate cancer have been associated with more aggressive disease, and it is possible that PTEN loss may be a key underlying molecular aberration driving poor prognosis in intraductal carcinoma. As noted earlier, the classification schemes to distinguish intraductal carcinoma from high-grade PIN on biopsy are fairly stringent to avoid overdiagnosis of IDC-P with subsequent overtreatment. Correspondingly, there is a subset of cases that will be diagnosed as borderline between high-grade PIN and IDC-P. PTEN loss in a minority of these borderline lesions may be consistent with IDC-P that is not morphologically recognized by current criteria. Future studies are needed to confirm the use of PTEN immunohistochemistry for distinguishing IDC-P from high-grade PIN in the prostate biopsy setting. All of the cited molecular studies support that IDC-P is a distinct lesion from high-grade PIN and represents a late event in prostate cancer evolution.

In summary, IDC-P on needle biopsy is frequently associated with high-grade cancer and poor prognostic parameters at radical prostatectomy as well as often advanced disease following other therapies. We recommend definitive therapy (i.e., radical prostatectomy or radiation therapy) for men with IDC-P on biopsy aggressively even in the absence of documented infiltrating cancer.

REFERENCES

1. Bostwick DG, Brawer MK. Prostatic intra-epithelial neoplasia and early invasion in prostate cancer. *Cancer.* 1987;59:788–794.
2. Drago JR, Mostofi FK, Lee F. Introductory remarks and workshop summary. *Urol.* 1989;34(suppl):2–3.
3. McNeal JE. Origin and development of carcinoma in the prostate. *Cancer.* 1969;23:24–34.
4. McNeal JE, Bostwick DG. Intraductal dysplasia: a premalignant lesion of the prostate. *Hum Pathol.* 1986;17:64–71.
5. Lee S, Han JS, Chang A, et al. Small cell-like change in prostatic intraepithelial neoplasia, intraductal carcinoma, and invasive prostatic carcinoma: a study of 7 cases. *Hum Pathol.* 2013;44:427–431.

6. Bostwick DG, Amin MB, Dundore P, et al. Architectural patterns of high-grade prostatic intraepithelial neoplasia. *Hum Pathol.* 1993;24:298–310.

7. Argani P, Epstein JI. Inverted (Hobnail) high-grade prostatic intraepithelial neoplasia (PIN): report of 15 cases of a previously undescribed pattern of high-grade PIN. *Am J Surg Pathol.* 2001;25:1534–1539.

8. Berman DM, Yang J, Epstein JI. Foamy gland high-grade prostatic intraepithelial neoplasia. *Am J Surg Pathol.* 2000;24:140–144.

9. Reyes AO, Swanson PE, Carbone JM, et al. Unusual histologic types of high-grade prostatic intraepithelial neoplasia. *Am J Surg Pathol.* 1997;21:1215–1222.

10. Zhao J, Epstein JI. High-grade foamy gland prostatic adenocarcinoma on biopsy or transurethral resection: a morphologic study of 55 cases. *Am J Surg Pathol.* 2009;33:583–590.

11. Cohen RJ, O'Brien BA, Wheeler TM. Desquamating apoptotic variant of high-grade prostatic intraepithelial neoplasia: a possible precursor of intraductal prostatic carcinoma. *Hum Pathol.* 2011;42:892–895.

12. Bostwick DG, Qian J. High-grade prostatic intraepithelial neoplasia. *Mod Pathol.* 2004;17:360–379.

13. Joniau S, Goeman L, Pennings J, et al. Prostatic intraepithelial neoplasia (PIN): importance and clinical management. *Eur Urol.* 2005;48:379–385.

14. McNeal JE, Villers A, Redwine EA, et al. Microcarcinoma in the prostate: its association with duct-acinar dysplasia. *Hum Pathol.* 1991;22:644–652.

15. Haggman MJ, Macoska JA, Wojno KJ, et al. The relationship between prostatic intraepithelial neoplasia and prostate cancer: critical issues. *J Urol.* 1997;158:12–22.

16. Bostwick DG, Pacelli A, Lopez-Beltran A. Molecular biology of prostatic intraepithelial neoplasia. *Prostate.* 1996;29:117–134.

17. Greene DR, Wheeler TM, Egawa S, et al. A comparison of the morphological features of cancer arising in the transition zone and in the peripheral zone of the prostate. *J Urol.* 1991;146:1069–1076.

18. Srodon M, Epstein JI. Central zone histology of the prostate: a mimicker of high-grade prostatic intraepithelial neoplasia. *Hum Pathol.* 2002;33:518–523.

19. Ayala AG, Srigley JR, Ro JY, et al. Clear cell cribriform hyperplasia of prostate. Report of 10 cases. *Am J Surg Pathol.* 1986;10:665–671.

20. Devaraj LT, Bostwick DG. Atypical basal cell hyperplasia of the prostate. Immunophenotypic profile and proposed classification of basal cell proliferations. *Am J Surg Pathol.* 1993;17:645–659.

21. Epstein JI, Armas OA. Atypical basal cell hyperplasia of the prostate. *Am J Surg Pathol.* 1992;16:1205–1214.

22. Hedrick L, Epstein JI. Use of keratin 903 as an adjunct in the diagnosis of prostate carcinoma. *Am J Surg Pathol.* 1989;13:389–396.

23. Epstein JI, Grignon DJ, Humphrey PA, et al. Interobserver reproducibility in the diagnosis of prostatic intraepithelial neoplasia. *Am J Surg Pathol.* 1995;19:873–886.

24. Kronz JD, Shaikh AA, Epstein JI. Atypical cribriform lesions on prostate biopsy. *Am J Surg Pathol.* 2001;25:147–155.

25. Kronz JD, Shaikh AA, Epstein JI. High-grade prostatic intraepithelial neoplasia with adjacent small atypical glands on prostate biopsy. *Hum Pathol.* 2001;32:389–395.

26. Jiang Z, Woda BA, Wu CL, et al. Discovery and clinical application of a novel prostate cancer marker: alpha-methylacyl CoA racemase (P504S). *Am J Clin Pathol.* 2004;122:275–289.

27. Wu CL, Yang XJ, Tretiakova M, et al. Analysis of alpha-methylacyl-CoA racemase (P504S) expression in high-grade prostatic intraepithelial neoplasia. *Hum Pathol.* 2004;35:1008–1013.

28. He H, Osunkoya AO, Carver P, et al. Expression of ERG protein, a prostate cancer specific marker, in high grade prostatic intraepithelial neoplasia (HGPIN): lack of utility to stratify cancer risks associated with HGPIN. *BJU Int.* 2012;110:E751–E755.

29. Zhang S, Pavlovitz B, Tull J, et al. Detection of TMPRSS2 gene deletions and translocations in carcinoma, intraepithelial neoplasia, and normal epithelium of the prostate by direct fluorescence in situ hybridization. *Diagn Mol Pathol.* 2010;19:151–156.

30. Christensen WN, Steinberg G, Walsh PC, et al. Prostatic duct adenocarcinoma. Findings at radical prostatectomy. *Cancer.* 1991;67:2118–2124.

31. Bostwick DG, Kindrachuk RW, Rouse RV. Prostatic adenocarcinoma with endometrioid features. Clinical, pathologic, and ultrastructural findings. *Am J Surg Pathol.* 1985;9: 595–609.

32. Epstein JI, Woodruff JM. Adenocarcinoma of the prostate with endometrioid features. A light microscopic and immunohistochemical study of ten cases. *Cancer.* 1986;57: 111–119.

33. Samaratunga H, Singh M. Distribution pattern of basal cells detected by cytokeratin 34 beta E12 in primary prostatic duct adenocarcinoma. *Am J Surg Pathol.* 1997;21: 435–40.

34. Tavora F, Epstein JI. High-grade prostatic intraepithelial neoplasialike ductal adenocarcinoma of the prostate: a clinicopathologic study of 28 cases. *Am J Surg Pathol.* 2008;32:1060–1067.

35. Hameed O, Humphrey PA. Stratified epithelium in prostatic adenocarcinoma: a mimic of high-grade prostatic intraepithelial neoplasia. *Mod Pathol.* 2006;19:899–906.

36. McNeal JE. Significance of duct-acinar dysplasia in prostatic carcinogenesis. *Urology.* 1989;34:9–15.

37. Epstein JI, Herawi M. Prostate needle biopsies containing prostatic intraepithelial neoplasia or atypical foci suspicious for carcinoma: implications for patient care. *J Urol.* 2006;175:820–834.

38. Egevad L, Allsbrook WC Jr, Epstein JI. Current practice of diagnosis and reporting of prostate cancer on needle biopsy among genitourinary pathologists. *Hum Pathol.* 2006;37:292–297.

39. Allam CK, Bostwick DG, Hayes JA, et al. Interobserver variability in the diagnosis of high-grade prostatic intraepithelial neoplasia and adenocarcinoma. *Mod Pathol.* 1996;9:742–751.

40. Chan TY, Epstein JI. Patient and urologist driven second opinion of prostate needle biopsies. *J Urol.* 2005;174:1390–1394; discussion 1394; author reply 1394.

41. Fowler JE Jr, Bigler SA, Lynch C, et al. Prospective study of correlations between biopsy-detected high grade prostatic intraepithelial neoplasia, serum prostate specific antigen concentration, and race. *Cancer.* 2001;91:1291–1296.

42. Ploussard G, Plennevaux G, Allory Y, et al. High-grade prostatic intraepithelial neoplasia and atypical small acinar proliferation on initial 21-core extended biopsy scheme: incidence and implications for patient care and surveillance. *World J Urol.* 2009;27:587–592.

43. Merrimen JL, Evans AJ, Srigley JR. Preneoplasia in the prostate gland with emphasis on high grade prostatic intraepithelial neoplasia. *Pathology.* 2013;45:251–263.

44. Alexander EE, Qian J, Wollan PC, et al. Prostatic intraepithelial neoplasia does not appear to raise serum prostate-specific antigen concentration. *Urology.* 1996;47:693–698.

45. Ronnett BM, Carmichael MJ, Carter HB, et al. Does high grade prostatic intraepithelial neoplasia result in elevated serum prostate specific antigen levels? *J Urol.* 1993;150: 386–389.

46. Merrimen JL, Jones G, Srigley JR. Is high grade prostatic intraepithelial neoplasia still a risk factor for adenocarcinoma in the era of extended biopsy sampling? *Pathology.* 2010;42:325–329.

47. Merrimen JL, Jones G, Walker D, et al. Multifocal high grade prostatic intraepithelial neoplasia is a significant risk factor for prostatic adenocarcinoma. *J Urol*. 2009;182:485–490.
48. De Nunzio C, Trucchi A, Miano R, et al. The number of cores positive for high grade prostatic intraepithelial neoplasia on initial biopsy is associated with prostate cancer on second biopsy. *J Urol*. 2009;181:1069–1074.
49. Netto GJ, Epstein JI. Widespread high-grade prostatic intraepithelial neoplasia on prostatic needle biopsy: a significant likelihood of subsequently diagnosed adenocarcinoma. *Am J Surg Pathol*. 2006;30:1184–1188.
50. Abdel-Khalek M, El-Baz M, Ibrahiem E. Predictors of prostate cancer on extended biopsy in patients with high-grade prostatic intraepithelial neoplasia: a multivariate analysis model. *BJU Int*. 2004;94:528–533.
51. Akhavan A, Keith JD, Bastacky SI, et al. The proportion of cores with high-grade prostatic intraepithelial neoplasia on extended-pattern needle biopsy is significantly associated with prostate cancer on site-directed repeat biopsy. *BJU Int*. 2007;99:765–769.
52. Lee MC, Moussa AS, Yu C, et al. Multifocal high grade prostatic intraepithelial neoplasia is a risk factor for subsequent prostate cancer. *J Urol*. 2010;184:1958–1962.
53. Bishara T, Ramnani DM, Epstein JI. High-grade prostatic intraepithelial neoplasia on needle biopsy: risk of cancer on repeat biopsy related to number of involved cores and morphologic pattern. *Am J Surg Pathol*. 2004;28:629–633.
54. Davidson D, Bostwick DG, Qian J, et al. Prostatic intraepithelial neoplasia is a risk factor for adenocarcinoma: predictive accuracy in needle biopsies. *J Urol*. 1995;154:1295–1299.
55. Kronz JD, Allan CH, Shaikh AA, et al. Predicting cancer following a diagnosis of high-grade prostatic intraepithelial neoplasia on needle biopsy: data on men with more than one follow-up biopsy. *Am J Surg Pathol*. 2001;25:1079–1085.
56. San Francisco IF, Olumi AF, Kao J, et al. Clinical management of prostatic intraepithelial neoplasia as diagnosed by extended needle biopsies. *BJU Int*. 2003;91:350–354.
57. Gao X, Li LY, Zhou FJ, et al. ERG rearrangement for predicting subsequent cancer diagnosis in high-grade prostatic intraepithelial neoplasia and lymph node metastasis. *Clin Cancer Res*. 2012;18:4163–4172.
58. Herawi M, Kahane H, Cavallo C, et al. Risk of prostate cancer on first re-biopsy within 1 year following a diagnosis of high grade prostatic intraepithelial neoplasia is related to the number of cores sampled. *J Urol*. 2006;175:121–124.
59. Lefkowitz GK, Sidhu GS, Torre P, et al. Is repeat prostate biopsy for high-grade prostatic intraepithelial neoplasia necessary after routine 12-core sampling? *Urology*. 2001;58:999–1003.
60. Lefkowitz GK, Taneja SS, Brown J, et al. Followup interval prostate biopsy 3 years after diagnosis of high grade prostatic intraepithelial neoplasia is associated with high likelihood of prostate cancer, independent of change in prostate specific antigen levels. *J Urol*. 2002;168:1415–1418.
61. Godoy G, Huang GJ, Patel T, et al. Long-term follow-up of men with isolated high-grade prostatic intra-epithelial neoplasia followed by serial delayed interval biopsy. *Urology*. 2011;77:669–674.
62. Kamoi K, Troncoso P, Babaian RJ. Strategy for repeat biopsy in patients with high grade prostatic intraepithelial neoplasia. *J Urol*. 2000;163:819–823.
63. Naya Y, Ayala AG, Tamboli P, et al. Can the number of cores with high-grade prostate intraepithelial neoplasia predict cancer in men who undergo repeat biopsy? *Urology*. 2004;63:503–508.
64. Park S, Shinohara K, Grossfeld GD, et al. Prostate cancer detection in men with prior high grade prostatic intraepithelial neoplasia or atypical prostate biopsy. *J Urol*. 2001;165:1409–1414.

65. Girasole CR, Cookson MS, Putzi MJ, et al. Significance of atypical and suspicious small acinar proliferations, and high grade prostatic intraepithelial neoplasia on prostate biopsy: implications for cancer detection and biopsy strategy. *J Urol.* 2006;175:929–933.

66. Pacelli A, Bostwick DG. Clinical significance of high-grade prostatic intraepithelial neoplasia in transurethral resection specimens. *Urology.* 1997;50:355–359.

67. Gaudin PB, Sesterhenn IA, Wojno KJ, et al. Incidence and clinical significance of high-grade prostatic intraepithelial neoplasia in TURP specimens. *Urology.* 1997;49:558–563.

68. Harvei S, Sander S, Tretli S, et al. Survival after transurethral and transvesical surgery in localized cancer of the prostate, Norway 1957–1981. *Cancer.* 1993;71:3966–3971.

69. Al-Hussain TO, Epstein JI. Initial high-grade prostatic intraepithelial neoplasia with carcinoma on subsequent prostate needle biopsy: findings at radical prostatectomy. *Am J Surg Pathol.* 2011;35:1165–1167.

70. Cohen RJ, McNeal JE, Baillie T. Patterns of differentiation and proliferation in intraductal carcinoma of the prostate: significance for cancer progression. *Prostate.* 2000;43:11–19.

71. McNeal JE, Reese JH, Redwine EA, et al. Cribriform adenocarcinoma of the prostate. *Cancer.* 1986;58:1714–1719.

72. McNeal JE, Yemoto CE. Spread of adenocarcinoma within prostatic ducts and acini. Morphologic and clinical correlations. *Am J Surg Pathol.* 1996;20:802–814.

73. Rubin MA, de La Taille A, Bagiella E, et al. Cribriform carcinoma of the prostate and cribriform prostatic intraepithelial neoplasia: incidence and clinical implications. *Am J Surg Pathol.* 1998;22:840–848.

74. Wilcox G, Soh S, Chakraborty S, et al. Patterns of high-grade prostatic intraepithelial neoplasia associated with clinically aggressive prostate cancer. *Hum Pathol.* 1998;29: 1119–1123.

75. Guo CC, Epstein JI. Intraductal carcinoma of the prostate on needle biopsy: histologic features and clinical significance. *Mod Pathol.* 2006;19:1528–1535.

76. Robinson BD, Epstein JI. Intraductal carcinoma of the prostate without invasive carcinoma on needle biopsy: emphasis on radical prostatectomy findings. *J Urol.* 2010; 184:1328–1333.

77. Oliai BR, Kahane H, Epstein JI. A clinicopathologic analysis of urothelial carcinomas diagnosed on prostate needle biopsy. *Am J Surg Pathol.* 2001;25:794–801.

78. Dawkins HJ, Sellner LN, Turbett GR, et al. Distinction between intraductal carcinoma of the prostate (IDC-P), high-grade dysplasia (PIN), and invasive prostatic adenocarcinoma, using molecular markers of cancer progression. *Prostate.* 2000;44:265–270.

79. Han B, Suleman K, Wang L, et al. ETS gene aberrations in atypical cribriform lesions of the prostate: implications for the distinction between intraductal carcinoma of the prostate and cribriform high-grade prostatic intraepithelial neoplasia. *Am J Surg Pathol.* 2010;34:478–485.

80. Lotan TL, Gumuskaya B, Rahimi H, et al. Cytoplasmic PTEN protein loss distinguishes intraductal carcinoma of the prostate from high-grade prostatic intraepithelial neoplasia. *Mod Pathol.* 2013;26:587–603.

6

DIAGNOSIS OF LIMITED ADENOCARCINOMA OF THE PROSTATE

DIAGNOSIS ON NEEDLE BIOPSY

General Principles in Diagnosing Prostate Cancer

There are two main issues in the diagnosis of limited cancer on needle biopsy of the prostate. The first is the recognition of limited carcinoma and the prevention of false-negative diagnoses, which is dealt with in this chapter. The second issue concerns lesions mimicking adenocarcinoma of the prostate and the prevention of false-positive diagnoses, which is discussed in Chapter 7.

The underdiagnosis of limited adenocarcinoma of the prostate on needle biopsy is one of the most frequent problems in prostate pathology. It is hard to obtain data on this phenomenon, because most institutions do not want for medicolegal reasons to go back and review old cases for potential missed cases of cancer. Some data come from one of the author's consultation practice, where we looked for lesions on needle biopsy that were missed by the contributor.[1] Of 1,840 patients that had all slides submitted in consultation and dotted by the referring pathologist, foci of prostatic adenocarcinoma were missed in 1.7% of cases.

Not everyone has the same threshold for diagnosing limited adenocarcinoma of the prostate on needle biopsy. Furthermore, everyone's threshold for diagnosing limited adenocarcinoma evolves over time and is influenced both by one's remote and recent experiences. It is expected that not everyone will feel equally comfortable in establishing a definitive diagnosis from some of the photographs of limited adenocarcinoma within this chapter. However, it is important to recognize these foci as atypical and suspicious for carcinoma so that further workup might lead to a more definitive diagnosis.

At the edge of most adenocarcinomas, scattered neoplastic glands infiltrate widely between larger benign glands (Fig. 6.1). It is therefore not uncommon to have several needle biopsy cores of prostatic tissue where there are only a few malignant glands. The importance of recognizing limited adenocarcinoma of the prostate is that there is often no correlation

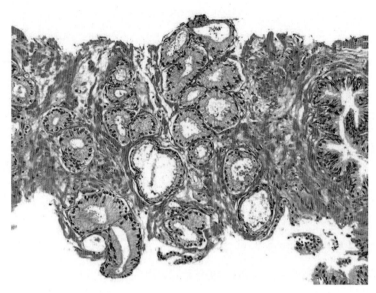

FIGURE 6.1 Adenocarcinoma composed of crowded glands with straight luminal borders.

between the amount of cancer seen on the needle biopsy and the amount of tumor present within the prostate. There may be only a few neoplastic glands in the core biopsy, despite significant tumor within the prostate gland (see Chapter 8).

Evaluating an atypical focus in a needle biopsy of the prostate should be a methodical process. When reviewing needle biopsies, one should develop a mental balance sheet where on one side of the column are features favoring the diagnosis of carcinoma and on the other side of the column are features against the diagnosis of cancer (Table 6.1). At the end of evaluating a case, hopefully all of the criteria are listed on one side of the column or the other such that a definitive diagnosis can be made. It is always helpful to first identify glands that you are confident are benign, and then compare these benign glands to the atypical glands that you are considering to diagnose as adenocarcinoma of the prostate. The greater the number of differences between the recognizable benign glands and the atypical glands, the more confidently a malignant diagnosis can be established. It will be stressed throughout this chapter that the diagnosis of cancer should be based on a constellation of features rather than relying on any one criterion by itself.

ARCHITECTURAL FEATURES IN THE DIAGNOSIS OF CANCER

It is important when examining needle biopsy specimens to gain an appreciation of what the overall architecture of the nonneoplastic prostate looks like. In order to identify limited amounts of cancer on needle biopsy material, one first has to identify the normal nonneoplastic prostate and

TABLE 6.1	Features More Common in Adenocarcinoma as Compared to Benign Glands

Nuclear
  Prominent nucleoli
  Enlarged nuclei
  Hyperchromatism
  Mitotic figures
  Apoptotic bodies
Cytoplasmic
  Amphophilic
  Sharp luminal border
  Lack of lipofuscin
Luminal contents
  Blue-tinged mucinous secretions
  Pink amorphous secretions
  Crystalloids
  Lack of corpora amylacea

(handwritten margin notes): — Crowded / — Small by large ? / — both sides / — linear

then look for glands that do not fit in. Although most prostates are relatively similar in their histologic appearance, some contain numerous small foci of crowded glands similar to adenosis. In such a case, the diagnosis of cancer based on a small focus of crowded glands with minimal cytologic atypia should be performed with caution. Other men's prostate glands are characterized by widespread atrophy; one should in these cases hesitate to diagnose cancer if the atypical glands have scant cytoplasm.

In general, scanning of prostate needle biopsies should be performed with either a 4× or 10× objective. Reviewing needle biopsies at lower magnifications runs the risk of overlooking limited foci of carcinoma. Evaluation of prostate needle biopsies at higher magnification is also nonproductive as glands with slight nuclear atypia taken out of context of their architectural pattern will often be erroneously confused with adenocarcinoma.

One pattern seen at low magnification that should raise a suspicion of carcinoma is the presence of a focus of crowded glands (Figs. 6.1 and 6.2, eFigs. 6.1 to 6.9). The second architectural pattern that is suspicious for adenocarcinoma of the prostate is the presence of small glands situated next to larger benign glands (Figs. 6.3 and 6.4, eFigs. 6.10 to 6.13). In most adenocarcinomas, the neoplastic glands are smaller than adjacent benign glands. Benign glands are recognized by their larger size, papillary infolding, and branching. Even if there are only a few small atypical glands, if they are crowded tightly in between benign glands, then they cannot be a tangential section off of high-grade prostatic intraepithelial neoplasia (PIN) (Fig. 6.5).

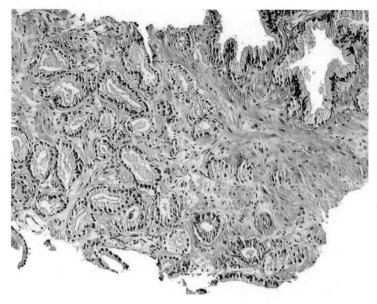

FIGURE 6.2 Crowded focus of adenocarcinoma glands with dense intraluminal pink secretions.

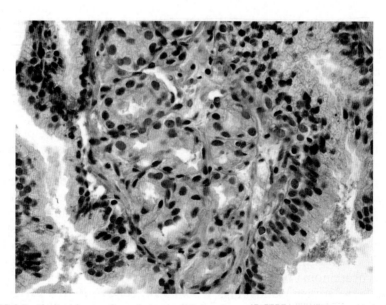

FIGURE 6.3 Limited focus of small glands with focally prominent nucleoli tucked in between benign glands.

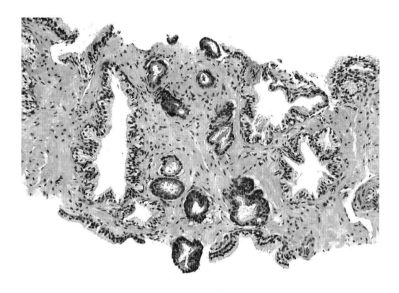

FIGURE 6.4 Adenocarcinoma with small glands with amphophilic cytoplasm in between larger benign glands.

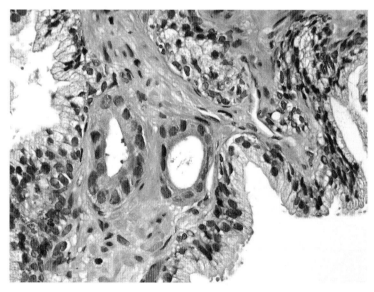

FIGURE 6.5 Very small focus of adenocarcinoma in between benign glands. Glands are small, have amphophilic cytoplasm, and have prominent nucleoli.

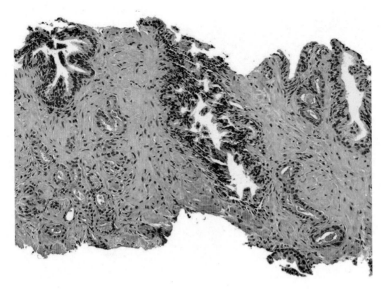

FIGURE 6.6 Small atypical glands on both sides of benign glands diagnostic of adenocarcinoma.

An infiltrative pattern, characterized by the presence of small atypical glands on both sides of a benign gland, is even more diagnostic of malignancy (Figs. 6.6 to 6.10, eFigs. 6.14 to 6.28). In contrast, mimickers of cancer will appear infiltrative as a collection of glands in between benign glands, but do not intercalate as isolated glands in between and around benign glands.

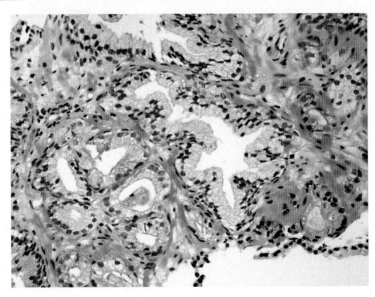

FIGURE 6.7 Small glands of adenocarcinoma with amphophilic cytoplasm, visible nucleoli, and intraluminal blue mucin on both sides of benign glands.

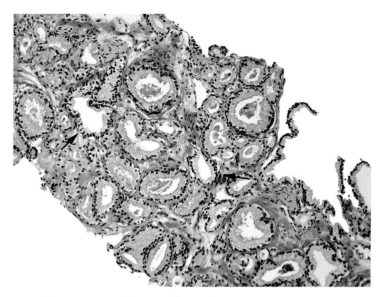

FIGURE 6.8 Subtler case of carcinoma with slightly more amphophilic cytoplasm infiltrating around benign glands (arrows).

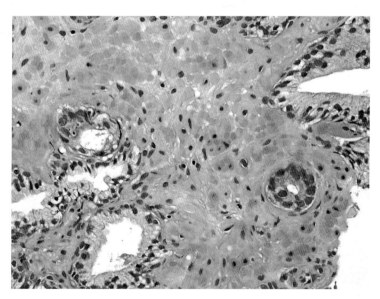

FIGURE 6.9 Two small atypical glands on different sides of benign glands, which along with the staining pattern (Fig. 6.10), is diagnostic of carcinoma. If only one gland is present, it would be atypical suspicious for carcinoma.

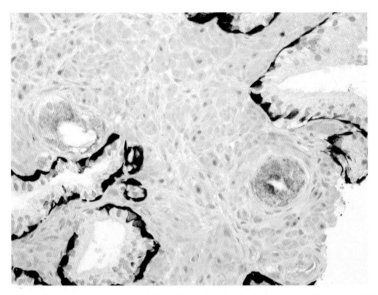

FIGURE 6.10   Same case as Figure 6.9 with both atypical glands positive for AMACR and negative for p63 and HMWCK.

Another characteristic pattern in prostate cancer is the finding of a linear row of atypical glands going either across the width of the core or along the edge of the core (Figs. 6.11 to 6.13). Linear growth is not a feature of mimickers of prostate adenocarcinoma.

In the evaluation of an atypical focus, the presence of several of the features can help establish a diagnosis of cancer even when limited tumor

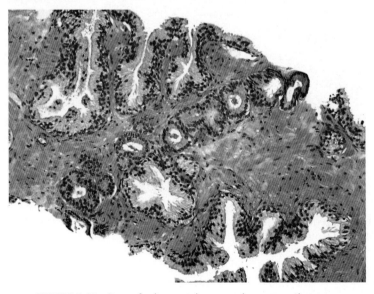

FIGURE 6.11   Row of adenocarcinoma going across the core.

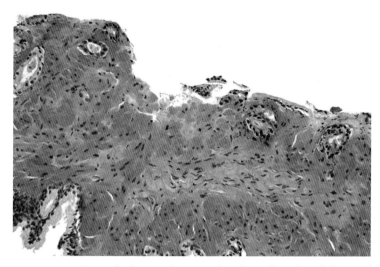

FIGURE 6.12   Row of adenocarcinoma going along the edge of the core.

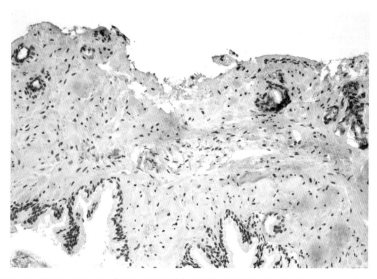

FIGURE 6.13   Same case as Figure 6.12 with small atypical glands along the edge positive for AMACR. Glands were also negative for basal cell markers (not shown).

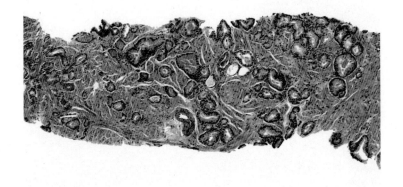

FIGURE 6.14   Numerous glands with an infiltrative pattern on needle biopsy.

is present. It is uncommon for the diagnosis of limited tumor to be solely based on the architectural pattern.[2] In these cases, when none of the features listed in Table 6.1 are present and the diagnosis is made on the architectural pattern, one should be extremely cautious and only diagnose cancer when the pattern is overtly malignant (Figs. 6.14 and 6.15).

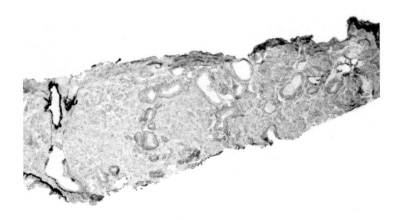

FIGURE 6.15   Same case as Figure 6.14 with all the glands negative for basal cell markers.

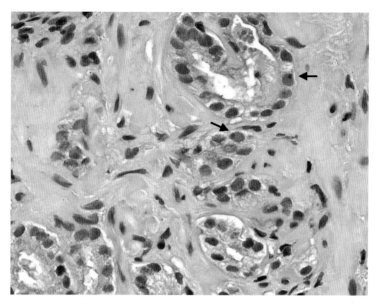

FIGURE 6.16   Small glands of adenocarcinoma with prominent nucleoli *(arrows).*

NUCLEAR FEATURES IN THE DIAGNOSIS OF CANCER

Prominent nucleoli, although important in the diagnosis of cancer on needle biopsy, should not be the sole criterion used to establish the diagnosis (Fig. 6.16, eFigs. 6.17 to 6.28). Reliance on prominent nucleoli for the diagnosis of prostate cancer will potentially lead both to an overdiagnosis as well as to an underdiagnosis of prostate cancer. Overdiagnosis of cancer can arise from prominent nucleoli being seen in various mimickers of cancer (see Chapter 7). Underdiagnosis of cancer relates to prominent nucleoli being seen in only 76% of cancers in consultation-based needle biopsy material, although more frequently present in routine biopsy material.[2,3] In addition, a significant minority of cancers may reveal only rare prominent nucleoli. In many of these cases, referring pathologists specifically noted that the lack of prominent nucleoli prevented them from definitively establishing a malignant diagnosis. The lack of prominent nucleoli in many of these cases probably reflected a sampling problem where areas of the tumor with prominent nucleoli were not biopsied. In other cases, overstained or thick sections obscured nuclear detail (Figs. 6.17 and 6.18). In some cases, greater nuclear detail can be seen on the immunostained sections, which tend to be cut thinner than the routine hematoxylin and eosin (H&E) sections (Figs. 6.19 and 6.20). If prominent nucleoli are relied upon to establish a diagnosis of limited prostate cancer on needle biopsy, a significant number of carcinomas will go underdiagnosed.

It has been stated that multiple nucleoli, especially those eccentrically located in the nucleus, are diagnostic of cancer.[3,4] In contrast to

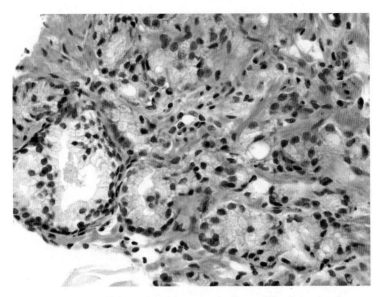

FIGURE 6.17   Thick section where nucleoli are difficult to visualize.

prior studies, we have analyzed not only cancer and benign tissue but a wide range of mimickers of cancer.[5] In our study, we found that multiple nucleoli was a rare (1%) finding in normal glands. It was most common in high-grade PIN (54%) and cancer (38%). Although the overall frequency of noneccentrically located nucleoli was higher than centrally positioned nucleoli in cancer and very uncommon in normal glands, various benign

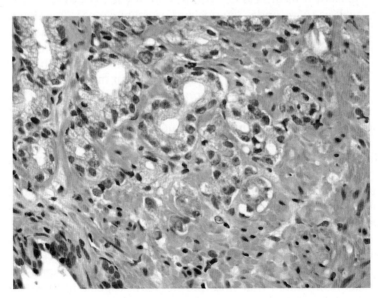

FIGURE 6.18   Same case as Figure 6.17 where thinner section reveals numerous prominent nucleoli.

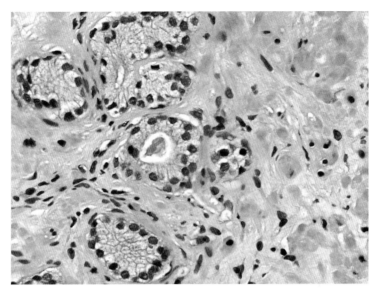

FIGURE 6.19   H&E section where nucleoli are not readily visible.

mimickers of prostate cancer had a sufficiently high frequency of multiple nucleoli and peripherally located nucleoli to render these features not useful in diagnostic practice. For example, in postatrophic hyperplasia, 37% of cases had more than one nucleolus per nucleus and 52% had some peripherally located nucleoli.

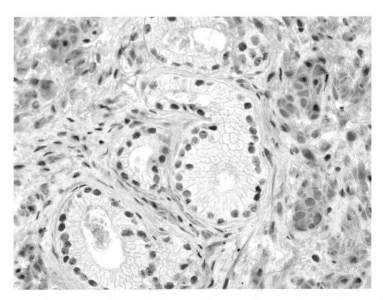

FIGURE 6.20   Same case as Figure 6.19 where the nucleoli are easily seen immunostained slide for HMWCK.

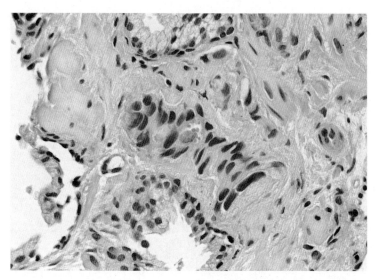

FIGURE 6.21   Adenocarcinoma with enlarged hyperchromatic nuclei.

Often, nuclear enlargement may be present when prominent nucleoli are not and is an important diagnostic feature.[2] Nuclear hyperchromasia is another cytologic feature that may help to distinguish cancerous from benign glands (Fig. 6.21, eFigs. 6.29 to 6.36).

Fewer works have examined the frequency of mitotic figures in prostate cancer (Fig. 6.22, eFigs. 6.37 and 6.38). We noted in a series of limited adenocarcinoma on needle biopsy that 11% contained mitotic figures.[2]

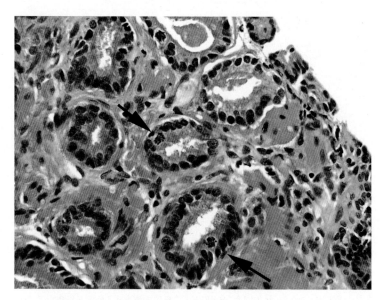

FIGURE 6.22   Adenocarcinoma with mitotic figures (arrows).

A comparable frequency of 10% was noted in a study of minimal volume cancers on biopsy by Iczkowski and Bostwick.[6] Vesalainen et al.[7] demonstrated that although mitotic figures were not uncommon in Gleason score 8–10 cancers, the mean number of mitotic figures per 10 high power fields was only 4.3 for Gleason score 5–7 tumors. Mitotic figures were also shown by Aihara et al.[8] to correlate with Gleason grade. In accordance with these studies, we found mitotic figures more commonly in high-grade PIN (12%) and cancer (13%) as compared to its infrequency (≤3%) in benign glandular mimickers of cancer with the exception of 6% of cases of benign glands with inflammation having mitoses.[5] Mitotic figures are, therefore, a helpful diagnostic feature that favors the diagnosis of prostate cancer, although its infrequency in focal Gleason score 6 cancer on needle biopsy limits its utility.

Most studies have found between 1% and 2% of benign prostate cells have apoptotic bodies using specialized techniques.[9,10] Identifying apoptotic bodies on routine H&E-stained sections, Montironi et al.[11] found that the frequency of apoptotic bodies increased from benign prostatic hyperplasia (BPH) (0.3%) to high-grade PIN (0.75%) to "small acinar carcinoma" (1.0%) to "cribriform cancer" (1.3%) to "solid carcinoma" (2.1%). Aihara et al.[8] also investigated the frequency of apoptotic bodies on H&E-stained sections and showed that the frequency increased across Gleason grade pattern 1 (0.04%), pattern 2 (0.15%), pattern 3 (0.3%), pattern 4 (0.5%), and pattern 5 (0.7%). Apoptotic bodies were rare in normal glands (0.07%).[8] We reported apoptotic bodies as being present or absent per small focus of cancer on needle biopsy and found that apoptotic bodies were fairly common in cancer, seen in 34% of small foci of cancer sent in for consultation. Apoptotic bodies were next most prevalent in high-grade PIN (13%). In contrast, apoptotic bodies were uncommon (≤3%) in normal glands and benign mimickers of cancer, such that the presence of apoptotic bodies is helpful in the diagnosis of challenging cases of prostate cancer on needle biopsy (Fig. 6.23, eFig. 6.39).[5]

Conventional prostate cancer, even when very high grade, typically consists of cells with relatively uniform nuclei. We have described rare cases on needle biopsy of prostate carcinoma with pleomorphic bizarre nuclei (Fig. 6.24, eFig. 6.40).[12] The presence of a more conventional prostatic adenocarcinoma component may clue one into the correct diagnosis once one realizes that prostate cancer can rarely display such prominent nuclear atypia. In cases where the conventional component is very poorly differentiated or absent, a battery of immunostains including melanoma, lymphoid, and epithelial markers, and antibodies against thrombomodulin, GATA3, and prostate-specific antigen (PSA), P501S, and NKX3.1 (see Chapter 15) should be performed. A further pitfall that must be recognized with evaluation of the immunohistochemical stains is that PSA is typically negative in the giant cell component and often only focal in the conventional adenocarcinoma component. Based on the limited number of cases in this study and other published studies, pleomorphic giant cell prostatic adenocarcinoma heralds a particularly aggressive clinical outcome.[12,13]

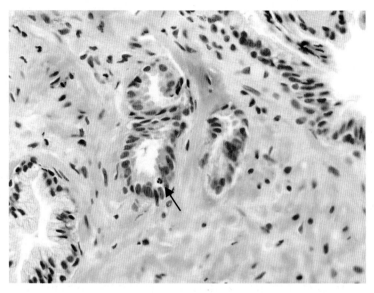

FIGURE 6.23   Apoptotic body *(arrow)* in adenocarcinoma.

CYTOPLASMIC FEATURES IN THE DIAGNOSIS OF CANCER

Although in the past there has been much less consideration paid to cytoplasmic features as compared to nuclear qualities, the nature of the cytoplasm may be critical in the diagnosis of some carcinomas. In some adenocarcinomas of the prostate, the cytoplasm of the malignant glands is

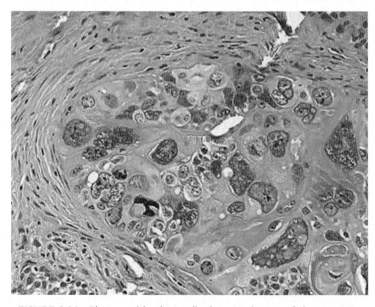

FIGURE 6.24   Pleomorphic giant cell adenocarcinoma of the prostate.

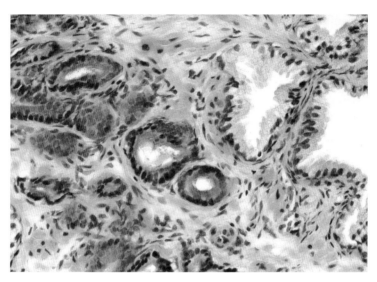

FIGURE 6.25   Adenocarcinoma with amphophilic cytoplasm.

more amphophilic than the surrounding benign glands that have pale to clear cytoplasm (Figs. 6.25 and 6.26, eFigs. 6.41 to 6.50). In order for this criterion to be helpful, the benign prostate glands must be appropriately stained such that they have a pale to clear appearance. In a study of consult cases, we found that in 32% of the cases, this criterion was not applicable since the benign glands also exhibited amphophilic cytoplasm.[2] Because this feature is helpful in a large number of cases, one's H&E stains

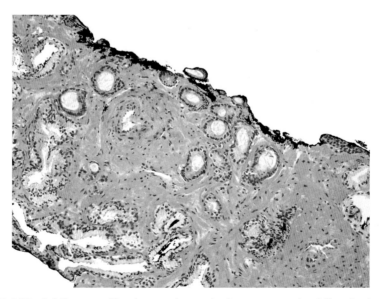

FIGURE 6.26   Subtle case with adenocarcinoma having more amphophilic cytoplasm and blue intraluminal mucin *(top)* compared to benign glands *(bottom)*.

should be adjusted so that the cytoplasm of the benign glands appears pale to clear.

The lack of lipofuscin in atypical prostatic glands suspicious for cancer, if there is prominent pigment in the surrounding benign glands, may help to establish a definitive diagnosis of cancer. Lipofuscin is uncommon in high-grade PIN and rare in cancer (eFigs. 6.51 to 6.55).[14]

Abundant cytoplasm with straight luminal borders in larger glands is also a feature of cancer, which is also described under the entity of "pseudohyperplastic cancer" (eFigs. 6.56 to 6.58). The only time benign prostate glands typically have straight luminal borders is when either the glands are small or large but with markedly atrophic cytoplasm.

INTRALUMINAL CONTENTS IN THE DIAGNOSIS OF CANCER

Prostatic crystalloids are dense eosinophilic crystal-like structures that appear in various geometric shapes such as rectangular, hexagonal, triangular, and rodlike structures (Figs. 6.27 and 6.28, eFigs. 6.59 to 6.62). Prostatic crystalloids have been reported in 25% of cancers seen on biopsy material, yet may also be seen in benign prostate acini.[2,15,16] The likelihood of finding crystalloids is dependent on the number of malignant glands present and the grade; crystalloids are inversely correlated with the Gleason grade. Crystalloids, although not diagnostic of carcinoma, are more frequently found in cancer than in benign glands.

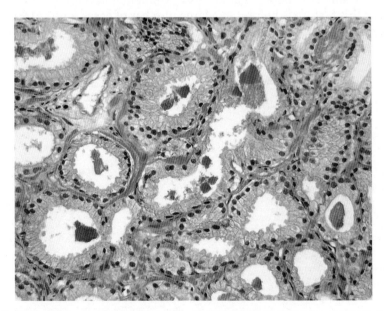

FIGURE 6.27 Adenocarcinoma with relatively straight luminal borders and intraluminal crystalloids.

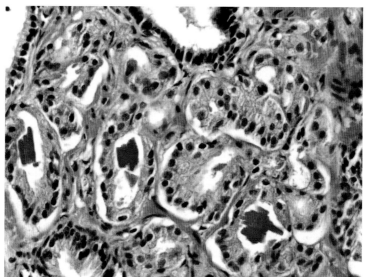

#1 blue
mucin

#2 cryth(of)

#3 Pink
stuff

FIGURE 6.28   Numerous crystalloids in adenocarcinoma.

The one condition that mimics cancer where crystalloids are frequently seen is adenosis, which consists of a lobule of pale-staining glands (see Chapter 7). Consequently, if crystalloids are seen in small glands with an infiltrative appearance in between benign glands, where adenosis is not in the differential, they may help to establish a diagnosis of cancer. The finding of prostatic crystalloids in benign glands does not indicate an increased risk of cancer on subsequent biopsy.[17]

Another diagnostic criterion relates to the nature of intraluminal secretions. Blue-tinged mucinous secretions seen on H&E-stained sections are mostly observed in carcinomas and only rarely identified in benign glands (Figs. 6.29 and 6.30)[2] (eFigs. 6.63 to 6.74). The prevalence of these blue-tinged secretions is in part influenced by the nature of the H&E stain. In some institutions' referral material, this feature appears to be fairly prevalent, whereas in other institutions, it is uncommonly seen or faint and wispy. Some laboratory's H&E stains are too basophilic, where even benign glands contain blue-tinged mucinous secretions. When normal colonic glands that are present on many prostate biopsies show an intense blue appearance, pathologists have to be cautious in placing too much weight on blue-tinged mucin in prostate glands as a diagnostic criterion for cancer. Although initial reports suggested that acid mucin stains could distinguish malignant from benign glands, subsequent articles demonstrated that acid mucin is variably present in mimickers of carcinoma, such as adenosis and atrophic glands.[18,19]

Another type of intraluminal secretion that may aid in the diagnosis of limited cancer is pink dense amorphous acellular secretions identified

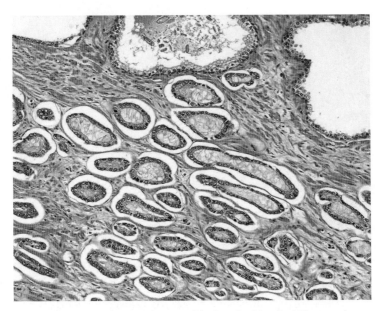

FIGURE 6.29 Adenocarcinoma with abundant luminal blue mucin.

in approximately half of cancers on needle biopsy and only occasionally seen in benign glands (Figs. 6.31 and 6.32, eFigs. 6.75 to 6.81).[2] These amorphous secretions should be distinguished from corpora amylacea, which are well-circumscribed round to oval structures with concentric lamellar rings that are prominent in benign glands and uncommonly

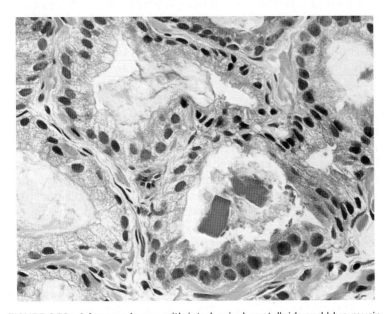

FIGURE 6.30 Adenocarcinoma with intraluminal crystalloids and blue mucin.

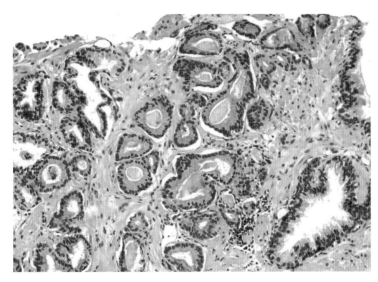

FIGURE 6.31   Dense pink amorphous secretions in adenocarcinoma.

seen in cancer (eFig. 6.82).[2,20,21] Both pink and blue secretions often co-exist in the same glands (Fig. 6.33, eFigs. 6.83 to 6.91). As with all of the criteria mentioned to this point, this feature is not specific for carcinoma. Rather, the presence of intraluminal secretions should be taken in context of the architectural pattern and the nuclear and cytoplasmic features.

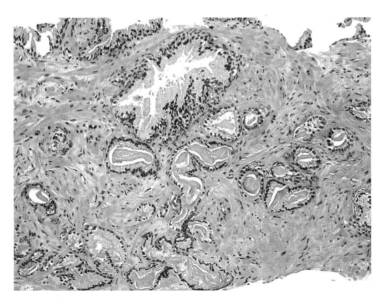

FIGURE 6.32   Small glands of adenocarcinoma with dense pink secretions.

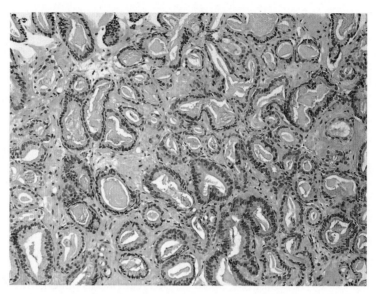

FIGURE 6.33   Adenocarcinoma with intraluminal dense pink and blue mucin secretions.

HISTOLOGIC FEATURES SPECIFIC FOR PROSTATE CANCER

There are three features that have not to date been identified in benign glands, and which are in and of themselves diagnostic of cancer (Table 6.2). These are mucinous fibroplasia (collagenous micronodules), glomerulations, and perineural invasion.

Occasionally, intraluminal mucinous secretions are so extensive that they become focally organized.[22,23] This lesion, known as either mucinous fibroplasia or collagenous micronodules, is typified by very delicate loose fibrous tissue with an ingrowth of fibroblasts (Figs. 6.34 and 6.35, eFigs. 6.92 to 6.111). Mucinous secretions can displace the epithelium, resulting in atrophic cytoplasm and small pyknotic nuclei, whereby these foci can be difficult to recognize as cancer (see Chapter 9 for grading).

Glomerulations consists of glands with a cribriform proliferation that is not transluminal (Fig. 6.36, eFigs. 6.112 to 6.119). Rather, these cribriform formations are attached to only one edge of the gland resulting in a structure superficially resembling a glomerulus (see Chapter 9 for grading).

TABLE 6.2 **Features Pathognomonic of Prostate Adenocarcinoma**
Perineural invasion
Mucinous fibroplasia (collagenous micronodules)
Glomerulations

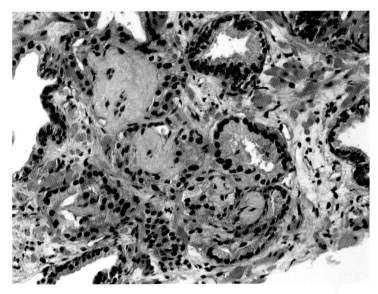

FIGURE 6.34 Mucinous fibroplasia in adenocarcinoma.

Perineural invasion is seen in approximately 20% of needle biopsies of the prostate showing adenocarcinoma.[24] In a difficult case where the diagnosis of carcinoma hinges on perineural invasion, the glands in question should circumferentially surround the nerve (eFigs. 6.120 to 6.125). Uncommonly, the only atypical glands in a case are those wrapping around

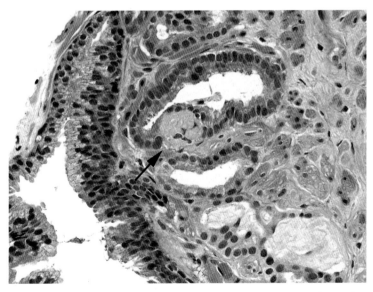

FIGURE 6.35 Small focus of adenocarcinoma with single gland with early mucinous fibroplasia *(arrow)*.

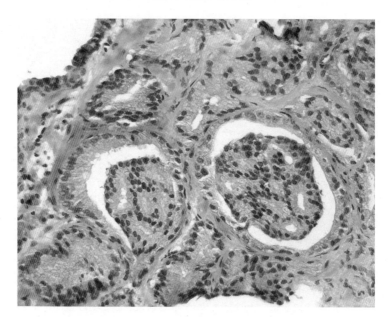

FIGURE 6.36   Glomerulations in adenocarcinoma.

a nerve.[22] Occasionally, cancer glands with perineural invasion have a peculiar proclivity to resemble a benign hyperplastic gland (Fig. 6.37). In other cases where there are some atypical features to the glands, perineural invasion can be diagnosed when the nerve is only partly encircled by the gland (Fig. 6.38). Perineural invasion must be distinguished

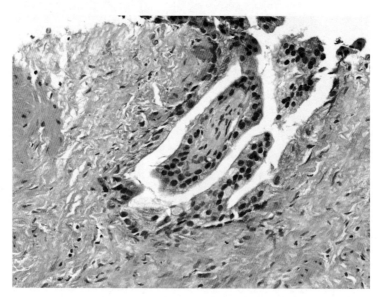

FIGURE 6.37   Adenocarcinoma wrapping around a nerve mimicking a benign hyperplastic gland.

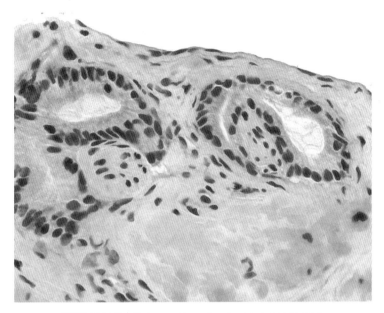

FIGURE 6.38 Perineural invasion by adenocarcinoma.

from perineural indentation by benign prostate glands[25,26] (eFigs. 6.126 to 6.133). The most common pattern of this phenomenon is perineural indentation by benign glands. We have called attention to other patterns of neural involvement by benign glands that are not as widely known, including intraneural and incomplete perineural involvement (Figs. 6.39

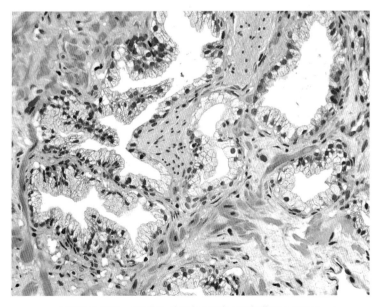

FIGURE 6.39 Benign glands partly encircling a nerve.

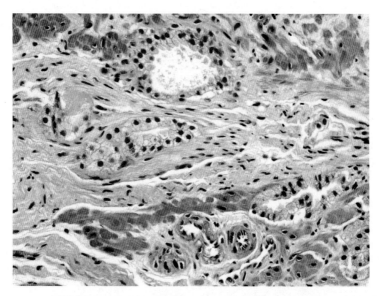

FIGURE 6.40   Intraneural involvement by benign glands.

and 6.40).[25] Complete circumferential wrapping was not observed in our cases as is often noted by cancerous acini, although one case did show up to 95% wrapping. Our study demonstrates that if one is going to use perineural involvement as the key *diagnostic* feature to establish malignancy in a given case, complete circumferential growth around the nerve is required especially if the glands have cytologic and architectural features more typically associated with benign glands. If the diagnosis of cancer is established based on other criteria, then the diagnosis of perineural invasion for *prognostic purposes* (see Chapter 8) can be made with less stringent criteria, including perineural tracking, intraneural involvement, and subtotal circumferential growth.

IDENTIFICATION OF BASAL CELLS ON HEMATOXYLIN AND EOSIN–STAINED SECTIONS

The problem of identifying basal cells on H&E-stained sections is that in cases of obvious carcinoma there may be cells that closely mimic basal cells. These cells when labeled with antibodies to high molecular weight keratin or p63 are negative and represent fibroblasts closely apposed to the neoplastic glands. Consequently, in a focus that is consistent with cancer architecturally and which has other features supportive of the diagnosis of carcinoma at higher power, a search for basal cells by light microscopy may be counterproductive. Because of the difficulty in distinguishing basal cells from fibroblasts as well as the problem with stratification of neoplastic nuclei due to tangential sectioning or thick sections, these authors usually do not search for basal cells in cases that satisfy the criteria for adenocarcinoma of the prostate (eFigs. 6.134 to 6.136).

DIAGNOSIS OF LIMITED HIGH-GRADE CARCINOMA

Occasionally, high-grade adenocarcinoma of the prostate may also be difficult to diagnose on needle biopsy. With an increase in the numbers of needle biopsies being performed for early disease detected by screening techniques, we are seeing an increase in the detection of small high-grade adenocarcinomas[27,28] (eFigs. 6.137 to 6.140). Although by itself not diagnostic, the presence of too many cells per unit area where the cells are not obvious inflammatory or stromal cells raises the question of a poorly differentiated prostate cancer. When labeled with antibodies to PSA, P501S, NKKX3.1, and pancytokeratin, these individual cells can be shown to be epithelial in nature. Given that there is no benign epithelial process with this pattern, the diagnosis of high-grade adenocarcinoma can be rendered. Despite the lack of cytologic atypia, a focus may be diagnostic of adenocarcinoma because of the lack of well-formed glands, inconsistent with a benign process.

CARCINOMAS MIMICKING BENIGN GLANDS

Just as there are benign mimickers of prostate cancer (Chapter 7), some cancers closely resemble benign prostate glands in their architectural pattern or cytology and may not be recognized as malignant. It may be necessary to verify these variants of prostate cancer with the use of immunohistochemistry for basal cell markers (see "Use of Immunohistochemistry Adjunctive Tests for Diagnosis of Cancer" for discussion of racemase immunoreactivity).

Foamy gland cancer must be recognized as carcinoma by its abundant foamy cytoplasm, its architectural pattern of crowded and/or infiltrative glands, and frequently present pink acellular intraluminal secretions[29] (Figs. 6.41 to 6.43, eFigs. 6.141 to 6.170). Although the cytoplasm has a xanthomatous appearance, it does not contain lipid, but rather empty vacuoles.[30] More typical features of adenocarcinoma such as nuclear enlargement and prominent nucleoli are frequently absent, which makes this lesion difficult to recognize as carcinoma. Characteristically, the nuclei in foamy gland carcinoma are small, round, and densely hyperchromatic. The nuclei in foamy gland carcinoma are actually rounder than those of benign prostatic secretory cells. Foamy gland cancers are typically Gleason score 6 or 7, although higher grade lesions exist (see Chapter 9 for grading).[31,32] Foamy gland carcinomas are typically admixed with usual adenocarcinoma of the prostate. Whereas on biopsy, one may see pure foamy gland carcinoma, which is difficult to diagnose; at radical prostatectomy, pure foamy gland cancer is uncommon.[31] Uncommon cases of foamy gland carcinoma have an extensive associated desmoplastic stromal

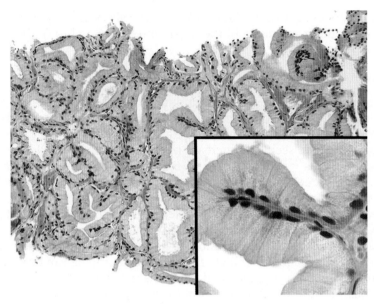

FIGURE 6.41 Foamy gland adenocarcinoma. *Inset* shows abundant xanthomatous-appearing cytoplasm with small bland nuclei.

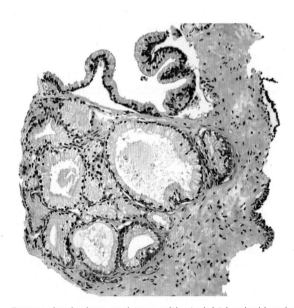

FIGURE 6.42 Foamy gland adenocarcinoma with straight luminal borders.

& gland dilatation

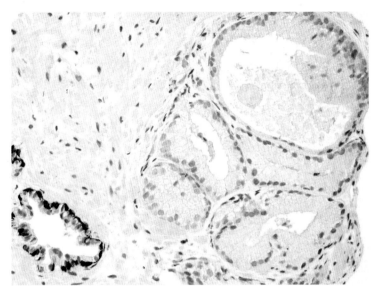

FIGURE 6.43   Same case as Figure 6.42, negative for p63 and HMWCK.

reaction, almost obscuring the carcinoma (Figs. 6.44 and 6.45). Another feature of foamy gland carcinoma, especially those of higher grade, is that occasional cells aberrantly express high molecular weight cytokeratin (HMWCK) staining in a nonbasal cell distribution.

Atrophic prostate cancers are rare and may be present on needle biopsy, usually unassociated with a prior history of hormonal therapy.[33,34]

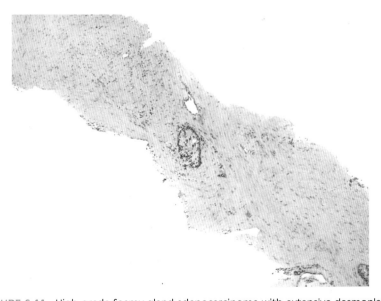

FIGURE 6.44   High-grade foamy gland adenocarcinoma with extensive desmoplasia.

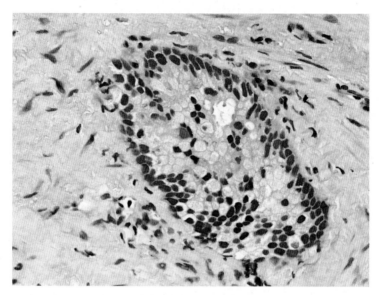

FIGURE 6.45   Same case as Figure 6.44 with higher magnification.

The diagnosis of carcinoma in these cases is made on (a) <u>a truly infiltrative process with individual small atrophic glands situated between larger benign glands</u> (Figs. 6.46 and 6.47), (b) the concomitant presence of ordinary less atrophic carcinoma, and (c) greater cytologic atypia than is seen in benign atrophy (Fig. 6.48, eFigs. 6.171 to 6.211).

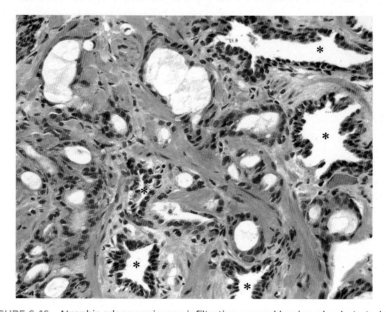

FIGURE 6.46   Atrophic adenocarcinoma infiltrating around benign glands *(asterisks)*.

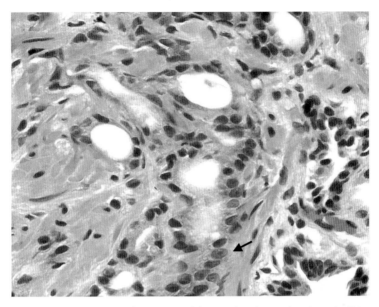

FIGURE 6.47 Same case as Figure 6.46 with occasional prominent nucleoli *(arrow)*.

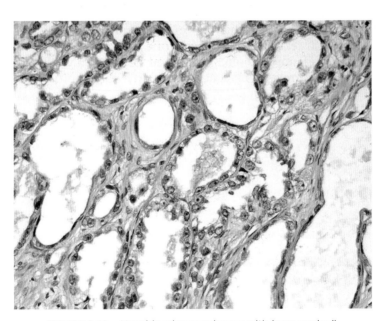

FIGURE 6.48 Atrophic adenocarcinoma with large nucleoli.

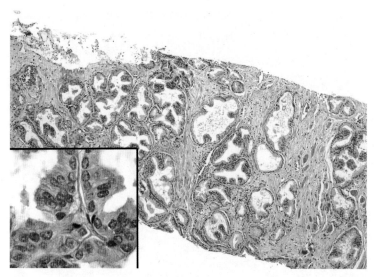

FIGURE 6.49   Pseudohyperplastic adenocarcinoma with prominent nucleoli *(inset).*

Pseudohyperplastic prostate cancer is characterized by the presence of larger glands with branching and papillary infolding[35,36] (Figs. 6.49 to 6.52, eFigs. 6.212 to 6.290). The recognition of cancer with this pattern is based on the architectural pattern of numerous closely packed glands as well as nuclear features more typical of carcinoma. A variant of pseudohyperplastic adenocarcinoma composed of markedly dilated glands with abundant cytoplasm may be particularly difficult to recognize as

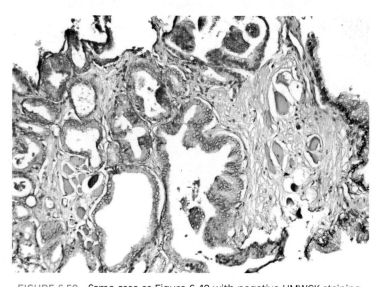

FIGURE 6.50   Same case as Figure 6.49 with negative HMWCK staining.

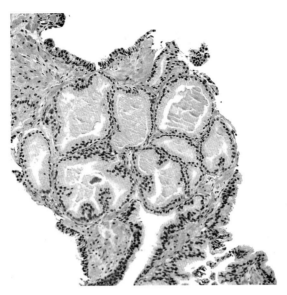

FIGURE 6.51 Small focus of pseudohyperplastic adenocarcinoma consisting of crowded large glands with papillary infolding.

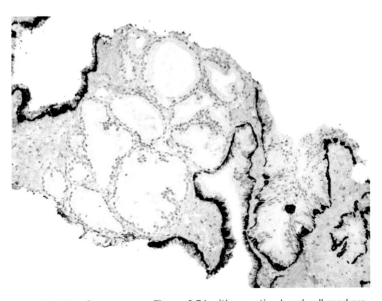

FIGURE 6.52 Same case as Figure 6.51 with negative basal cell markers.

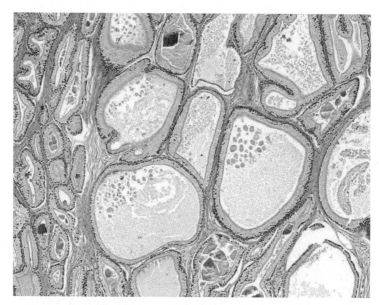

FIGURE 6.53 Pseudohyperplastic adenocarcinoma with large glands with abundant cyto-plasm and straight luminal borders.

malignant. This form of cancer can be recognized by the appearance of numerous large glands that are almost back-to-back with straight even luminal borders and abundant cytoplasm (Fig. 6.53). Comparably sized benign glands either have papillary infolding or are atrophic. The presence of cytologic atypia in some of these glands further distinguishes them from benign glands. Although a variant of pseudohyperplastic carcinoma, some have considered this pattern a unique entity termed *pseudocystic* prostate carcinoma. As with foamy gland cancer, pseudohyperplastic cancer, despite its benign appearance, may be associated with intermediate grade cancer and can exhibit aggressive behavior (i.e., extraprostatic extension) (see Chapter 9 for grading).

DIAGNOSIS OF CANCER ON TRANSURETHRAL RESECTION

Whereas nuclear features play a prominent role in the diagnosis of adeno-carcinoma of the prostate on needle biopsy material, they are often not as helpful in diagnosing low-grade adenocarcinoma on transurethral resec-tion specimens. Often, low-grade adenocarcinomas of the prostate lack enlarged nuclei and prominent nucleoli, and mitoses are rarely found.[37] Cytoplasmic features are often not very helpful because they are often pale-clear, similar to benign glands. The most useful feature in diagnos-ing low-grade adenocarcinoma on transurethral resection material is the recognition of cancer's architectural growth pattern as seen at relatively low magnification.

Many of the following illustrated examples are somewhat repetitive in that they demonstrate the same abnormal growth pattern of low-grade prostate carcinoma. This repetition is intentional because it is difficult to convey with words concepts such as "infiltrative," "haphazard," or "growing in an irregular fashion," which are features better depicted by numerous visual examples (Figs. 6.54 to 6.57, eFigs. 6.291 to 6.322).

Benign prostatic glands tend to grow either as circumscribed nodules within BPH or radiate in columns out from the urethra in a linear fashion. In contrast, adenocarcinoma of the prostate grows in a haphazard fashion. Although low-grade carcinoma tends to be fairly well circumscribed, the glands infiltrate for a short distance in different directions out into the prostatic stroma. Glands oriented perpendicular to each other and glands separated by bundles of smooth muscle are indicative of an infiltrative process. Another feature used to diagnose adenocarcinoma of the prostate is the appearance of glands splitting the muscle fibers in an infiltrative fashion. Although this pattern is suggestive of adenocarcinoma, occasionally benign glands can also be seen in between large smooth muscle bundles. Another feature associated with cancer is that some of the vessels among the cancer may show a proliferation of cells resembling glomus cells[38] (eFig. 6.323).

In some cases, comparison of the neoplastic glands to the surrounding benign glands is helpful in that there are certain features that are more frequent in adenocarcinoma as compared to benign glands. These features

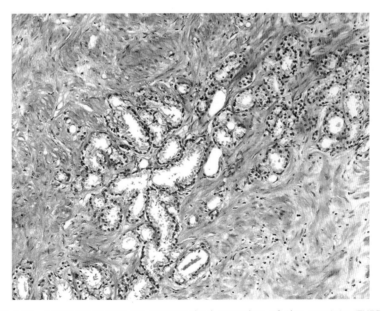

FIGURE 6.54 Adenocarcinoma on transurethral resection of the prostate (TURP) with gland infiltrating perpendicular to each other as opposed to a lobular growth seen in benign glands.

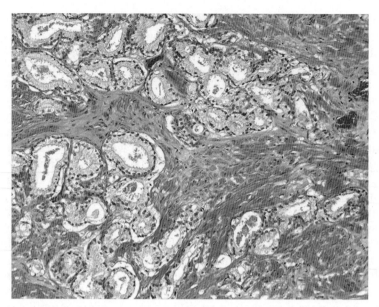

FIGURE 6.55 Adenocarcinoma with infiltrative pattern of splitting large smooth muscle bundles.

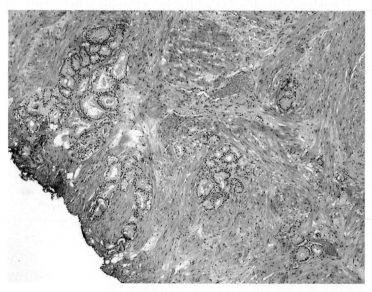

FIGURE 6.56 Scattered foci of adenocarcinoma separated by smooth muscle.

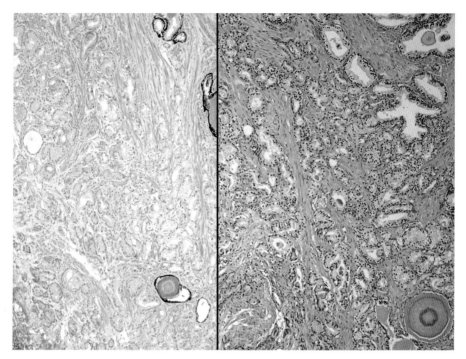

FIGURE 6.57 Crowded glands of adenocarcinoma **(right)** which are difficult to diagnose solely on the H&E stain. The lacks of basal cell staining in all the small glands **(left)** is diagnostic of adenocarcinoma.

have been discussed earlier in the chapter and are listed in Table 6.1. The finding of apical snouts is not helpful in distinguishing benign versus malignant glands as they can be seen in both.

A problem unique to material removed by transurethral resection is cautery artifact (eFig. 6.324). Extensive cautery artifact in a suspicious focus may prevent a definitive diagnosis of carcinoma. However, even in some cases with extensive cautery artifact, the presence of solid sheets of cells with high nuclear to cytoplasmic ratios and nuclear hyperchromasia could be nothing else but that of carcinoma. There are also some cases of better differentiated gland-forming carcinomas with extensive cautery artifact that, based on a pattern of numerous back-to-back glands, is also diagnostic of carcinoma.

USE OF IMMUNOHISTOCHEMICAL ADJUNCTIVE TESTS FOR DIAGNOSIS OF CARCINOMA

There are cases which some pathologists may not feel comfortable diagnosing as adenocarcinoma on the H&E-stained sections where immunohistochemistry for basal cell markers may resolve the diagnosis. The most commonly used antibody to label basal cells in benign mimickers of prostate cancer is HMWCK (34βE12, cytokeratin 5/6 [ck5/6])[39–44] (eFigs. 6.325 to 6.328). HMWCK immunoreactivity in benign glands is localized to the cytoplasm of basal cells and is negative in prostate cancer. Antibodies to p63 also label the nuclei of basal cells in benign prostatic lesions.[45–47] p40, which is an isoform of p63, shows less aberrant p63 immunoreactivity in adenocarcinoma of the prostate but also has more nonspecific cytoplasmic staining compared to p63. In general, p63 and p40 are comparable.[48]

Several studies comparing HMWCK and p63 have showed p63 to be slightly superior.[45,46] One study demonstrated that ck5/6 was superior to 34βE12, although only a minority of pathologists use ck5/6.[49] The use of a double cocktail combining HMWCK and p63 can increase the sensitivity of basal cell detection with a decrease in staining variability.[50–52]

The use of HMWCK or p63 in a focus with only a few atypical glands is not as diagnostic, since benign glands may not show uniform positivity with these markers.[41] Negative staining for basal cell markers is most diagnostic when more than a few glands are present for evaluation and the morphologic features are very suspicious for carcinoma. The immunohistochemical detection of basal cells is sometimes more diagnostic on transurethral resection, as there are a greater number of glands available for evaluation (eFigs. 6.329 to 6.333). Cautery can result in false-negative staining for HMWCK, such that before interpreting a negative result as diagnostic of cancer, benign glands on the same chip should be immunoreactive as an internal positive control. Rather than used to establish a diagnosis of cancer, we use these antibodies to help verify a suspicious focus as cancer. If we favor, although are not sure, that a focus is benign and the basal cell stains are negative, we will diagnose it as atypical rather than as cancer. In a small focus of atypical glands on prostate biopsy, negative staining for HMWCK should not necessarily lead to a definitive malignant diagnosis in all cases, as almost half of these biopsies on follow-up sampling are benign.[53] If we are confident the focus is benign and stains performed at an outside institution are negative in a small focus of glands, we will still diagnose the focus as benign because certain mimickers of prostate cancer may not react with these antibodies (see Chapter 7).

Uncommonly, one can see occasional cancer cells that are positive for antibodies to HMWCK and less likely p63, yet as long as these cells are not in a basal cell distribution, these cells represent aberrant expression of the antigen in cancer (Figs. 6.58 to 6.61, eFigs. 6.334 to 6.344). Uncommonly, one can have prostate adenocarcinoma where most or all of the tumor aberrantly expresses p63 (Fig. 6.62).[54,55] The majority of these cases have distinctive histology with glands, nests, and cords with atrophic cytoplasm, hyperchromatic nuclei, and visible nucleoli. Despite poor gland formation, limited data indicates that these tumors may not be as aggressive as their architectural pattern suggests. Rare lesions with the appearance of prostate cancer show HMWCK staining in a basal cell

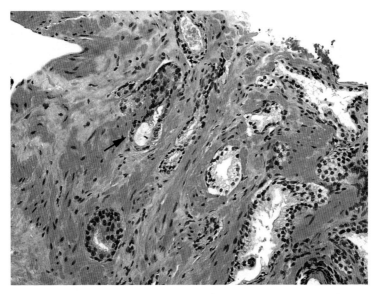

FIGURE 6.58 Small glands of adenocarcinoma *(left)* with amphophilic cytoplasm compared to larger benign glands with pale cytoplasm *(lower right)*. Note cancer gland with *arrow.*

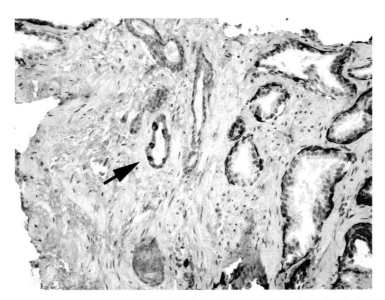

FIGURE 6.59 Same case as Figure 6.58 labeled with HMWCK. Benign glands *(lower right)* show immunoreactivity in flattened basal cells beneath negative secretory cells. Same cancer gland highlighted in Figure 6.58 *(arrow)* with tumor cells positive for HMWCK not in a basal cell distribution.

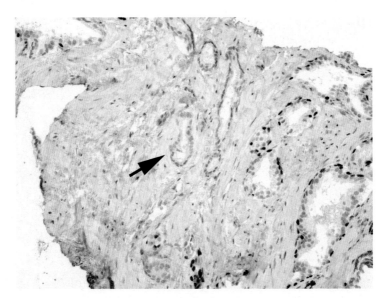

FIGURE 6.60   Same case as Figures 6.58 and 6.59 labeled with p63. Benign glands *(lower right)* have basal cells and all the cancer glands including the one gland that nonspecifically stained with HMWCK *(arrow)* are negative for p63.

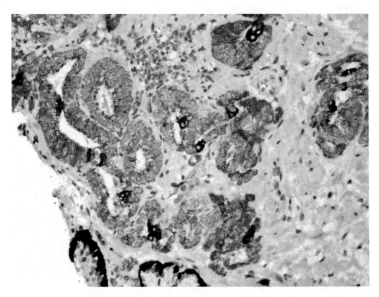

FIGURE 6.61   Triple cocktail stain with p63 (nuclei—*brown*), HMWCK (cytoplasm—*brown*), and AMACR *(red)*. Benign glands *(lower left)* have basal cells labeled with HMWCK and p63. Cancer with AMACR positivity shows brown staining of scattered tumor cells in a nonbasal cell distribution. Note positive tumor cells show cytoplasmic staining only, indicating nonspecific positivity for HMWCK and not p63.

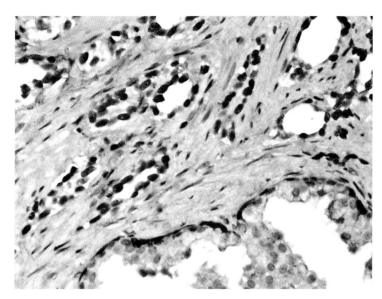

FIGURE 6.62 Adenocarcinoma with aberrant p63 staining. Note only nuclear positivity in small glands of carcinoma *(top)* compared to both nuclear and cytoplasmic immuno-reactivity in basal cells of benign gland *(bottom)*.

distribution either from retention of basal cells by early invasive cancer or from high-grade PIN outpouching. The lack of adjacent PIN in some cases and the large ratio of small atypical glands to PIN glands argue against high-grade PIN outpouching as the sole explanation. In cases with adjacent high-grade PIN, a comparison of the proximity and number of the small, atypical, infiltrative-appearing glands to high-grade PIN is helpful. The diagnosis of prostate cancer in the face of positive HMWCK basal cell staining should be made with extreme caution, only in the face of unequivocal cancer on the H&E stain.[56] Pitfalls in the use of immuno-histochemistry for the diagnosis of prostate carcinoma are summarized in the review article by Brimo and Epstein.[55]

Alpha-methylacyl-CoA-racemase (AMACR), an enzyme involved in the β-oxidation of branched-chain fatty acids, is significantly upregu-lated in prostate cancer. Antibodies have been developed against its gene product, P504S protein.[50,57–59] By immunohistochemistry, the majority of prostate cancers are positive for AMACR, the sensitivity varying amongst studies from 82% to 100%[59–65] (eFigs. 6.345 to 6.405). Often, the staining is fine dot-like and luminal. Although the data is somewhat conflicting, some studies have shown relative decrease AMACR immunoreactivity in foamy gland, atrophic, and pseudohyperplastic prostate cancers.[62,64,66] AMACR staining of PIN and mimickers of prostate cancer is discussed in Chapters 5 and 7, respectively. As negative staining for basal cell markers especially in a small focus of atypical glands is not necessarily diagnostic of prostate cancer, positive staining for AMACR can increase the level of confidence in establishing a definitive malignant diagnosis.[67] Two studies have shown that if a case is still considered atypical by a uropathology expert after negative basal cell staining, positive staining for AMACR can help establish in 50% of these cases a definitive diagnosis of cancer.[67,68] There does not appear to be a difference between polyclonal and monoclonal P504S, in the sensitivity of labeling prostate cancer.[69] Negative AMACR staining in small suspicious glands is not necessarily sufficient for a benign diagnosis. Conversely, positive staining for AMACR is not diagnostic of prostatic adenocarcinoma as it can be seen to varying degrees with mimickers of prostate cancer (see Chapter 7). AMACR immunohistochemical result can be helpful in establishing a diagnosis of limited prostate cancer on needle biopsy, although AMACR positivity must be taken in context of the lesion's histology.

Different cocktails have been investigated combining antibodies for AMACR and basal cell specific markers. One combination is with antibodies to p63 that label basal cell nuclei of benign glands and AMACR that stains cytoplasm of cancer.[70–72] Although these authors have reported that this cocktail is essentially equal to each antibody used separately, in our experience, a problem with this cocktail is that in some cases stains for p63 show some background staining of the cytoplasm in benign glands, which can be confused with AMACR immunoreactivity. With small foci of atypical glands, the lesion may not survive sectioning to do separate stains for basal cell markers and AMACR on different slides.[73] A triple stain cocktail using a brown chromogen for HMWCK and p63 and a red chromogen for AMACR optimizes the preservation of tissue for immunohistochemistry and has been shown to be better than basal cell markers by themselves.[74] In cases where there is no more tissue within the paraffin block and where there are at least two H&E sections with the lesion, a technique has been developed to transfer tissue from one of the H&E slides to charged slides so that the triple stain can be performed; an equivalent sensitivity compared to performing immunohistochemistry off of the paraffin block can be achieved.[75]

The latest marker that has been proposed as an aid to the diagnosis of limited adenocarcinoma of the prostate is ERG. Fusions between the androgen-regulated transmembrane protease serine 2 (*TMPRSS2*) gene and the *ERG* gene are present in approximately 40% to 50% of prostate adenocarcinomas. This gene fusion is highly specific for prostate cancer, with the exception that 16% to 20% of high-grade PIN also show the gene fusion. *TMPRSS2-ERG* gene fusions monoclonal anti-ERG antibodies are available that correlate well with fusion-positive cancer (see Chapter 19). ERG antibodies have been shown to be negative in postatrophic hyperplasia, partial atrophy, and adenosis.[76–78] Rare benign glands can express ERG.[76,79] As an internal control, ERG labels endothelium. The major limitation of ERG as a diagnostic test is its low sensitivity, such that a negative stain does not exclude prostate carcinoma. Other weakness of this marker is that in 16% to 28% of cancers, there is heterogeneous ERG expression, further contributing to false-negative staining on biopsy.[80–83] In 16% to 20% of cases that are ERG positive, staining is also weak.[80,84] Cocktails have also been developed for p63/ERG and ERG/AMACR/HMWCK/p63.[80,84] There are conflicting studies on the diagnostic use of ERG. Shah et al.[84] claimed that ERG helped establish a diagnosis of prostate cancer in 28% of cases that otherwise would have been diagnosed as "atypical, suspicious for carcinoma" using immunohistochemistry for basal cell markers and AMACR. He et al.,[76] however, reported that ERG immunohistochemistry was not discriminatory in helping to stratify which "atypical foci" were likely to be associated with prostate cancer on rebiopsy.[76] We have not adopted ERG immunostaining in our routine workup of atypical foci.

In general, the use of immunohistochemistry for PSA and other prostate markers is not helpful in distinguishing benign versus malignant glandular lesions of the prostate because both conditions are positive. Some situations where it may be helpful in establishing the diagnosis of prostatic adenocarcinoma is in the setting of poorly preserved individual cells or sheets of cauterized cells, where these markers can identify these cells as being of prostatic origin and thus diagnostic of prostatic carcinoma.

REFERENCES

1. Kronz JD, Milord R, Wilentz R, et al. Lesions missed on prostate biopsies in cases sent in for consultation. *Prostate.* 2003;54:310–314.
2. Epstein JI. Diagnostic criteria of limited adenocarcinoma of the prostate on needle biopsy. *Hum Pathol.* 1995;26:223–229.
3. Varma M, Lee MW, Tamboli P, et al. Morphologic criteria for the diagnosis of prostatic adenocarcinoma in needle biopsy specimens. A study of 250 consecutive cases in a routine surgical pathology practice. *Arch Pathol Lab Med.* 2002;126:554–561.
4. Helpap B. Observations on the number, size and localization of nucleoli in hyperplastic and neoplastic prostatic disease. *Histopathology.* 1988;13:203–211.
5. Aydin H, Zhou M, Herawi M, et al. Number and location of nucleoli and presence of apoptotic bodies in diagnostically challenging cases of prostate adenocarcinoma on needle biopsy. *Hum Pathol.* 2005;36:1172–1177.
6. Iczkowski KA, Bostwick DG. Criteria for biopsy diagnosis of minimal volume prostatic adenocarcinoma: analytic comparison with nondiagnostic but suspicious atypical small acinar proliferation. *Arch Pathol Lab Med.* 2000;124:98–107.
7. Vesalainen S, Lipponen P, Talja M, et al. Mitotic activity and prognosis in prostatic adenocarcinoma. *Prostate.* 1995;26:80–86.
8. Aihara M, Truong LD, Dunn JK, et al. Frequency of apoptotic bodies positively correlates with Gleason grade in prostate cancer. *Hum Pathol.* 1994;25:797–801.
9. Colombel M, Vacherot F, Diez SG, et al. Zonal variation of apoptosis and proliferation in the normal prostate and in benign prostatic hyperplasia. *Br J Urol.* 1998;82:380–385.
10. Kyprianou N, Tu H, Jacobs SC. Apoptotic versus proliferative activities in human benign prostatic hyperplasia. *Hum Pathol.* 1996;27:668–675.

11. Montironi R, Magi Galluzzi C, Scarpelli M, et al. Occurrence of cell death (apoptosis) in prostatic intra-epithelial neoplasia. *Virchows Arch A Pathol Anat Histopathol.* 1993; 423:351–357.

12. Parwani AV, Herawi M, Epstein JI. Pleomorphic giant cell adenocarcinoma of the prostate: report of 6 cases. *Am J Surg Pathol.* 2006;30:1254–1259.

13. Lopez-Beltran A, Eble JN, Bostwick DG. Pleomorphic giant cell carcinoma of the prostate. *Arch Pathol Lab Med.* 2005;129:683–685.

14. Brennick JB, O'Connell JX, Dickersin GR, et al. Lipofuscin pigmentation (so-called "melanosis") of the prostate. *Am J Surg Pathol.* 1994;18:446–454.

15. Holmes EJ. Crystalloids of prostatic carcinoma: relationship to Bence-Jones crystals. *Cancer.* 1977;39:2073–2080.

16. Ro JY, Ayala AG, Ordonez NG, et al. Intraluminal crystalloids in prostatic adenocarcinoma. Immunohistochemical, electron microscopic, and x-ray microanalytic studies. *Cancer.* 1986;57:2397–2407.

17. Henneberry JM, Kahane H, Humphrey PA, et al. The significance of intraluminal crystalloids in benign prostatic glands on needle biopsy. *Am J Surg Pathol.* 1997;21: 725–728.

18. Epstein JI, Fynheer J. Acidic mucin in the prostate: can it differentiate adenosis from adenocarcinoma? *Hum Pathol.* 1992;23:1321–1325.

19. Goldstein NS, Qian J, Bostwick DG. Mucin expression in atypical adenomatous hyperplasia of the prostate. *Hum Pathol.* 1995;26:887–891.

20. Christian JD, Lamm TC, Morrow JF, et al. Corpora amylacea in adenocarcinoma of the prostate: incidence and histology within needle core biopsies. *Mod Pathol.* 2005;18: 36–39.

21. Humphrey PA, Vollmer RT. Corpora amylacea in adenocarcinoma of the prostate; prevalence in 100 prostatectomies and clinicopathologic correlations. *Surg Pathol.* 1990; 3:133–141.

22. Baisden BL, Kahane H, Epstein JI. Perineural invasion, mucinous fibroplasia, and glomerulations: diagnostic features of limited cancer on prostate needle biopsy. *Am J Surg Pathol.* 1999;23:918–924.

23. McNeal JE, Alroy J, Villers A, et al. Mucinous differentiation in prostatic adenocarcinoma. *Hum Pathol.* 1991;22:979–988.

24. Bastacky SI, Walsh PC, Epstein JI. Relationship between perineural tumor invasion on needle biopsy and radical prostatectomy capsular penetration in clinical stage B adenocarcinoma of the prostate. *Am J Surg Pathol.* 1993;17:336–341.

25. Ali TZ, Epstein JI. Perineural involvement by benign prostatic glands on needle biopsy. *Am J Surg Pathol.* 2005;29:1159–1163.

26. Carstens PH. Perineural glands in normal and hyperplastic prostates. *J Urol.* 1980;123: 686–688.

27. Fine SW, Epstein JI. Minute foci of Gleason score 8–10 on prostatic needle biopsy: a morphologic analysis. *Am J Surg Pathol.* 2005;29:962–968.

28. Yang XJ, Lecksell K, Potter SR, et al. Significance of small foci of Gleason score 7 or greater prostate cancer on needle biopsy. *Urology.* 1999;54:528–532.

29. Nelson RS, Epstein JI. Prostatic carcinoma with abundant xanthomatous cytoplasm. Foamy gland carcinoma. *Am J Surg Pathol.* 1996;20:419–426.

30. Tran TT, Sengupta E, Yang XJ. Prostatic foamy gland carcinoma with aggressive behavior: clinicopathologic, immunohistochemical, and ultrastructural analysis. *Am J Surg Pathol.* 2001;25:618–623.

31. Hudson J, Cao D, Vollmer R, et al. Foamy gland adenocarcinoma of the prostate: incidence, Gleason grade, and early clinical outcome. *Hum Pathol.* 2012;43:974–979.

32. Zhao J, Epstein JI. High-grade foamy gland prostatic adenocarcinoma on biopsy or transurethral resection: a morphologic study of 55 cases. *Am J Surg Pathol.* 2009;33: 583–590.

33. Cina SJ, Epstein JI. Adenocarcinoma of the prostate with atrophic features. *Am J Surg Pathol.* 1997;21:289–295.

34. Egan AJ, Lopez-Beltran A, Bostwick DG. Prostatic adenocarcinoma with atrophic features: malignancy mimicking a benign process. *Am J Surg Pathol.* 1997;21:931–935.

35. Levi AW, Epstein JI. Pseudohyperplastic prostatic adenocarcinoma on needle biopsy and simple prostatectomy. *Am J Surg Pathol.* 2000;24:1039–1046.

36. Humphrey PA, Kaleem Z, Swanson PE, et al. Pseudohyperplastic prostatic adenocarcinoma. *Am J Surg Pathol.* 1998;22:1239–1246.

37. Kramer CE, Epstein JI. Nucleoli in low-grade prostate adenocarcinoma and adenosis. *Hum Pathol.* 1993;24:618–623.

38. Garcia FU, Taylor CA, Hou JS, et al. Increased cellularity of tumor-encased native vessels in prostate carcinoma is a marker for tumor progression. *Mod Pathol.* 2000;13:717–722.

39. Goldstein NS, Underhill J, Roszka J, et al. Cytokeratin 34 beta E-12 immunoreactivity in benign prostatic acini. Quantitation, pattern assessment, and electron microscopic study. *Am J Clin Pathol.* 1999;112:69–74.

40. Brawer MK, Peehl DM, Stamey TA, et al. Keratin immunoreactivity in the benign and neoplastic human prostate. *Cancer Res.* 1985;45:3663–3667.

41. Hedrick L, Epstein JI. Use of keratin 903 as an adjunct in the diagnosis of prostate carcinoma. *Am J Surg Pathol.* 1989;13:389–396.

42. O'Malley FP, Grignon DJ, Shum DT. Usefulness of immunoperoxidase staining with high-molecular-weight cytokeratin in the differential diagnosis of small-acinar lesions of the prostate gland. *Virchows Arch A Pathol Anat Histopathol.* 1990;417:191–196.

43. Shah IA, Schlageter MO, Stinnett P, et al. Cytokeratin immunohistochemistry as a diagnostic tool for distinguishing malignant from benign epithelial lesions of the prostate. *Mod Pathol.* 1991;4:220–224.

44. Wojno KJ, Epstein JI. The utility of basal cell-specific anti-cytokeratin antibody (34 beta E12) in the diagnosis of prostate cancer. A review of 228 cases. *Am J Surg Pathol.* 1995; 19:251–260.

45. Shah RB, Zhou M, LeBlanc M, et al. Comparison of the basal cell-specific markers, 34betaE12 and p63, in the diagnosis of prostate cancer. *Am J Surg Pathol.* 2002;26: 1161–1168.

46. Weinstein MH, Signoretti S, Loda M. Diagnostic utility of immunohistochemical staining for p63, a sensitive marker of prostatic basal cells. *Mod Pathol.* 2002;15:1302–1308.

47. Parsons JK, Gage WR, Nelson WG, et al. p63 protein expression is rare in prostate adenocarcinoma: implications for cancer diagnosis and carcinogenesis. *Urology.* 2001; 58:619–624.

48. Sailer V, Stephan C, Wernert N, et al. Comparison of p40 (DeltaNp63) and p63 expression in prostate tissues—which one is the superior diagnostic marker for basal cells? *Histopathology.* 2013;63:50–56.

49. Abrahams NA, Ormsby AH, Brainard J. Validation of cytokeratin 5/6 as an effective substitute for keratin 903 in the differentiation of benign from malignant glands in prostate needle biopsies. *Histopathology.* 2002;41:35–41.

50. Rubin MA, Zhou M, Dhanasekaran SM, et al. alpha-Methylacyl coenzyme A racemase as a tissue biomarker for prostate cancer. *JAMA.* 2002;287:1662–1670.

51. Shah RB, Kunju LP, Shen R, et al. Usefulness of basal cell cocktail (34betaE12 + p63) in the diagnosis of atypical prostate glandular proliferations. *Am J Clin Pathol.* 2004; 122:517–523.

52. Zhou M, Shah R, Shen R, et al. Basal cell cocktail (34betaE12 + p63) improves the detection of prostate basal cells. *Am J Surg Pathol.* 2003;27:365–371.

53. Halushka MK, Kahane H, Epstein JI. Negative 34betaE12 staining in a small focus of atypical glands on prostate needle biopsy: a follow-up study of 332 cases. *Hum Pathol.* 2004;35:43–46.

54. Osunkoya AO, Hansel DE, Sun X, et al. Aberrant diffuse expression of p63 in adenocarcinoma of the prostate on needle biopsy and radical prostatectomy: report of 21 cases. *Am J Surg Pathol.* 2008;32:461–467.

55. Brimo F, Epstein JI. Immunohistochemical pitfalls in prostate pathology. *Hum Pathol.* 2012;43:313–324.

56. Oliai BR, Kahane H, Epstein JI. Can basal cells be seen in adenocarcinoma of the prostate?: an immunohistochemical study using high molecular weight cytokeratin (clone 34betaE12) antibody. *Am J Surg Pathol.* 2002;26:1151–1160.

57. Zhou M, Chinnaiyan AM, Kleer CG, et al. Alpha-Methylacyl-CoA racemase: a novel tumor marker over-expressed in several human cancers and their precursor lesions. *Am J Surg Pathol.* 2002;26:926–931.

58. Luo J, Zha S, Gage WR, et al. Alpha-methylacyl-CoA racemase: a new molecular marker for prostate cancer. *Cancer Res.* 2002;62:2220–2226.

59. Jiang Z, Woda BA, Rock KL, et al. P504S: a new molecular marker for the detection of prostate carcinoma. *Am J Surg Pathol.* 2001;25:1397–1404.

60. Jiang Z, Wu CL, Woda BA, et al. P504S/alpha-methylacyl-CoA racemase: a useful marker for diagnosis of small foci of prostatic carcinoma on needle biopsy. *Am J Surg Pathol.* 2002;26:1169–1174.

61. Jiang Z, Wu CL, Woda BA, et al. Alpha-methylacyl-CoA racemase: a multi-institutional study of a new prostate cancer marker. *Histopathology.* 2004;45:218–225.

62. Beach R, Gown AM, De Peralta-Venturina MN, et al. P504S immunohistochemical detection in 405 prostatic specimens including 376 18-gauge needle biopsies. *Am J Surg Pathol.* 2002;26:1588–1596.

63. Magi-Galluzzi C, Luo J, Isaacs WB, et al. Alpha-methylacyl-CoA racemase: a variably sensitive immunohistochemical marker for the diagnosis of small prostate cancer foci on needle biopsy. *Am J Surg Pathol.* 2003;27:1128–1133.

64. Zhou M, Jiang Z, Epstein JI. Expression and diagnostic utility of alpha-methylacyl-CoA-racemase (P504S) in foamy gland and pseudohyperplastic prostate cancer. *Am J Surg Pathol.* 2003;27:772–778.

65. Kunju LP, Rubin MA, Chinnaiyan AM, et al. Diagnostic usefulness of monoclonal antibody P504S in the workup of atypical prostatic glandular proliferations. *Am J Clin Pathol.* 2003;120:737–745.

66. Farinola MA, Epstein JI. Utility of immunohistochemistry for alpha-methylacyl-CoA racemase in distinguishing atrophic prostate cancer from benign atrophy. *Hum Pathol.* 2004;35:1272–1278.

67. Jiang Z, Iczkowski KA, Woda BA, et al. P504S immunostaining boosts diagnostic resolution of "suspicious" foci in prostatic needle biopsy specimens. *Am J Clin Pathol.* 2004;121:99–107.

68. Zhou M, Aydin H, Kanane H, et al. How often does alpha-methylacyl-CoA-racemase contribute to resolving an atypical diagnosis on prostate needle biopsy beyond that provided by basal cell markers? *Am J Surg Pathol.* 2004;28:239–243.

69. Kunju LP, Chinnaiyan AM, Shah RB. Comparison of monoclonal antibody (P504S) and polyclonal antibody to alpha methylacyl-CoA racemase (AMACR) in the work-up of prostate cancer. *Histopathology.* 2005;47:587–596.

70. Molinie V, Fromont G, Sibony M, et al. Diagnostic utility of a p63/alpha-methyl-CoA-racemase (p504s) cocktail in atypical foci in the prostate. *Mod Pathol.* 2004;17:1180–1190.

71. Hameed O, Sublett J, Humphrey PA. Immunohistochemical stains for p63 and alpha-methylacyl-CoA racemase, versus a cocktail comprising both, in the diagnosis of prostatic carcinoma: a comparison of the immunohistochemical staining of 430 foci in radical prostatectomy and needle biopsy tissues. *Am J Surg Pathol*. 2005;29:579–587.

72. Sanderson SO, Sebo TJ, Murphy LM, et al. An analysis of the p63/alpha-methylacyl coenzyme A racemase immunohistochemical cocktail stain in prostate needle biopsy specimens and tissue microarrays. *Am J Clin Pathol*. 2004;121:220–225.

73. Browne TJ, Hirsch MS, Brodsky G, et al. Prospective evaluation of AMACR (P504S) and basal cell markers in the assessment of routine prostate needle biopsy specimens. *Hum Pathol*. 2004;35:1462–1468.

74. Jiang Z, Li C, Fischer A, et al. Using an AMACR (P504S)/34betaE12/p63 cocktail for the detection of small focal prostate carcinoma in needle biopsy specimens. *Am J Clin Pathol*. 2005;123:231–236.

75. Hameed O, Humphrey PA. p63/AMACR antibody cocktail restaining of prostate needle biopsy tissues after transfer to charged slides: a viable approach in the diagnosis of small atypical foci that are lost on block sectioning. *Am J Clin Pathol*. 2005;124:708–715.

76. He H, Magi-Galluzzi C, Li J, et al. The diagnostic utility of novel immunohistochemical marker ERG in the workup of prostate biopsies with "atypical glands suspicious for cancer." *Am J Surg Pathol*. 2011;35:608–614.

77. Green WM, Hicks JL, De Marzo A, et al. Immunohistochemical evaluation of TMPRSS2-ERG gene fusion in adenosis of the prostate. *Hum Pathol*. 2013;44:1895–1901.

78. Cheng L, Davidson DD, Maclennan GT, et al. Atypical adenomatous hyperplasia of prostate lacks TMPRSS2-ERG gene fusion. *Am J Surg Pathol*. 2013;37:1550–1554.

79. Tomlins SA, Palanisamy N, Siddiqui J, et al. Antibody-based detection of ERG rearrangements in prostate core biopsies, including diagnostically challenging cases: ERG staining in prostate core biopsies. *Arch Pathol Lab Med*. 2012;136:935–946.

80. Yaskiv O, Zhang X, Simmerman K, et al. The utility of ERG/P63 double immunohistochemical staining in the diagnosis of limited cancer in prostate needle biopsies. *Am J Surg Pathol*. 2011;35:1062–1068.

81. Minner S, Gartner M, Freudenthaler F, et al. Marked heterogeneity of ERG expression in large primary prostate cancers. *Mod Pathol*. 2013;26:106–116.

82. Mertz KD, Horcic M, Hailemariam S, et al. Heterogeneity of ERG expression in core needle biopsies of patients with early prostate cancer. *Hum Pathol*. 2013;44:2727–2735.

83. Mosquera JM, Mehra R, Regan MM, et al. Prevalence of TMPRSS2-ERG fusion prostate cancer among men undergoing prostate biopsy in the United States. *Clin Cancer Res*. 2009;15:4706–4711.

84. Shah RB, Tadros Y, Brummell B, et al. The diagnostic use of ERG in resolving an "atypical glands suspicious for cancer" diagnosis in prostate biopsies beyond that provided by basal cell and alpha-methylacyl-CoA-racemase markers. *Hum Pathol*. 2013;44: 786–794.

7

MIMICKERS OF ADENOCARCINOMA OF THE PROSTATE

MIMICKERS OF GLEASON SCORE 2 TO 6 ADENOCARCINOMA

Adenosis

There are several mimickers of Gleason 2 to 6 adenocarcinoma (Table 7.1). One of the most common lesions that may be confused with carcinoma is adenosis.[1-7]

The other commonly used term for adenosis is *atypical adenomatous hyperplasia* (AAH). We prefer the term *adenosis*, as prefacing *adenomatous hyperplasia* with *atypical* has adverse consequences both in terms of practical patient management and in our theoretical framework of this entity. As outlined in the following text, there are very little data in support of a relation between adenosis and carcinoma. By designating these lesions as atypical, many patients will be subjected to unnecessary repeat biopsies. Conceptually, as has happened in the past, use of the term atypical adenomatous hyperplasia will result in this entity being considered with prostatic intraepithelial neoplasia (PIN) as precursors to carcinoma of the prostate. Whereas there is strong evidence that PIN is a precursor to some prostate cancers, this evidence is lacking in adenosis.

There is a wide spectrum in the literature in terms of the reported incidence of adenosis on transurethral resection of the prostate (TURP), ranging from 2.2% to 19.6%.[8] The reason for this broad range is different thresholds for diagnosing a focus of crowded glands as adenosis. Included within the lower threshold are prostate specimens with foci of crowded glands, which could be considered a minimal example of adenosis, although they do not closely mimic adenocarcinoma. Crowded benign glands that have absent or patchy staining for basal cell markers and/ or positive racemase immunoreactivity are one of the more frequent mimickers of prostate cancer.[9] At the other extreme, seen in 1.6% of benign TURPs performed at The Johns Hopkins Hospital, adenosis closely mimics adenocarcinoma of the prostate. The diagnosis of adenosis should be restricted to cases with a sufficiently atypical growth pattern that one has to seriously consider the diagnosis of low-grade cancer. This gradual spectrum within adenosis from a crowded focus of obviously benign glands

TABLE 7.1 Benign Mimickers of Gleason Score 2 to 6 Adenocarcinoma
• Atrophy (T = N)
• Radiation atypia (T = N)
• Verumontanum mucosal gland hyperplasia (T = N)
• Adenosis (atypical adenomatous hyperplasia) (T > N)
• Basal cell hyperplasia (T > N)
• Nephrogenic adenoma (T > N)
• Seminal vesicles (N > T)
• Mesonephric hyperplasia (T)
• Colonic mucosa (N)
• Cowper gland (N)

T, likelihood of seeing in transurethral resection specimens; N, likelihood of seeing in needle biopsy specimens.

to lesions that share similar features, yet more closely resemble cancer, supports the concept that adenosis is a hyperplastic rather than neoplastic lesion. Because adenosis preferentially occurs within the transition zone, it is more frequently seen on TURP as an incidental finding than on needle biopsy. However, in approximately 0.8% of needle biopsies, adenosis may be identified. This incidence is infrequent enough that many pathologists do not consider it in the differential diagnosis of small glandular lesions on needle biopsy. However, the frequency of adenosis on needle biopsy is sufficiently high that there is a good chance that one will see this lesion in one's practice with the potential to overdiagnose it as adenocarcinoma.

The distinction of adenosis from low-grade adenocarcinoma is based on architectural and cytologic features (Table 7.2). In order to minimize

TABLE 7.2 Diagnostic Criteria of Adenosis	
Adenosis	Cancer
Lobular	Haphazard growth pattern
Small glands share features with admixed larger glands	Small glands differ from adjacent benign glands
Pale to clear cytoplasm	Occasionally amphophilic cytoplasm
Medium-sized nucleoli	Occasionally large nucleoli
Blue mucinous secretions rare	Blue mucinous secretions common
Corpora amylacea common	Corpora amylacea rare
Basal cells present	Basal cells absent

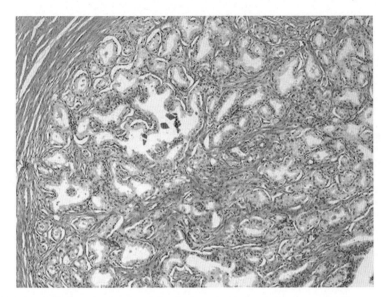

FIGURE 7.1   Well-circumscribed nodule of adenosis. Note admixed more benign–appearing glands with branching and papillary infolding adjacent to smaller crowded glands suspicious for cancer.

misdiagnoses, the constellation of histologic features seen in a lesion should outweigh the significance of any one diagnostic feature (eFigs. 7.1 to 7.115). At scanning magnification, adenosis is characterized by a lobular proliferation of small glands (Figs. 7.1 to 7.5). In contrast, low-grade carcinoma has a haphazard, irregular, infiltrative growth pattern. Despite the overall lobular pattern seen in adenosis, 19% of cases reveal minimal infiltration of glands into the surrounding stroma (Fig. 7.4).

Probably the most important differentiating feature of adenosis seen on hematoxylin and eosin (H&E) stain is that within a nodule of adenosis there are elongated glands with papillary infolding and branching lumina typical of more benign glands, yet in their nuclear and cytoplasmic features, they look similar to the adjacent small glands suspicious for carcinoma (Figs. 7.6 and 7.7). Another common feature seen is the budding off of glands of adenosis from obviously benign glands. Glands of adenocarcinoma, even in the unusual case when the tumor is fairly lobular, shows a pure population of small crowded glands without benign architectural features that do not merge in with adjacent larger benign glands.

At higher power, adenosis is typically composed of small glands with pale to clear cytoplasm, as opposed to some carcinomas, which have more amphophilic cytoplasm (Figs. 7.7 to 7.9). In order for this feature to be diagnostically useful, the cytoplasm of benign prostate glands should appear pale or clear on routinely stained slides. A diagnosis of carcinoma should not be rendered based on what appears to be either a few individual cells or poorly formed glands within a nodule that is otherwise

(text continues on p. 137)

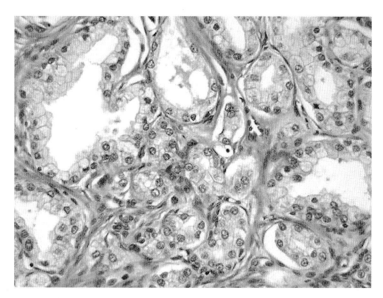

FIGURE 7.2 Medium magnification of Figure 7.1 with small glands merging in with more recognizably benign glands.

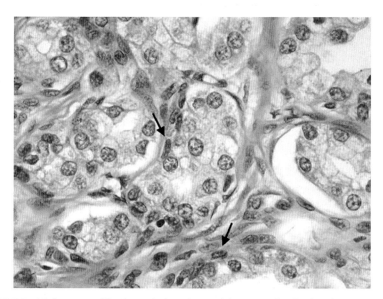

FIGURE 7.3 Higher magnification of Figure 7.1 with some glands showing recognizable basal cells *(arrows)*. Note adenosis may contain small visible nucleoli.

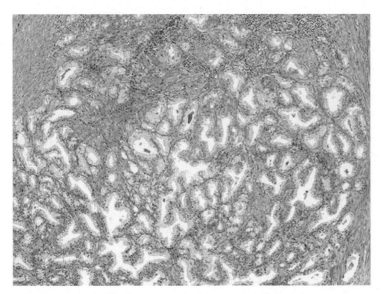

FIGURE 7.4 Adenosis which appears circumscribed in some areas *(right)* yet somewhat more infiltrative in others *(top)*. Note admixture of more benign–appearing glands with papillary infolding and branching adjacent to smaller crowded glands.

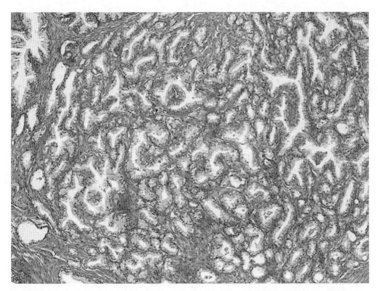

FIGURE 7.5 Well-circumscribed nodule of adenosis containing benign-appearing glands with papillary infolding and branching mixed with smaller crowded glands resembling cancer.

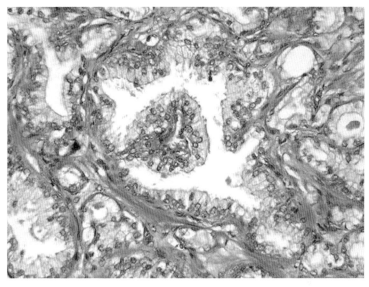

FIGURE 7.6 Medium magnification of Figure 7.5 where small glands of adenosis share identical nuclear and cytoplasmic features to adjacent more benign–appearing gland.

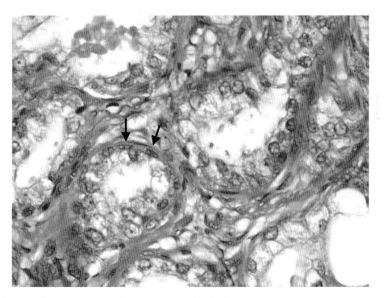

FIGURE 7.7 Higher magnification of Figure 7.5 of adenosis showing occasional glands with recognizable basal cell layer *(arrows)*. Note small but visible nucleoli.

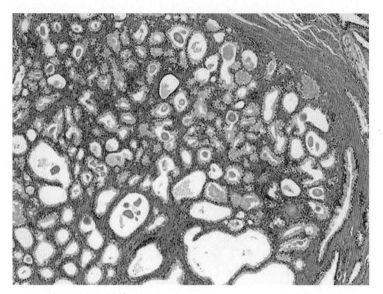

FIGURE 7.8 Well-circumscribed nodule of adenosis.

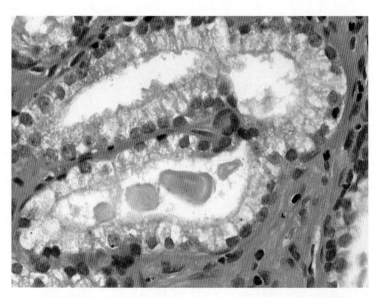

FIGURE 7.9 Adenosis with some visible nucleoli. Note corpora amylacea (same case as Fig. 7.8).

TABLE 7.3   Features Shared in Adenosis and Cancer
• Crowded glands
• Crystalloids
• Medium sized nucleoli
• Scattered poorly formed glands and singles
• Minimal infiltration at periphery
• AMACR immunoreactivity

AMACR, alpha-methylacyl-coenzyme A racemase.

typical of adenosis. Occasional single cells or poorly formed glands are not uncommon in a nodule of adenosis and probably represent tangential sections of small glands (Table 7.3).

Usually, adenosis has been described as having totally bland-appearing nuclei without nucleoli. This is generally valid; most (60%) lesions contain no or at most rare prominent nucleoli. In the other 40%, fairly prominent (>1.6 microns) nucleoli are present, which should not lead to the diagnosis of carcinoma (Fig. 7.9).[10]

In another study, 18% contained nucleoli larger than 1 micron.[1] Only huge nucleoli (>3 microns) are incompatible with a diagnosis of adenosis. In contrast, the majority (70%) of foci of low-grade adenocarcinoma have occasional or frequent large nucleoli. The remaining low-grade carcinomas have either no prominent or at most rare prominent nucleoli. These findings emphasize that, although nucleoli are generally helpful in differentiating adenosis from adenocarcinoma, there is overlap between the two entities.

The luminal contents also may be useful in this differential diagnosis. Corpora amylacea are commonly seen in adenosis and are rare in carcinoma. Only 2% of cases of adenosis contain blue intraluminal secretions visible on H&E-stained sections, a feature common in low-grade carcinomas. It is not helpful to perform special stains for mucin. Despite earlier studies' claims that acid mucin was diagnostic of carcinoma, a later work found that 54% of foci of adenosis contained acid mucin secretions.[11] Crystalloids are intraluminal structures that have been touted as distinguishing adenosis from carcinoma. However, 18% to 39% of foci of adenosis contain crystalloids, sometimes in great number (Fig. 7.10). Crystalloids should not be used to differentiate adenosis and carcinoma (Table 7.3).

The presence of basal cells is the one feature seen in adenosis that is typically not seen in carcinoma. Although basal cells may be difficult to identify within many of the glands, a flattened basal cell layer can be seen in at least some of the glands. As long as the glands with a basal cell layer are otherwise identical to the glands where a basal cell layer cannot be identified, then the entire lesion is benign. It is important to distinguish basal cells from adjacent fibroblasts. Although fibroblasts have elongated,

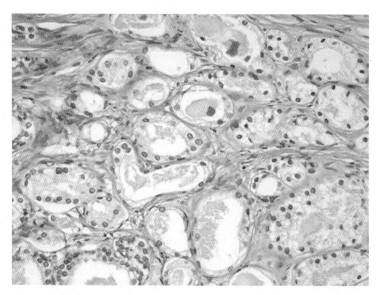

FIGURE 7.10 Adenosis consisting of glands with pale to clear cytoplasm, benign-appearing nuclei, and scattered crystalloids.

pointed, hyperchromatic nuclei, basal cell nuclei that are recognizable in routine sections have a more cigar-shaped ovoid contour with chromatin similar to that of the overlying secretory cells (Fig. 7.7). Basal cells may sometimes be apparent as a cluster of cells with scant cytoplasm polarized at the edge of a gland. In foci of glandular crowding where all of the features are typical of adenosis and there is no cytologic atypia, adenosis can be diagnosed without immunohistochemical stains even if basal cells are not visible on routine sections.

In cases where the architectural pattern favors adenosis yet there are visible nucleoli, the diagnosis can be clarified using immunohistochemistry for basal cells. The use of a basal cell specific antibodies to high molecular weight keratin or p63 is helpful since some glands will show a thin rim of keratin immunoreactivity beneath the cuboidal or columnar secretory cells.[2,3,12] As few as 10% of the glands in a nodule of adenosis may be labeled with antibodies to basal cell markers, although usually more than half of the glands will show some staining. The stain is also patchy within a given gland, with sometimes only one to two basal cells identified (Figs. 7.11 and 7.12). If some glands suspicious for adenosis lack high molecular weight cytokeratin or p63 immunoreactivity, yet are otherwise indistinguishable from adjacent glands that demonstrate basal cell immunoreactivity, the absence of a basal cell layer in some glands should not be used to diagnose the lesion as carcinoma. Some of the variability in basal cell immunoreactivity within adenosis and other lesions may be caused by tissue fixation because more uniform immunoreactivity has been observed in frozen tissue. In addition to the patchy staining in adenosis, another

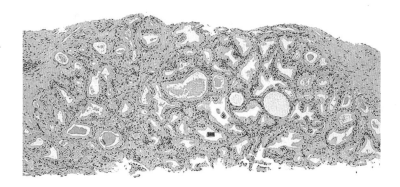

FIGURE 7.11 Crowded glands of adenosis on needle biopsy. Note admixture of more benign–appearing glands with papillary infolding.

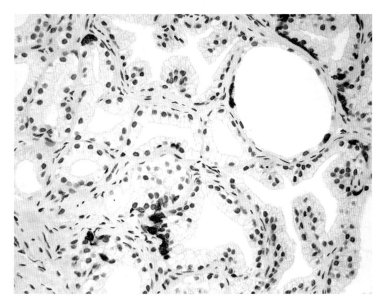

FIGURE 7.12 Adenosis may contain only patchy basal cells around a minority of the glands with immunostains for basal cell markers. However, the negatively stained glands are identical to those that show a patchy basal cell layer (same case as Fig. 7.11).

immunohistochemical pitfall in the interpretation of these lesions is that they express racemase, a marker preferentially expressed in prostatic adenocarcinoma. In one study, 10% of cases demonstrated focal racemase positivity with 7.5% showing diffuse immunoreactivity.[13]

Adenosis often appears to be multifocal. In a few cases on TURP, foci are so numerous that, if misdiagnosed as carcinoma, they would be classified as stage T1b, leading to unwarranted radical therapy. The distinction between adenosis and low-grade adenocarcinoma in even a single focus may be critical, because diagnosis of even a single focus of carcinoma on TURP in a relatively young man may lead to aggressive surgery.

The diagnosis of adenosis on needle biopsy is more difficult, since it is more difficult to appreciate the architectural pattern on needle biopsy. Adenosis on needle biopsy appears as a relatively well-localized nodule of closely packed glands with pale to clear cytoplasm (Figs. 7.11 to 7.13). In only 7% of foci is the entire lobular lesion visualized on needle biopsy.[3] In 45% of foci, one edge of the nodule can be appreciated and is circumscribed, yet the other side is not visible because the lesion is bisected by one edge of the needle biopsy. The remaining 48% of foci are transected in the middle of the nodule of adenosis such that the lesion extends to both edges of the needle biopsy. Although in these cases assessment of circumscription is difficult, in all but a few cases foci of adenosis occupy a small portion of the core length, uncommonly measuring more than 3 mm of the core length. Other than not having an entire nodule available for evaluation, the histologic features of adenosis on needle biopsy are the same as

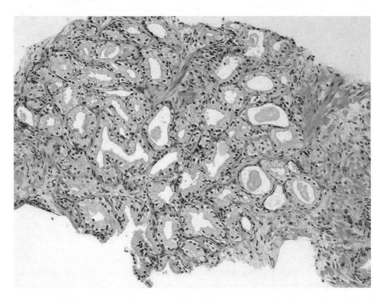

FIGURE 7.13 Nodule of adenosis on needle biopsy containing luminal undulations and some containing corpora amylacea typical of benign glands.

on TURP. On needle biopsy, due to the limited number of glands in question, basal cell specific antibodies must be interpreted with caution. Because basal cell staining may be patchy in adenosis, negative staining in a small focus of glands is not necessarily indicative of malignancy. However, if some of the glands within a crowded glandular focus on needle biopsy demonstrate a basal cell layer, then adenosis can be diagnosed. Because of the difficulty in diagnosing adenosis on needle biopsy, it is useful to verify the diagnosis with high molecular weight cytokeratin or p63 antibodies. In the evaluation of a nodule of adenosis, it is difficult to determine where the smaller crowded glands, where one is considering the diagnosis of cancer, end and the more obviously benign glands begin, because the small glands of adenosis merge in with the surrounding more recognizable benign glands. In contrast, with cancer, one should be able to identify each gland in question as malignant based on cytologic and/or architectural differences compared to adjacent benign glands. Whereas the immunohistochemical staining pattern in adenosis shows a few glands with patchy basal cell staining, cancer glands are negative and adjacent benign glands show circumferential complete basal cell immunoreactivity (Figs. 7.14 to 7.21).

Although adenosis mimics carcinoma, there is no conclusive evidence suggesting that patients with adenosis have an increased risk of harboring or developing adenocarcinoma of the prostate. In one series of adenosis, 14% of the transurethral resection (TUR) specimens examined also contained incidental foci of adenocarcinoma of the prostate.[2] This is similar to the reported frequency of incidental adenocarcinomas found in

(text continues on p. 145)

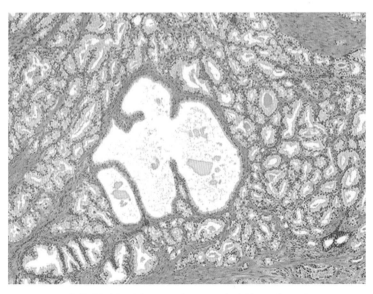

FIGURE 7.14   Adenocarcinoma mimicking adenosis.

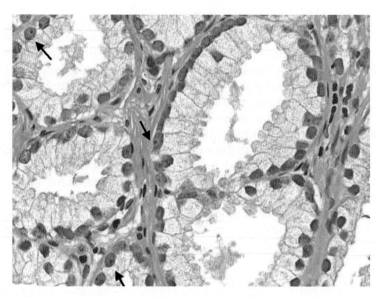

FIGURE 7.15 Adenocarcinoma mimicking adenosis. Multiple prominent nucleoli *(arrows)* raise the question of adenocarcinoma (same case as Fig. 7.14).

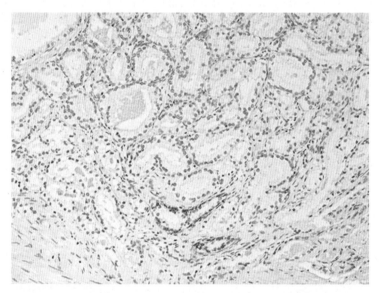

FIGURE 7.16 All of the atypical glands are negative for high molecular weight cytokeratin. Only positive glands are entrapped benign glands, which stain uniformly in contrast to patchy basal cell staining seen with adenosis (same case as Fig. 7.14).

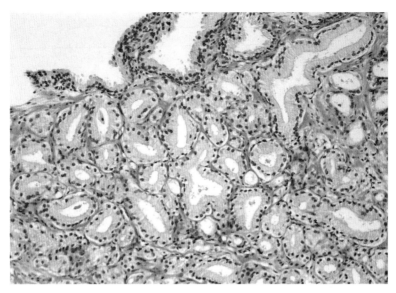

FIGURE 7.17 Adenocarcinoma mimicking adenosis, although the small glands do not merge in with the more obvious benign glands at the *top*.

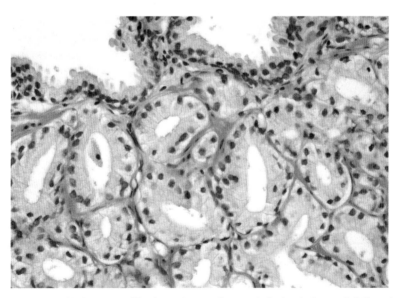

FIGURE 7.18 At higher magnification, the small crowded glands have slightly enlarged nuclei relative to the benign glands at the *top* (same case as Fig. 7.17).

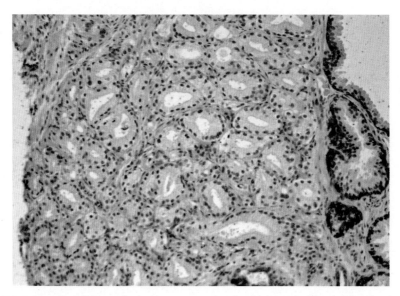

FIGURE 7.19 All of the small glands are negative for high molecular weight cytokeratin diagnostic of carcinoma (same case as Fig. 7.17).

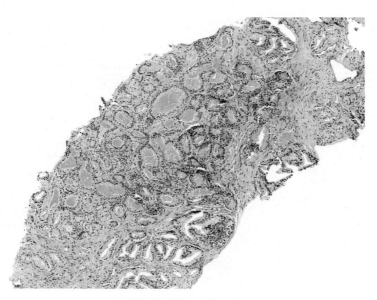

FIGURE 7.20 Adenosis.

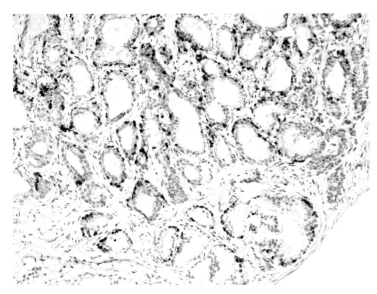

FIGURE 7.21   Adenosis with triple cocktail stain showing patchy brown basal cell staining for high molecular weight cytokeratin, p63 and red cytoplasmic staining for AMACR (same case as Fig. 7.20).

TURs performed for clinically benign disease. Prior reports of transitions between adenosis and carcinoma were not verified with the use of basal cell specific antibodies and may have been adenosis with foci of individual cells, minimal infiltration, or visible nucleoli. Another argument that has been raised to suggest that adenosis is a precursor to prostate cancer is that the two entities share certain morphologic features. Several studies have shown that adenosis may contain acid mucin, crystalloids, nucleoli, racemase, and have a patchy basal cell layer. Rather than proving a relation between adenosis and carcinoma, these findings demonstrate that any one of these features, by itself, is not specific for carcinoma. For example, acid mucin may be seen in atrophy a patchy basal cell layer in clear cell cribriform hyperplasia, racemase in partial atrophy, and nucleoli in basal cell hyperplasia.[9,11,14,15] None of these lesions is considered a precursor to prostate cancer. The interpretation of these features must be made in the context of the totality of a lesion's architectural and cytologic features. Those studies suggesting a higher risk of carcinoma in men with adenosis have defined it differently, including many examples of what most authorities would call carcinoma.[16] Adenosis is closer to benign prostatic hyperplasia than carcinoma in terms of its proliferation rate.[17,18] There have been a limited number of studies looking at the genetic findings in adenosis. Qian et al.,[19] using fluorescence in situ hybridization (FISH) analysis, demonstrated chromosomal anomalies in only 9% of cases of adenosis as compared to 55% of carcinomas. There was also no relationship between the chromosomal anomalies seen in adenosis and matched foci of carcinoma. In another study by the same group, Cheng et al.[20] noted allelic imbalances in 7 of 15 (47%) cases of adenosis. A subsequent study by Doll et al.,[21] however, found allelic imbalances in only 12% of cases of adenosis. One potential difference between the two studies was that the cases with foci of adenosis in the study by Doll et al.[21] lacked associated carcinomas. Also, Doll et al.[21] used the more stringent allelic imbalance criteria of a 50% reduction of allelic intensity in adenosis samples as compared to the patient-matched normal samples, whereas Cheng et al.[20] used a 30% reduction criterion. Bettendorf et al.,[22] using comparative genomic hybridization, found that adenosis uncommonly had allelic imbalances and concluded that adenosis is not closely linked to prostatic carcinoma. These cumulative results suggest that genetic alterations in adenosis may be infrequent.

In a more recent study by Cheng et al.,[23] *TMPRSS2-ERG* gene fusion (see Chapter 19), a common chromosomal rearrangement that occurs early in the development of invasive adenocarcinoma of the prostate and is present in 50% of adenocarcinomas and in 20% of high-grade prostate intraepithelial lesions, were assessed in adenosis by FISH and immunohistochemistry techniques. None of the 55 prostatic adenosis specimens that were investigated showed evidence of *TMPRSS2-ERG* alteration by either technique.[23] Similar results were also found by our group.[24] Formalin-fixed, paraffin-embedded tissue sections of adenosis from cases of prostate biopsies ($n = 30$), TURPs ($n = 12$), and radical prostatectomies ($n = 3$) were analyzed using immunohistochemistry for ERG. None of the foci of adenosis were positive for ERG protein expression. In comparison, in 40 cases of Gleason score 6 adenocarcinoma on a tissue microarray, 22 (55%) were positive for ERG protein. The findings in both studies support the notion that adenosis is not a precursor lesion of adenocarcinoma. Moreover, it suggests that immunohistochemistry for ERG expression could be a useful tool to differentiate adenosis from adenocarcinoma.[24]

The most critical issue in terms of patient management is whether patients with adenosis on histologic examination are at increased risk of subsequently being diagnosed with adenocarcinoma. In the only study to address this issue, Renedo et al.[25] studied 24 men with foci of adenosis compared to 61 men with benign prostatic hyperplasia. Men with adenosis were followed on average 6.5 years. There was no difference in the subsequent development of adenocarcinoma between the two groups. When diagnosing adenosis, we include the following statement, "Adenosis, although mimicking cancer, has not been shown to be associated with an increased risk of prostate cancer."

DIFFUSE ADENOSIS OF THE PERIPHERAL ZONE

We have observed a group of typically younger patients with multiple foci of small, nonlobular, crowded, but relatively bland acini on needle biopsy as well as in prostatectomy specimens.[26] The architectural pattern can mimic low-grade adenocarcinoma especially in the subset of cases that may display rare acini with cytologic atypia. It is unclear whether this architectural pattern, which we have termed *diffuse adenosis of the peripheral zone* (DAPZ), is simply a crowded glandular variant of normal prostate morphology or whether it represents a precursor or a risk factor for the development of prostatic carcinoma. Men with DAPZ tend to be younger (mean age: 49 years; range: 34 to 73 years) than the average age of men with prostate cancer. We evaluated 60 such cases on needle biopsy. Over half of the men on rebiopsy cases (57%) were subsequently diagnosed with carcinoma. Although the majority of tissue sampled in a typical DAPZ case had no cytologic atypia, in two-thirds of cases there were admixed rare foci of atypical glands with prominent nucleoli comprising less than 1% of submitted tissue. Patients with a subsequent diagnosis of carcinoma were more likely to have had DAPZ with focal atypia. DAPZ should be considered a risk factor for prostate cancer and that patients with such finding should be followed closely and rebiopsied (Fig. 7.22).[26]

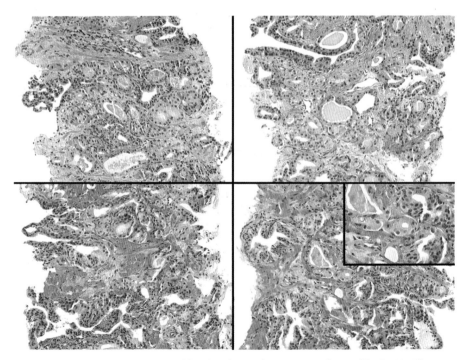

FIGURE 7.22 Four needle core biopsies from the same patient with DAPZ. All cores demonstrate small, crowded acinar foci with minimal cytologic atypia in a nonlobular distribution throughout the biopsies. *Inset* shows minimal nuclear enlargement yet no prominent nucleoli.

ATROPHY

Typically considered to be a process affecting the elderly, atrophy has been demonstrated in at least 70% of 19- to 29-year-old men.[27] Atrophy may result in prostatic induration or give rise to a hypoechoic lesion on transrectal ultrasound and may be biopsied as a lesion suspicious for cancer.

There are distinct histologic variants of atrophy, which can be classified as simple atrophy, postatrophic hyperplasia (PAH), and partial atrophy.[28] At low magnification, glands of simple atrophy appear basophilic, which reflects relative lack of cytoplasm both apically and laterally compared to normal epithelium. Simple atrophy glands are of relatively normal caliber and are generally spaced apart in a configuration similar to that of normal epithelium. In simple atrophy with cyst formation, the acini are rounded and appear cyst-like. Many of the acini in this pattern are arranged in a back-to-back configuration with little intervening stroma. Simple atrophy does not pose diagnostic difficulties.

PAH also often appears basophilic at low power. It consists of acini that are small and mostly round that are arranged in a lobular distribution.[29] Often, these acini appear to be surrounding a somewhat dilated "feeder" duct (Figs. 7.23 to 7.25). Many of these lesions frequently resemble normal-appearing resting breast lobules and are referred to by some authors as lobular atrophy. The lesions appear hyperplastic because the close packing of multiple small acini suggests that there is an increase in their number compared to normal tissue. PAH glands have a much higher proliferation rate than nonatrophic benign glands, and in some cases,

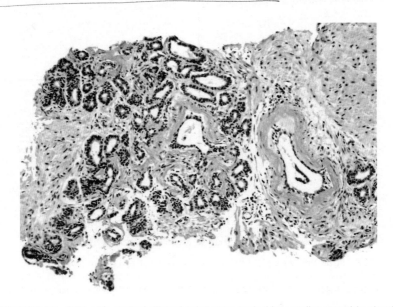

FIGURE 7.23 PAH with central dilated acini surrounded by smaller atrophic glands.

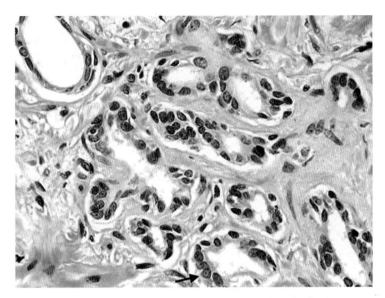

FIGURE 7.24   Sclerotic atrophy. Note occasional nucleoli *(arrow)*.

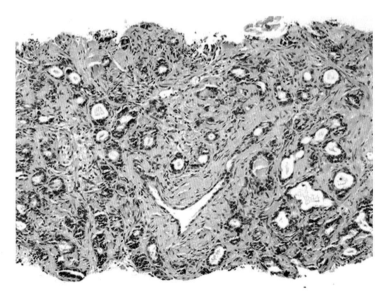

FIGURE 7.25   PAH with central dilated acinus surrounded by sclerosis and smaller atrophic glands.

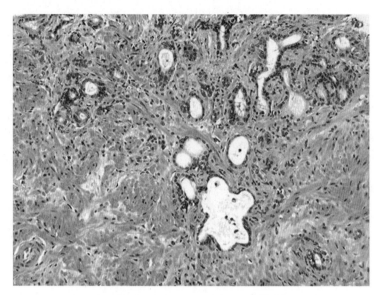

FIGURE 7.26   Postatrophic hyperplasia.

mitotic figures can be identified (Figs. 7.26 and 7.27).[30] Although the glands may appear infiltrative, they appear invasive as a patch not as individual glands infiltrating in between larger benign glands. The basophilic appearance of glands of atrophy is due to their scant cytoplasm and crowded nuclei such that at low magnification one is merely seeing a

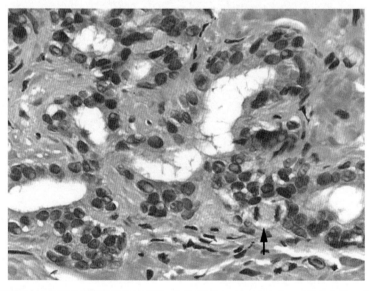

FIGURE 7.27   Higher magnification of Figure 7.26 showing atrophy with occasional nucleoli and a mitotic figure (arrow).

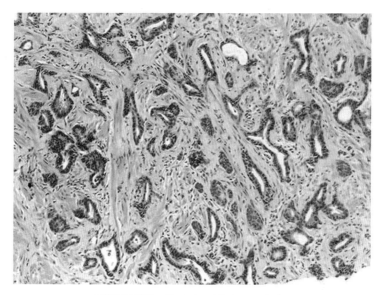

FIGURE 7.28   Postatrophic hyperplasia.

nuclear outline of the gland (Figs. 7.28 and 7.29, eFigs. 7.116 to 7.149). Longitudinal tangential sections of atrophic glands results in cords of cells that can further mimic cancer (Fig. 7.30, eFigs. 7.150 to 7.152). In some cases, there may be associated fibrosis, which gives the atrophic glands a more infiltrative appearance that has been termed in the past as *sclerotic*

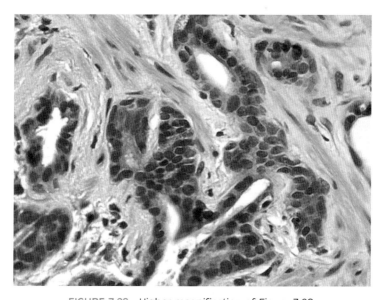

FIGURE 7.29   Higher magnification of Figure 7.28.

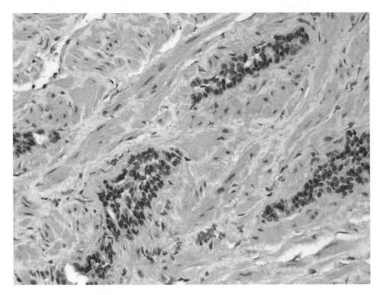

FIGURE 7.30 Tangential section of benign atrophic glands.

atrophy (Fig. 7.31). Whether one uses the term *postatrophic hyperplasia* or merely *benign prostate tissue with atrophy* in one's diagnostic reports is a matter of personal preference.

Compared to atrophy, gland-forming adenocarcinomas of the prostate typically have a greater amount of cytoplasm so that at low magnification,

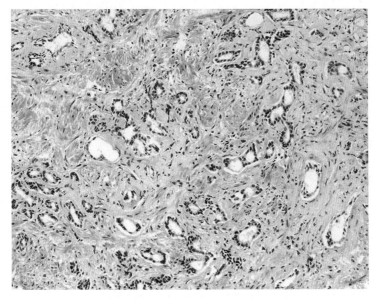

FIGURE 7.31 Sclerotic atrophy.

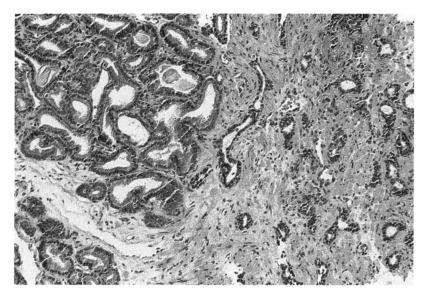

FIGURE 7.32 Atrophy *(right)* contrasted amphophilic cancer *(left)*.

the neoplastic glands are not as basophilic. Atrophy's very basophilic appearance is distinctive even when compared to adenocarcinoma with very amphophilic cytoplasm (Fig. 7.32). Atrophy may show enlarged nuclei and prominent nucleoli, although not the huge eosinophilic nucleoli seen in some prostate cancers. Although prominent nucleoli are more common in atrophic glands associated with inflammation, we have also seen prominent nucleoli in atrophy without inflammation. Furthermore, the inflammation associated with atrophy may be trivial and chronic in nature but still give rise to significant nuclear atypia. In deciding whether an atypical focus represents carcinoma, the presence of atrophic cytoplasm should, in general, make one cautious in diagnosing carcinoma. When there are concerns as to whether a focus represents PAH or adenocarcinoma, immunohistochemistry with antibodies to high molecular weight cytokeratin or p63 can be performed to resolve the issue, as PAH uniformly labels with basal cell markers (Fig. 7.33). As opposed to partial atrophy (see the following text), PAH uncommonly expresses racemase.[31,32]

Rarely, carcinoma with an atrophic appearance may be present on needle biopsy. The diagnosis of carcinoma in these cases is made on (a) a truly infiltrative process with individual small atrophic glands situated between larger benign glands; (b) the concomitant presence of ordinary, less atrophic carcinoma; and (c) greater cytologic atypia than is seen in benign atrophy (see Chapter 6).[31]

Another variant of atrophy, the most common mimicker of prostate cancer that causes confusion with carcinoma, is "partial atrophy"[9,33]

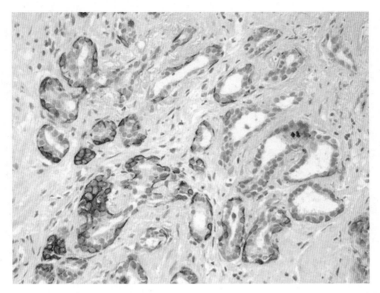

FIGURE 7.33 PAH with diffuse positivity for high molecular weight cytokeratin.

(eFigs. 7.153 to 7.201). Partial atrophy may still retain the lobular pattern of PAH, or as seen in Figures 7.34 and 7.35, have more of a disorganized diffuse appearance. Partial atrophy lacks the basophilic appearance of fully developed atrophy (simple atrophy, PAH) as the nuclei are more spaced apart (Figs. 7.36 to 7.38). The presence of crowded glands with pale

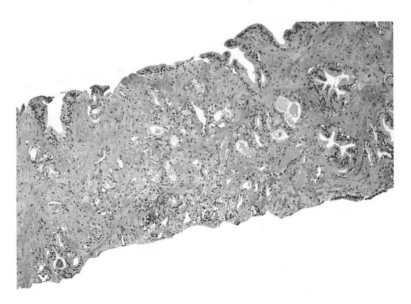

FIGURE 7.34 Partial atrophy.

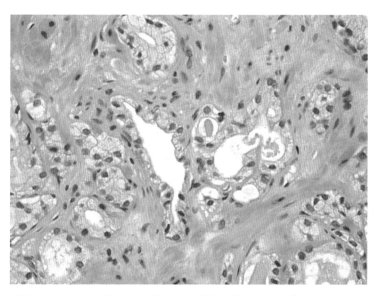

FIGURE 7.35 Higher magnification of Figure 7.34 with glands of partial atrophy having scant apical cytoplasm and subtle luminal infoldings.

cytoplasm may lead to an overdiagnosis of low-grade adenocarcinoma. At higher power, however, the glands have benign features characterized by undulating luminal surfaces with papillary infolding. Most carcinomas have more straight, even luminal borders. In addition, the glands are partially atrophic with nuclei in areas reaching the full height of the

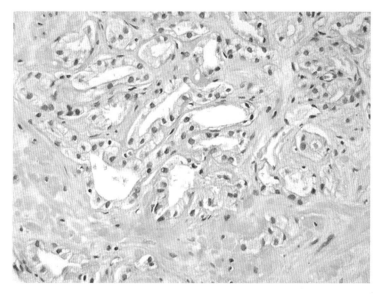

FIGURE 7.36 Partial atrophy.

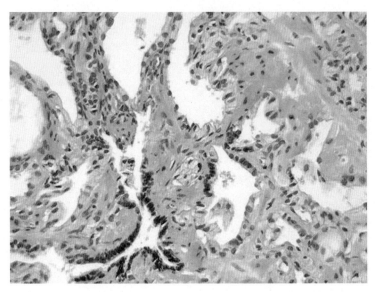

FIGURE 7.37   Partial atrophy merging in with fully developed atrophy *(lower left).*

cytoplasm. The nuclear features in partial atrophy tend to be relatively benign without prominent nucleoli, although nuclei may appear slightly enlarged with small nucleoli. One should hesitate diagnosing cancer when the nuclei occupy almost the full cell height and the cytoplasm has the same appearance as surrounding more obvious benign glands. As with

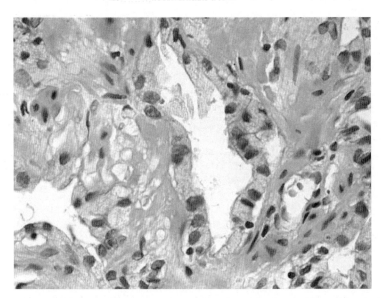

FIGURE 7.38   Higher magnification of Figure 7.37 showing glands of partial atrophy with scant apical yet abundant lateral cytoplasm and minimally enlarged nuclei.

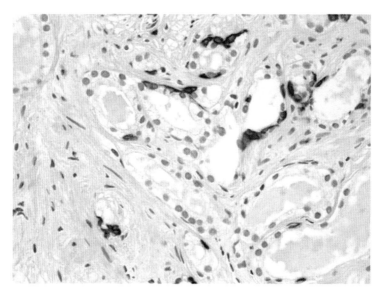

FIGURE 7.39 Case of Figures 7.37 and 7.38 with patchy basal cells staining for high molecular weight cytokeratin.

adenosis, partial atrophy typically has a patchy basal cell layer and express racemase (Fig. 7.39).[9]

There is emerging data that atrophy and associated inflammation are linked with prostate carcinogenesis.[34] However, the hypothesis is that these factors are involved in the initiation of prostate cancer and are not proximately related to cancer by the time atrophy is identified on needle biopsy. Atrophy of all morphologic types are very common on needle biopsy and are not associated with an increased risk of cancer or PIN on subsequent biopsy.[35]

BASAL CELL HYPERPLASIA

A spectrum of basaloid lesions ranging from hyperplasia to carcinoma exists in the prostate. Basal cell hyperplasia may resemble prostate acini seen in the fetus, accounting for the synonyms "fetalization" and "embryonal hyperplasia" of the prostate.

The most common form of basal cell hyperplasia consists of tubules or glands with piling up of the basal cell layer.[36–38] Although they are often overlooked, small glands with basal cell hyperplasia are not uncommonly found focally within nodules of benign prostatic hyperplasia (Fig. 7.40). Glandular-stromal nodules in which a majority of glands show basal cell hyperplasia may also be identified. In these cases, there is usually no confusion with carcinoma given the well-circumscribed nature of the lesion, the abundant stroma, as well as the intermingling of the glands of basal cell hyperplasia with normal glands.

Basal cell hyperplasia may be more florid in some cases, whereby it may be confused with prostatic adenocarcinoma (eFigs. 7.202 to 7.240)

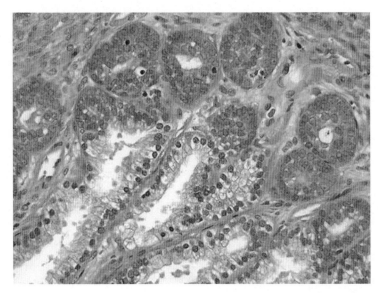

FIGURE 7.40   Basal cell hyperplasia composed of glands with multilayered round nuclei and atrophic cytoplasm.

(Table 7.4). In some cases of florid basal cell hyperplasia, the basal cell proliferation still retains a lobular configuration. In other instances, the lobular configuration may either be lost or not appreciated because of the fragmented nature of the TUR specimen (Figs. 7.41 and 7.42). Even at low magnification, basal cell hyperplasia can be distinguished from carcinoma by its very basaloid appearance. The glands appear basophilic at low power due to multilayering of the basal cells that have scant cytoplasm. In contrast, gland-forming adenocarcinomas of the prostate almost always have more abundant

TABLE 7.4   Features of Basal Cell Hyperplasia Not Typically Seen in Carcinoma

- Multilayering of cells
- Solid nests
- Cells with scant cytoplasm
- Glandular lumina with atrophic luminal cytoplasm
- Pseudocribriform glands
- Well-formed lamellar calcifications
- Intracytoplasmic eosinophilic globules
- Positivity for high molecular weight cytokeratin and p63
- Negative AMACR immunoreactivity

AMACR, alpha-methylacyl-coenzyme A racemase.

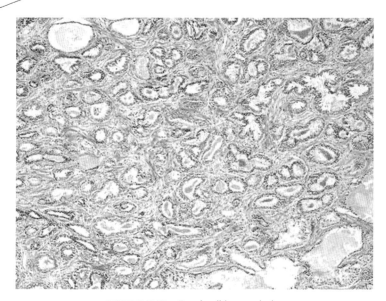

FIGURE 7.41   Basal cell hyperplasia.

cytoplasm resulting in a more eosinophilic appearance to the glands at low magnification. Within basal cell hyperplasia, there is piling up of the nuclei within the lumen ranging from a double cell layer in a few glands, to three to four cells thick in other glands, to solid nests of epithelium (Figs. 7.43 and 7.44). Basal cell hyperplasia may reveal focal cribriform and more commonly pseudocribriform glands. Pseudocribriform hyperplasia consists

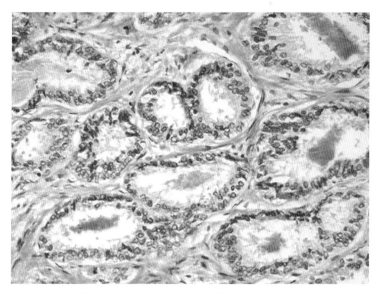

FIGURE 7.42   Basal cell hyperplasia with minimal piling up of nuclei (same case as Fig. 7.41).

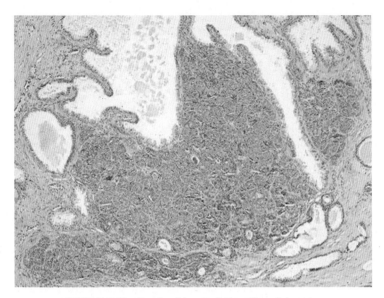

FIGURE 7.43   Basal cell hyperplasia with solid nests.

of back-to-back small round glands of basal cell hyperplasia rather than a solid nest of cells with punched out lumina that characterize true cribriform glands (Fig. 7.45).[39] Adjacent to cribriform and pseudocribriform basal cell hyperplasia are usually more typical individual glands of basal cell hyperplasia. Basal cell hyperplasia is also one of the few prostatic entities that

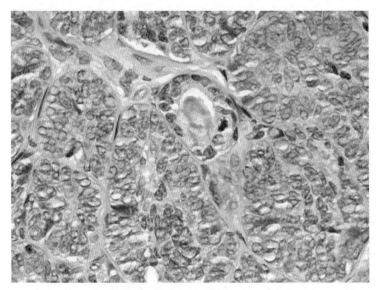

FIGURE 7.44   Higher magnification of Figure 7.43 with solid nests of basal cell hyperplasia showing nuclei with visible nucleoli and a mitotic figure.

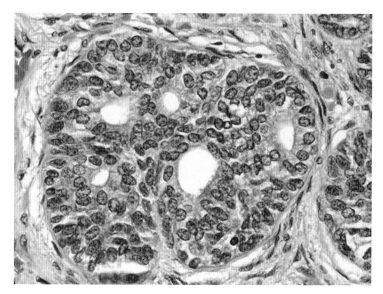

FIGURE 7.45   Basal cell hyperplasia with focal pseudocribriform formation, glands appear more back-to-back than true cribriform.

contain intraluminal calcifications (Fig. 7.46). These calcifications consist of well-formed lamellar calcifications. Carcinomas rarely contain calcifications, and when present, usually consist of fine calcified grains usually within central necrosis in high-grade cancers or intraductal carcinoma (eFigs. 7.241 to 7.244).[39] Another unique feature seen within the cells of basal cell hyperplasia

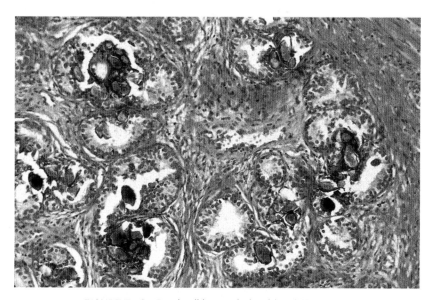

FIGURE 7.46   Basal cell hyperplasia with calcifications.

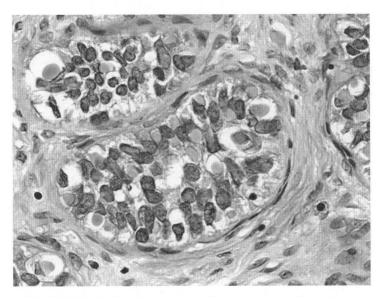

FIGURE 7.47   Basal cell hyperplasia with numerous hyaline globules.

is the presence of intracytoplasmic eosinophilic globules (Fig. 7.47, eFigs. 7.245 to 7.252).[39] Squamous features can also be seen in a minority of cases of basal cell hyperplasia, which tend to have more prominent fibrous stroma between the basaloid nests than normal prostatic stroma.[39] With the exception of basal cell hyperplasia with squamous features, basal cell hyperplasia lacks an associated desmoplastic response. In between the glands of basal cell hyperplasia is relatively unremarkable smooth muscle or on occasion a minimally myxoid stroma.

Basal cell lesions are preferentially located in the transition zone and are usually seen on TURP. Basal cell hyperplasia less frequently occurs in the peripheral zone, where it can be sampled on needle biopsy (eFigs. 7.253 to 7.268).[40,41] A unique difficulty of recognizing basal cell hyperplasia on needle biopsy is that the lobular growth pattern often seen on TURP or enucleation is not apparent when nodules of basal cell hyperplasia are transected on needle biopsy. In a series of basal cell hyperplasia seen on needle biopsy, the most common patterns were either individual glands or solid nests. The presence of solid nests of cells helps to rule out adenocarcinoma. However, basal cell hyperplasia with retention of glandular lumina further mimics cancer. Although occasionally adenocarcinomas of the prostate appear to consist of glands with multilayering, the multilayered glands typically occupy only a minority of the cancerous glands. In contrast, all of the glands in basal cell hyperplasia have multilayering. Glands of basal cell hyperplasia also tend to have more atrophic cytoplasm than adenocarcinoma. Other potential worrisome features that can be seen in basal cell hyperplasia on needle biopsy include cribriform and pseudocribriform formation, prominent nucleoli, mitoses, and an infiltrative pattern between benign prostate glands.[41]

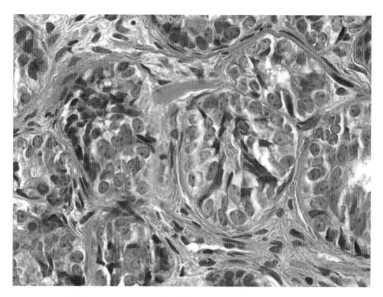

FIGURE 7.48   Basal cell hyperplasia with nucleoli.

If by light microscopy there is difficulty in distinguishing basal cell hyperplasia from prostatic adenocarcinoma, utilization of immunohisto-chemistry with a basal cell specific antibody can differentiate between the two lesions (Figs. 7.48 and 7.49). On the average, over 80% of the glands of basal cell hyperplasia are immunoreactive with these antibodies and

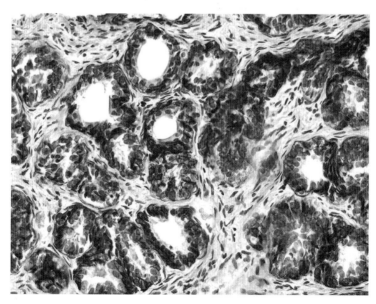

FIGURE 7.49   High molecular weight cytokeratin positivity in basal cell hyperplasia seen in Figure 7.48.

often the staining is very intense.[12,37,42,43] Racemase is typically negative in basal cell hyperplasia.[38,41]

Basal cell hyperplasia may have prominent nucleoli but is otherwise identical to ordinary basal cell hyperplasia[15,44] (Fig. 7.48, eFigs. 7.269 to 7.276). In the past, these cases were referred to as atypical basal cell hyperplasia. As these lesions are not associated with an adverse prognosis, we have dropped the word *atypical* so as not to cause undue concern for clinicians or patients. The enlarged nucleoli in general are seen diffusely throughout the lesion. In some cases of basal cell hyperplasia with prominent nucleoli, nuclei are seen undermining the overlying secretory cells that are cytologically normal. Other features usually attributable to carcinoma that may be seen in basal cell hyperplasia with prominent nucleoli are nuclear hyperchromasia, rare mitotic figures, nuclear enlargement, individual cell necrosis, necrotic intraluminal secretions, and blue-tinged mucinous secretions. Basal cell hyperplasia with prominent nucleoli is distinguished from acinar adenocarcinoma by the multilayering of its nuclei, solid nests, and atrophic cytoplasm. There is no known association between basal cell hyperplasia showing prominent nucleoli and either acinar adenocarcinoma or basal cell carcinoma. Distinguishing basal cell hyperplasia with prominent nucleoli from PIN is more difficult (see Chapter 5).

When a well-formed distinct nodule of basaloid nests is formed, the term *basal cell adenoma* or *adenoid basal cell tumor* is sometimes employed, although it is preferable to consider these lesions as more pronounced examples of basal cell hyperplasia (eFig. 7.277).[37,45,46]

COLONIC MUCOSA

Rarely, distorted fragments of colonic mucosa on transrectal biopsies of the prostate can be confused with adenocarcinoma of the prostate (Fig. 7.50, eFigs. 7.278 to 7.286).[47] In addition to the distorted architecture, features mimicking prostate cancer include (a) blue-tinged intraluminal mucinous secretions, (b) prominent nucleoli, (c) mitotic activity, (d) extracellular mucin, and (e) infrequently adenomatous changes of the rectal tissue. Immunohistochemical results further mimic prostate cancer with negative stains for the basal cell markers and positive stains for racemase. Diagnostic clues to recognizing that these foci are distorted rectal fragments are the presence of (a) lamina propria in the focus, (b) the rectal tissue located on a detached fragment of tissue, (c) associated inflammation, (d) goblet cells, and (e) muscularis propria. Assessing the colonic mucosa can also be helpful in diagnosing limited prostate cancer on biopsy. In some cases, the H&E stain is so basophilic that the colonic mucosa has a blue hue, such that the significance of blue-tinged mucinous secretions in atypical prostatic glands is not as discriminatory as in cases where the H&E stain is not as basophilic.

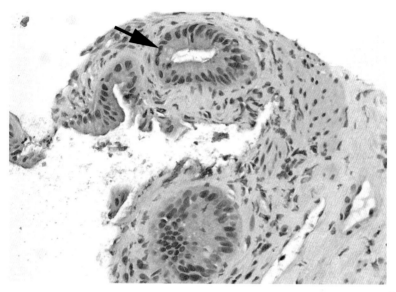

FIGURE 7.50 Colonic mucosa mimicking prostate adenocarcinoma. Note rare goblet cell *(arrow)*.

COWPER GLANDS

Initially, Cowper glands were identified on TUR as a potential pitfall in the diagnosis of prostate cancer. Subsequently, it was noted that they may be sampled on needle biopsy.[48] Cowper glands particularly resembles foamy gland carcinoma, which typically has bland cytology (Figs. 7.51 and 7.52, eFigs. 7.287 to 7.300).[49] The presence of glands in skeletal muscle may further mimic cancer if the lesion is not recognized as Cowper glands. The diagnosis of Cowper glands rests on the recognition of a noninfiltrative lobular pattern of a dimorphic population of ducts and mucinous acini in Cowper glands with the caveat that the ducts may not be obvious in all foci. Cowper glands have distended rounded cells that are expanded to the point that glandular lumina are often totally or subtotally occluded. In contrast, foamy gland cancers lack globoid cells and have well-formed open lumina often with dense pink secretions. The presence of abundant mucin-filled cytoplasm also distinguishes this lesion from carcinoma. Although prostate cancer cytoplasm may contain neutral mucinous secretions, they lack abundant intracytoplasmic mucin.

In difficult cases where ducts in Cowper glands may not be obvious, immunohistochemistry with a panel of antibodies may be useful.[48,50] Prostate-specific acid phosphatase (PSAP) is negative in all cases, although the abundant cytoplasm of the acinar cells may stain focally with prostate-specific antigen (PSA) in a heterogeneous "clumped" fashion. Ductal epithelium fails to react with either antibody. High molecular weight

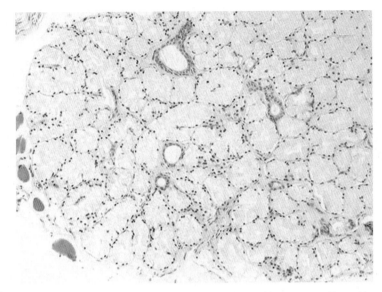

FIGURE 7.51 Cowper gland. Note muscle *(left)* and dimorphic pattern with scattered atrophic ducts among acini lined by mucinous cells.

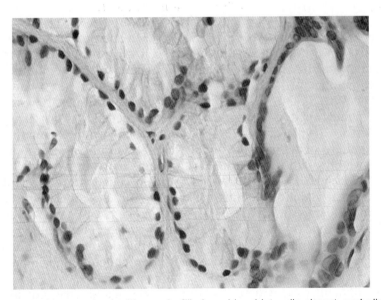

FIGURE 7.52 Cowper gland with mucin-filled ovoid goblet cells almost occluding the lumina of the acini.

cytokeratin decorates the ductal epithelium, hybrid cells, and an attenuated basal layer at the periphery of acini. Muscle-specific actin may be positive in a basal distribution, in contrast to negative staining in prostate cancer.

MESONEPHRIC REMNANT HYPERPLASIA

Mesonephric remnant hyperplasia in the prostate is a very rare benign mimicker of prostate adenocarcinoma that is identical to the lesion seen in the female genital tract (Fig. 7.53).[51,52] They are negative for PSA and prostate-specific acid phosphatase (eFigs. 7.301 to 7.308).

The anatomic location and histologic spectrum and their immuno-histochemical profile using current prostatic diagnostic markers have been addressed in a recent series from our group.[53] The latter included 10 cases of mesonephric remnant hyperplasia involving the prostate and periprostatic tissue, including 8 cases seen in radical prostatectomy specimens and 2 TURP specimens performed for obstruction. One patient underwent prostatectomy because of the misdiagnosis of mesonephric remnant hyperplasia on TUR as carcinoma. Patients ranged in age from 48 to 70 years (mean age: 60 years). The distribution of prostatic mesonephric hyperplasia was concentrated in two areas: (a) the anterior fibromuscular stroma and adjacent anterolateral periprostatic tissue (75%) and (b) the base posteriorly and posterolaterally either within or exterior to the prostate and around the seminal vesicle (50%). Histologic patterns observed included in order of frequency: small- to medium-sized acini or tubules with a lobular distribution (all cases); cysts either in clusters or scattered containing secretions; small or ill-formed glands with an infiltrative growth;

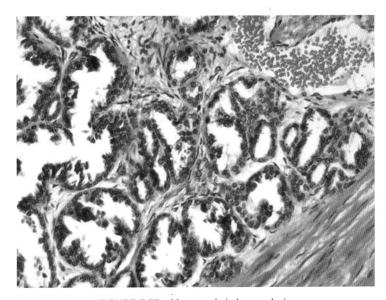

FIGURE 7.53 Mesonephric hyperplasia.

glands with papillary infoldings or micropapillary tufts; and two cases exceptionally displayed nodules of ill-formed small glands intermixed with spindle cells, mimicking sclerosing adenosis or Gleason pattern 5 prostate cancer. Most cases had florid hyperplasia and harbored three or more growth patterns. All cases were negative for PSA. High molecular weight cytokeratin was diffusely positive in almost half of the cases and showed focal immunoreactivity in the remaining cases. Except for occasional focal positivity seen in 4 of 7 cases, p63 was largely negative. Racemase was also focally positive in 4 of 7 cases. Importantly, small glands with an infiltrative growth pattern, the most difficult pattern to distinguish from cancer, were negative or only focally positive for high molecular weight cytokeratin, negative for p63, and only focally positive for racemase. All cases examined in the study were diffusely positive for PAX8, a marker that is very helpful in the differential diagnosis especially in cases where basal cell marker and racemase expression may overlap with that of prostate cancer. Lack of PSA is another helpful distinguishing feature.[53]

NEPHROGENIC ADENOMA

Nephrogenic adenoma can rarely affect the prostatic urethra. Extension of small tubules of nephrogenic adenoma into the underlying prostatic fibromuscular stroma can lead to the misdiagnosis of low-grade prostatic adenocarcinoma in TUR specimens and rarely on prostate biopsies. As this lesion is mainly associated with the prostatic urethra, it is discussed in Chapter 18.

RADIATION ATYPIA

Radiation changes in benign prostate glands can mimic adenocarcinoma of the prostate. This subject is discussed in Chapter 14 along with other manifestations of therapy-related morphologic changes.

SEMINAL VESICLES

The incidence of TUR material containing seminal vesicle epithelium in our institution is approximately 3%. There are differences in the literature as to the clinical significance of resecting seminal vesicle epithelium. In one study, there was a high incidence of postoperative epididymitis, whereas there was no significant morbidity in another study.[54,55] Although the overdiagnosis of seminal vesicles as carcinoma is less likely in TUR material given the greater amount of tissue to evaluate, there are some instances where seminal vesicle epithelium is composed of closely packed glands resembling adenocarcinoma (Figs. 7.54 to 7.56, eFigs. 7.309 to 7.323). Occasionally, seminal vesicles sampled on needle biopsy can also be a source of overdiagnosing prostatic adenocarcinoma. The recognition of seminal vesicle rests on appreciating its architectural as well as

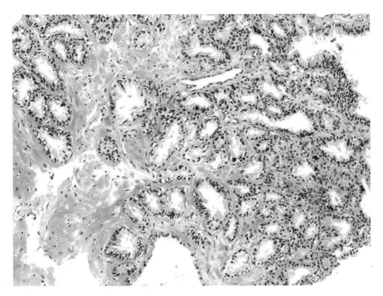

FIGURE 7.54 Seminal vesicles on biopsy with lumen toward right and outpouchings of seminal vesicles surrounding lumen.

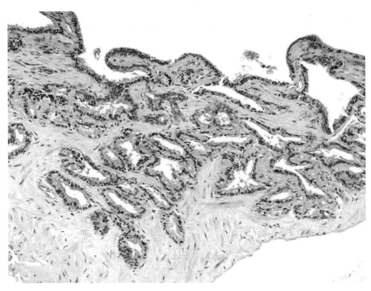

FIGURE 7.55 Seminal vesicle on needle biopsy. Note lumina of seminal vesicle *(top)* with outpouchings off of seminal vesicle *(bottom)*.

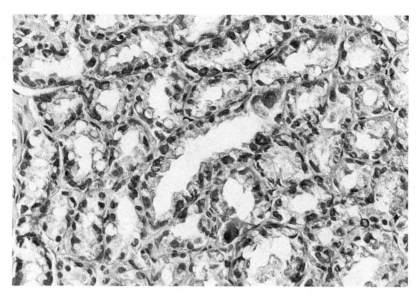

FIGURE 7.56 Seminal vesicle epithelium with scattered markedly atypical hyperchromatic degenerative-appearing nuclei. Note abundant lipofuscin pigment.

cytologic features. Seminal vesicles are characterized by a central large dilated lumina with numerous small glands clustered around the periphery. Often, the glands appear to bud off from the central lumen. Although on needle biopsy it may be difficult to recognize the architectural pattern of seminal vesicles due to the limited tissue, certain features may be present. A common finding on needle biopsy of the seminal vesicle is the dilated irregular lumen of the seminal vesicle seen at the edge of the tissue core, where the core has fragmented as it entered the seminal vesicle lumen. Surrounding this dilated structure are clusters of smaller glands (Fig. 7.55). Recognition that the small glands suspicious for carcinoma are all clustered around this dilated glandular structure is the first step in not overdiagnosing seminal vesicle epithelium as carcinoma. Verification that one is dealing with seminal vesicle epithelium can readily be accomplished at higher magnification examination. Seminal vesicle epithelium characteristically have scattered cells showing prominent nuclear atypia.[56] These nuclei are markedly enlarged with bizarre shapes and have marked hyperchromasia that often obscures nuclear details (Fig. 7.56). Despite these pleomorphic features, these nuclei lack mitotic activity. The atypia appears degenerative in nature, similar to that which is seen with radiation atypia. The common finding within seminal vesicles of markedly atypical nuclei present within well-formed glandular structures differs from prostate cancer in which gland-forming well- to moderately differentiated carcinomas have only slight to moderate nuclear atypia. Even in poorly differentiated prostatic carcinoma that lacks glandular differentiation, one rarely sees the severe atypia that is present within scattered seminal vesicle epithelial cells. Prominent globular golden brown lipofuscin granules are typical of seminal vesicle epithelium. Benign prostate tissue, high-grade PIN, and rarely carcinoma may contain lipofuscin pigment, but it differs in that the granules are smaller and more red-orange or blue (eFigs. 7.324 to 7.328).[57] If there still exists questions as to whether the lesion is seminal vesicle epithelium or prostatic adenocarcinoma, immunohistochemistry for high molecular weight cytokeratin will label basal cells surrounding seminal vesicle epithelium, whereas basal cells are absent in prostate adenocarcinoma. Although not commonly used in practice, antibodies to MUC6 label seminal vesicle ejaculatory duct epithelium and are negative in prostate cancer.[58] Caution must be used with immunohistochemistry using antibodies to PSA and PSAP, because it may label seminal vesicle tissue.[59]

VERUMONTANUM MUCOSAL GLAND HYPERPLASIA

Gagucas et al.[60] reported the presence of a distinctive small acinar proliferation in radical prostatectomy specimens involving the verumontanum and adjacent posterior urethra. This lesion, termed *verumontanum mucosal gland hyperplasia* (VMGH), is a potential mimic of adenocarcinoma and should be included in the differential diagnosis of small acinar proliferations of the prostate (Fig. 7.57, eFigs. 7.329 to 7.339). Similar lesions may be rarely encountered in prostatic needle biopsy specimens.[61]

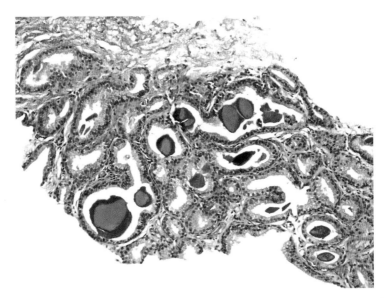

FIGURE 7.57 VMGH on needle biopsy with crowded glands with gray-green intraluminal concretions.

The verumontanum is situated along the posterior prostatic urethral wall and is the point at which the utricle and ejaculatory ducts merge with the prostatic urethra. The mimicry of adenocarcinoma that is produced by VMGH is particularly evident at low magnification. Here, the small size and crowded nature of verumontanum mucosal glands may simulate low-grade prostatic adenocarcinoma. Further confusion with carcinoma may arise from the presence of VMGH in multiple cores or from extensive involvement (i.e., >50%) of a single biopsy core. The glands of VMGH lack the infiltrative and haphazard arrangement of the glands typically found in prostatic adenocarcinoma. Moreover, the glands of prostatic adenocarcinoma are often found infiltrating between benign prostatic glands, a feature that is absent in VMGH. In addition, VMGH is characteristically identified adjacent to and often contiguous with urothelium. Contents of these mucosal glands are sufficiently distinct to allow discrimination from prostatic adenocarcinoma. Unlike prostatic adenocarcinoma, corpora amylacea are a feature typical of VMGH. Also, in VMGH, one characteristically finds distinctive brown-orange-green concretions. Verumontanum mucosal glands are immunophenotypically similar to prostatic acini; thus, the secretory cells of these mucosal glands stain positively with antibodies to PSA, whereas the basal cells stain with antibodies to high molecular weight cytokeratin and p63.

MIMICKERS OF GLEASON SCORE 7 TO 10 ADENOCARCINOMA

Clear Cell Cribriform Hyperplasia

One of the mimickers of Gleason score 7 to 10 adenocarcinoma is clear cell cribriform hyperplasia, which occurs within the transition zone and is mostly seen in TURP specimens removed for urinary obstructive symptoms and rarely seen on needle biopsy (Table 7.5). It is considered by some to be a cribriform variant of benign prostatic hyperplasia (BPH).

TABLE 7.5 Benign Mimickers of Gleason Score 7 to 10 Adenocarcinoma

Entity	Predominant Mode of Sampling
Nonspecific granulomatous prostatitis	TURP = Needle
Paraganglia	TURP = Needle
Clear cell cribriform hyperplasia	TURP > Needle
Sclerosing adenosis	TURP >> Needle
Xanthoma	Needle > TURP
Signet ring cell lymphocytes	TURP

TURP, transurethral resection of the prostate.

Although its classification within a conceptual framework is unresolved, it remains useful from the practical standpoint to consider it as a distinct entity, because it may be confused with either PIN or adenocarcinoma of the prostate.

In its most readily recognized form, clear cell cribriform hyperplasia is composed of numerous cribriform glands separated from one another by a modest amount of stroma in a pattern of nodular hyperplasia.[14] In florid cases, the glands infiltrate the stroma more diffusely and can have back-to-back glands (Figs. 5.20 and 5.21, eFig. 7.340 to 7.362). If it were to be misdiagnosed as adenocarcinoma, it would be classified as cribriform Gleason score $4 + 4 = 8$. The epithelial cells have distinctive clear cytoplasm and small bland nuclei with inconspicuous or small nucleoli. Around many of the glands of clear cell cribriform hyperplasia is a strikingly prominent basal cell layer, consisting of a row of cuboidal darkly stained cells beneath the clear cells (Fig. 5.22). The basal cells may form small knots at the periphery of some of the glands. Occasionally, the basal cells may have small nucleoli. The basal cell layer may be incomplete and in some glands may be invisible in routine sections. Tangential sections can also result in the appearance of occasional nests of clear cells without cribriform architecture or basal cells. Although usually unnecessary, immunostains for high molecular weight cytokeratin can highlight the basal cell layer.

The distinction between clear cell cribriform hyperplasia and cribriform PIN may be difficult (see Chapter 5). The distinction between clear cell cribriform hyperplasia and infiltrating cribriform carcinoma is easier. The presence of basal cells around some of the glands in clear cell cribriform hyperplasia rules out carcinoma, even though some glands with identical nuclear and cytoplasmic features may not have an apparent basal cell layer. The glands in clear cell cribriform hyperplasia lack cytologic atypia, in contrast to infiltrating cribriform carcinoma. Also, it is uncommon to see cribriform carcinoma unaccompanied by small infiltrating neoplastic glands.

Clear cell cribriform hyperplasia is uncommon, and its natural history is unknown. Although 3 of 25 reported cases were associated with adenocarcinoma of the prostate, there were no areas of transition from clear cell cribriform hyperplasia to carcinoma of the prostate.[14,62] Taking into account prostate cancer's high incidence in elderly men, it is felt that clear cell cribriform hyperplasia is unrelated to adenocarcinoma of the prostate.

NONSPECIFIC GRANULOMATOUS PROSTATITIS

One of the principle entities that can be confused with high-grade prostate cancer is nonspecific granulomatous prostatitis (NSGP).[63] Although discussed in general in Chapter 4, it is discussed here in the context of its differentiation from adenocarcinoma. NSGP can closely mimic cancer clinically. In a series of cases on needle biopsy, prostatic carcinoma was suspected or considered prior to biopsy in 55% of cases.[64] PSA levels greater than 4 ng/mL were seen in 84% of NSGP and digital rectal exam was frequently abnormal.

Although most cases of NSGP seen on needle biopsy do not histologically resemble prostate cancer, 4% of cases can closely resemble cancer. These cases of NSGP consists of sheets of epithelioid histiocytes, some with prominent nucleoli with abundant granular cytoplasm (Figs. 7.58 and 7.59, eFigs. 7.363 to 7.370). Reactive cribriform nonneoplastic prostatic glands further mimicking cancer may be seen in 7% of NSGP cases on biopsy. The key feature to avoid a misdiagnosis of cancer is to recognize the other inflammatory cells in NSGP, such as scattered neutrophils, lymphocytes, plasma cells, and eosinophils. The presence of scattered multinucleated giant cells may also aid in the diagnosis of NSGP. However, despite its name, approximately 50% of cases of NSGP lack multinucleated giant cells on needle biopsy.[64] In contrast, most adenocarcinomas of the prostate lack an associated inflammatory component.[65] Although it may be difficult to appreciate on needle biopsy specimens, NSGP initially is localized around ruptured ducts and acini. As seen in Figure 7.59, the epithelioid cells are not present diffusely throughout the needle biopsy core but surround an acinus or duct with attenuated partially disrupted epithelium. If this were carcinoma, the epithelioid cells would show no relationship to acini and ducts but would infiltrate throughout the core.

If there are difficulties in distinguishing NSGP from poorly differentiated adenocarcinoma, immunohistochemistry can be utilized. These

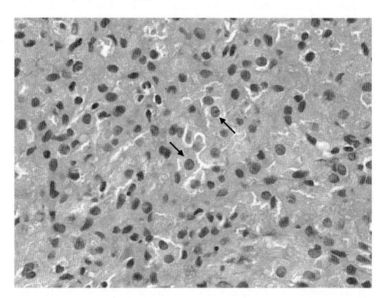

FIGURE 7.58　NSGP mimicking prostate cancer. Sheets of epithelioid cells some with nuclei showing prominent nucleoli (arrows).

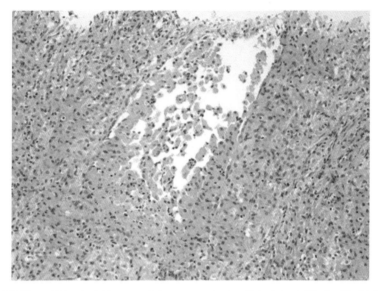

FIGURE 7.59   NSGP mimicking prostate cancer. Note dilated duct filled with histiocytes which ruptured giving rise to surrounding NSGP.

epithelioid cells will be negative for PSA, PSAP, and pancytokeratin and positive for various histiocytic markers.[66] Just as isolated architecturally atypical glands can be seen on H&E stains in a heavily inflamed prostate, there may be focal architectural abnormalities when evaluating sections labeled with PSA, PSAP, or pancytokeratin. Out of context, focal collections of individual immunoreactive epithelial cells may be suspicious for cancer. However, these foci are localized and the vast majority of epithelioid cells are negative for epithelial markers indicating that these areas represent ruptured ducts and acini.

PARAGANGLIA

Paraganglia have been identified in 8% of radical prostatectomies.[67] They are usually present in the posterolateral soft tissue exterior to the prostate. Uncommonly, they may be found in the lateral prostatic stroma or in the bladder neck smooth muscle. Rarely, paraganglia may be seen on TURP or on needle biopsy where their distinction from carcinoma must be made.[68] They consist of clusters of clear or amphophilic cells with fine cytoplasmic granules and a prominent vascular pattern, often intimately related to nerves (Fig. 7.60, eFigs. 7.371 to 7.376). Nucleoli are occasionally prominent, and when present, nuclear atypia is usually degenerative in appearance as seen in endocrine lesions. Paraganglia are situated in smooth muscle, not admixed with benign prostate glands. Although this lesion closely mimics high-grade adenocarcinoma of the

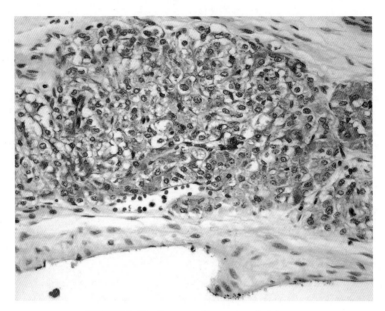

FIGURE 7.60   Paraganglia on needle biopsy.

prostate, the highly vascular setting and degenerative atypia are clues to prevent a misdiagnosis. Also before diagnosing a small focus of high-grade carcinoma on TURP or needle biopsy, where the atypical focus appears entirely extraprostatic, paraganglia should be considered in the differential diagnosis. Verification of the diagnosis can be accomplished with positive immunostaining for neuroendocrine markers diffusely and S100 labeling sustentacular cells and negative reactivity for PSA and PSAP.

SCLEROSING ADENOSIS

Lesions with the morphology of sclerosing adenosis were first reported in 1983 as an adenomatoid prostatic tumor.[69] The preferred term is *sclerosing adenosis* as their histogenesis is unrelated to adenomatoid tumors seen elsewhere.[70–72] In one series, sclerosing adenosis was found in approximately 2% of prostatic specimens. In most cases, lesions are discovered incidentally in TURs performed for urinary obstructive symptoms. Usually, only one or two small foci are present, although in one report, as many as 10 prostatic chips contained the lesion. As with any lesion seen on TUR, true multifocality as opposed to multiple sections through a single lesion cannot be distinguished. Very rarely, sclerosing adenosis may be seen on needle biopsy.[7,73] The major differential diagnosis rests between sclerosing adenosis and adenocarcinoma. Sclerosing adenosis consists of a mixture of well-formed glands, single cells, and a cellular spindle cell component (Fig. 7.61, eFigs. 7.377 to 7.403).

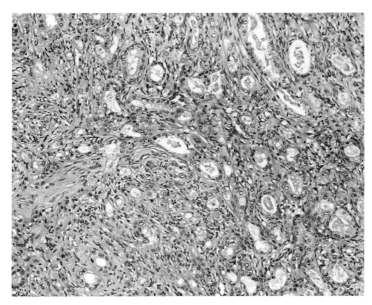

FIGURE 7.61 Sclerosing adenosis with mixture of well-formed glands and cellular spindle cell proliferation.

There are several features that should prevent a misdiagnosis of malignancy:

1. Adenocarcinomas of the prostate composed of an admixture of glands, poorly formed glandular structures, and single cells would be assigned a high Gleason score (7 or 8). Prostatic adenocarcinomas with these scores are only rarely seen as limited foci within a TURP. The finding of only one or several small foci of a cellular lesion suspicious for high-grade carcinoma should prompt a consideration of sclerosing adenosis or paraganglia. Furthermore, although sclerosing adenosis may be minimally infiltrative at its perimeter, the lesion is still relatively circumscribed in contrast to high-grade prostate adenocarcinoma.

2. The glandular structures in sclerosing adenosis resemble those seen in ordinary adenosis. They are composed of cells with pale to clear cytoplasm and relatively benign-appearing nuclei. In many of the glandular structures, a basal cell layer can be identified on H&E-stained sections that may be focally prominent and contains dense amphophilic cytoplasm.[73] This contrasts to carcinoma where basal cells are absent.

3. Sclerosing adenosis contains a dense spindle cell component that is typically lacking in adenocarcinomas (Figs. 7.61 and 7.62) the stromal cells are plump fusiform cells with amphophilic cytoplasm. The stroma occasionally displays a characteristic myxoid appearance.[73] Usually, adenocarcinomas of the prostate show no apparent stromal response or at most a hypocellular fibrotic reaction.

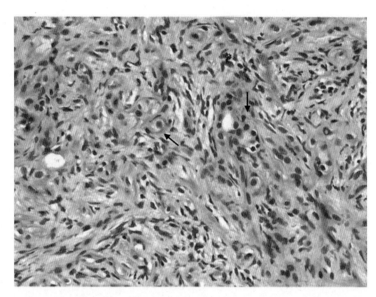

FIGURE 7.62 Sclerosing adenosis on needle biopsy. Note hyaline sheath around some of the glands and individual cells (arrows).

4. A rather unique feature of sclerosing adenosis is the presence of a hyaline sheath–like structure around some of the glands (Figs. 7.62 and 7.63). The glands in ordinary adenocarcinoma lack such a col-larette and have a "naked" appearance as they infiltrate the stroma.

5. The relatively bland cytology may also help in distinguishing scleros-ing adenosis from adenocarcinoma, although some nuclei within sclerosing adenosis may be moderately enlarged and contain promi-nent nucleoli.

These light microscopic features are classic for sclerosing adenosis, and it is usually not necessary to perform immunohistochemistry to clarify the diagnosis. However, immunohistochemistry is definitive in difficult cases. Ordinary adenocarcinomas of the prostate of all grades lack basal cells. Sclerosing adenosis contains a basal cell layer around most of the glandular structures as well as among the individual cells and cords of cells. The basal cells within sclerosing adenosis, however, are distinctive in their immuno-phenotypical staining and differ from ordinary basal cells. Ordinary basal cells of the prostate show no myoepithelial cell differentiation. They lack staining for muscle-specific actin and ultrastructurally do not show con-tractile elements. Within sclerosing adenosis, the basal cells show muscle-specific actin positivity and may also show S100 positivity consistent with myoepithelial cell differentiation (Fig. 7.64).[69,72,73] The dense spindle cell component in sclerosing adenosis also shows partial staining with keratin and muscle-specific actin and occasionally S100 consistent with myoepi-thelial cell differentiation.[73] Ultrastructural examination of several of these

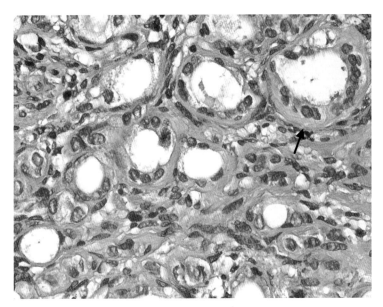

FIGURE 7.63 Sclerosing adenosis with hyaline sheath around some of the glands *(arrow)*. Note cellular stroma in between glands.

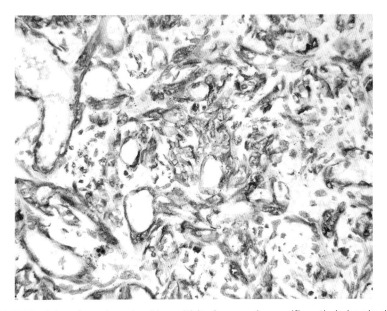

FIGURE 7.64 Sclerosing adenosis with positivity for muscle-specific actin in basal cells and focally in intervening stroma.

cases has verified their myoepithelial differentiation.[70] There is no known association between sclerosing adenosis and adenocarcinoma of the prostate.

SIGNET RING LYMPHOCYTES

TURP specimens may frequently show aggregates of degenerated lymphocytes with a signet ring cell appearance.[74] This finding results from thermal injury and is not seen in needle biopsy or open prostatectomy specimens. Only rarely are these changes so prominent to be confused with signet ring cell carcinoma (Fig. 7.65, eFigs. 7.404 to 7.407).

XANTHOMA

Although rare, prostatic xanthoma can be a source of diagnostic confusion, particularly with small tissue fragments such as those obtained from needle biopsies (Fig. 7.66, eFigs. 7.408 to 7.428).[75,76] Most cases contain only one focus of prostatic xanthoma, which are 0.5 mm or smaller. Exceptionally, xanthomas may range up to 2.5 mm. Xanthoma cells have small uniform, benign-appearing nuclei; small inconspicuous nucleoli; and abundant vacuolated, foamy cytoplasm with no mitotic figures. Although most xanthomas are arranged in a circumscribed solid nodular pattern, xanthomas can form cords and individual cells infiltrating the prostatic stroma, further mimicking high-grade prostate carcinoma. Careful attention to morphology with adjunctive use of CD68 (positive) and CAM5.2 (negative) immunohistochemical stains are helpful in the diagnosis of prostatic xanthoma, especially in difficult cases with an infiltrative pattern.

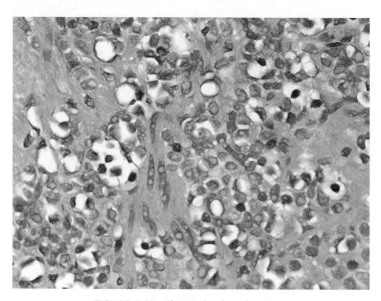

FIGURE 7.65 Signet ring lymphocytes.

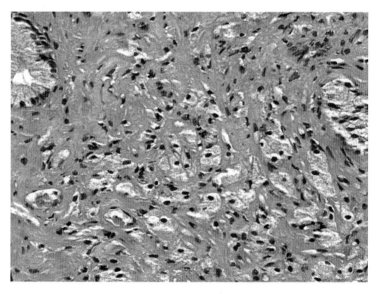

FIGURE 7.66   Xanthoma.

REFERENCES

1. Bostwick DG, Srigley J, Grignon D, et al. Atypical adenomatous hyperplasia of the prostate: morphologic criteria for its distinction from well-differentiated carcinoma. *Hum Pathol.* 1993;24:819–832.

2. Gaudin PB, Epstein JI. Adenosis of the prostate. Histologic features in transurethral resection specimens. *Am J Surg Pathol.* 1994;18:863–870.

3. Gaudin PB, Epstein JI. Adenosis of the prostate. Histologic features in needle biopsy specimens. *Am J Surg Pathol.* 1995;19:737–747.

4. Harik LR, O'Toole KM. Nonneoplastic lesions of the prostate and bladder. *Arch Pathol Lab Med.* 2012;136:721–734.

5. Montironi R, Scarpelli M, Mazzucchelli R, et al. The spectrum of morphology in non-neoplastic prostate including cancer mimics. *Histopathology.* 2012;60:41–58.

6. Hameed O, Humphrey PA. Pseudoneoplastic mimics of prostate and bladder carcinomas. *Arch Pathol Lab Med.* 2010;134:427–443.

7. Berney DM, Fisher G, Kattan MW, et al. Pitfalls in the diagnosis of prostatic cancer: retrospective review of 1791 cases with clinical outcome. *Histopathology.* 2007;51: 452–457.

8. Mittal BV, Amin MB, Kinare SG. Spectrum of histological lesions in 185 consecutive prostatic specimens. *J Postgrad Med.* 1989;35:157–161.

9. Herawi M, Parwani AV, Irie J, et al. Small glandular proliferations on needle biopsies: most common benign mimickers of prostatic adenocarcinoma sent in for expert second opinion. *Am J Surg Pathol.* 2005;29:874–880.

10. Kramer CE, Epstein JI. Nucleoli in low-grade prostate adenocarcinoma and adenosis. *Hum Pathol.* 1993;24:618–623.

11. Epstein JI, Fynheer J. Acidic mucin in the prostate: can it differentiate adenosis from adenocarcinoma? *Hum Pathol.* 1992;23:1321–1325.

12. Hedrick L, Epstein JI. Use of keratin 903 as an adjunct in the diagnosis of prostate carcinoma. *Am J Surg Pathol.* 1989;13:389–396.

13. Yang XJ, Wu CL, Woda BA, et al. Expression of alpha-Methylacyl-CoA racemase (P504S) in atypical adenomatous hyperplasia of the prostate. *Am J Surg Pathol.* 2002;26:921–925.

14. Ayala AG, Srigley JR, Ro JY, et al. Clear cell cribriform hyperplasia of prostate. Report of 10 cases. *Am J Surg Pathol.* 1986;10:665–671.

15. Epstein JI, Armas OA. Atypical basal cell hyperplasia of the prostate. *Am J Surg Pathol.* 1992;16:1205–1214.

16. Brawn PN. Adenosis of the prostate: a dysplastic lesion that can be confused with prostate adenocarcinoma. *Cancer.* 1982;49:826–833.

17. Haussler O, Epstein JI, Amin MB, et al. Cell proliferation, apoptosis, oncogene, and tumor suppressor gene status in adenosis with comparison to benign prostatic hyperplasia, prostatic intraepithelial neoplasia, and cancer. *Hum Pathol.* 1999;30: 1077–1086.

18. Helpap B. Cell kinetic studies on prostatic intraepithelial neoplasia (PIN) and atypical adenomatous hyperplasia (AAH) of the prostate. *Pathol Res Pract.* 1995;191:904–907.

19. Qian J, Jenkins RB, Bostwick DG. Chromosomal anomalies in atypical adenomatous hyperplasia and carcinoma of the prostate using fluorescence in situ hybridization. *Urology.* 1995;46:837–842.

20. Cheng L, Shan A, Cheville JC, et al. Atypical adenomatous hyperplasia of the prostate: a premalignant lesion? *Cancer Res.* 1998;58:389–391.

21. Doll JA, Zhu X, Furman J, et al. Genetic analysis of prostatic atypical adenomatous hyperplasia (adenosis). *Am J Pathol.* 1999;155:967–971.

22. Bettendorf O, Schmidt H, Eltze E, et al. Cytogenetic changes and loss of heterozygosity in atypical adenomatous hyperplasia, in carcinoma of the prostate and in non-neoplastic prostate tissue using comparative genomic hybridization and multiplex-PCR. *Int J Oncol.* 2005;26:267–274.

23. Cheng L, Davidson DD, Maclennan GT, et al. Atypical adenomatous hyperplasia of prostate lacks TMPRSS2-ERG gene fusion. *Am J Surg Pathol.* 2013;37:1550–1554.

24. Green WM, Hicks JL, De Marzo A, et al. Immunohistochemical evaluation of TMPRSS2-ERG gene fusion in adenosis of the prostate. *Hum Pathol.* 2013;44: 1895–1901.

25. Renedo D, Poy E, Wojno K. Clinical significance and distinction of adenosis from low-grade adenocarcinoma of the prostate on TURP. *Mod Pathol.* 1995;8:82A.

26. Lotan TL, Epstein JI. Diffuse adenosis of the peripheral zone in prostate needle biopsy and prostatectomy specimens. *Am J Surg Pathol.* 2008;32:1360–1366.

27. Gardner WA Jr, Culberson DE. Atrophy and proliferation in the young adult prostate. *J Urol.* 1987;137:53–56.

28. de Marzo AM, Platz EA, Epstein JI, et al. A working group classification of focal prostate atrophy lesions. *Am J Surg Pathol.* 2006;30:1281–1291.

29. Amin MB, Tamboli P, Varma M, et al. Postatrophic hyperplasia of the prostate gland: a detailed analysis of its morphology in needle biopsy specimens. *Am J Surg Pathol.* 1999;23:925–931.

30. Ruska KM, Sauvageot J, Epstein JI. Histology and cellular kinetics of prostatic atrophy. *Am J Surg Pathol.* 1998;22:1073–1077.

31. Farinola MA, Epstein JI. Utility of immunohistochemistry for alpha-methylacyl-CoA racemase in distinguishing atrophic prostate cancer from benign atrophy. *Hum Pathol.* 2004;35:1272–1278.

32. Beach R, Gown AM, De Peralta-Venturina MN, et al. P504S immunohistochemical detection in 405 prostatic specimens including 376 18-gauge needle biopsies. *Am J Surg Pathol.* 2002;26:1588–1596.

33. Oppenheimer JR, Wills ML, Epstein JI. Partial atrophy in prostate needle cores: another diagnostic pitfall for the surgical pathologist. *Am J Surg Pathol.* 1998;22:440–445.

34. Palapattu GS, Sutcliffe S, Bastian PJ, et al. Prostate carcinogenesis and inflammation: emerging insights. *Carcinogenesis.* 2005;26:1170–1181.

35. Postma R, Schroder FH, van der Kwast TH. Atrophy in prostate needle biopsy cores and its relationship to prostate cancer incidence in screened men. *Urology.* 2005;65: 745–749.

36. Cleary KR, Choi HY, Ayala AG. Basal cell hyperplasia of the prostate. *Am J Clin Pathol.* 1983;80:850–854.

37. Grignon DJ, Ro JY, Ordonez NG, et al. Basal cell hyperplasia, adenoid basal cell tumor, and adenoid cystic carcinoma of the prostate gland: an immunohistochemical study. *Hum Pathol.* 1988;19:1425–1433.

38. Yang XJ, Tretiakova MS, Sengupta E, et al. Florid basal cell hyperplasia of the prostate: a histological, ultrastructural, and immunohistochemical analysis. *Hum Pathol.* 2003; 34:462–470.

39. Rioux-Leclercq NC, Epstein JI. Unusual morphologic patterns of basal cell hyperplasia of the prostate. *Am J Surg Pathol.* 2002;26:237–243.

40. Thorson P, Swanson PE, Vollmer RT, et al. Basal cell hyperplasia in the peripheral zone of the prostate. *Mod Pathol.* 2003;16:598–606.

41. Hosler GA, Epstein JI. Basal cell hyperplasia: an unusual diagnostic dilemma on prostate needle biopsies. *Hum Pathol.* 2005;36:480–485.

42. Brawer MK, Peehl DM, Stamey TA, et al. Keratin immunoreactivity in the benign and neoplastic human prostate. *Cancer Res.* 1985;45:3663–3667.

43. Shah IA, Schlageter MO, Stinnett P, et al. Cytokeratin immunohistochemistry as a diagnostic tool for distinguishing malignant from benign epithelial lesions of the prostate. *Mod Pathol.* 1991;4:220–224.

44. Devaraj LT, Bostwick DG. Atypical basal cell hyperplasia of the prostate. Immunophenotypic profile and proposed classification of basal cell proliferations. *Am J Surg Pathol.* 1993;17:645–659.

45. Ronnett BM, Epstein JI. A case showing sclerosing adenosis and an unusual form of basal cell hyperplasia of the prostate. *Am J Surg Pathol.* 1989;13:866–872.

46. Lin JI, Cohen EL, Villacin AB, et al. Basal cell adenoma of prostate. *Urology.* 1978;11: 409–410.

47. Schowinsky JT, Epstein JI. Distorted rectal tissue on prostate needle biopsy: a mimicker of prostate cancer. *Am J Surg Pathol.* 2006;30:866–870.

48. Cina SJ, Silberman MA, Kahane H, Epstein JI. Diagnosis of Cowper's glands on prostate needle biopsy. *Am J Surg Pathol.* 1997;21:550–555.

49. Nelson RS, Epstein JI. Prostatic carcinoma with abundant xanthomatous cytoplasm. Foamy gland carcinoma. *Am J Surg Pathol.* 1996;20:419–426.

50. Saboorian MH, Huffman H, Ashfaq R, et al. Distinguishing Cowper's glands from neoplastic and pseudoneoplastic lesions of prostate: immunohistochemical and ultrastructural studies. *Am J Surg Pathol.* 1997;21:1069–1074.

51. Bostwick DG, Qian J, Ma J, et al. Mesonephric remnants of the prostate: incidence and histologic spectrum. *Mod Pathol.* 2003;16:630–635.

52. Gikas PW, Del Buono EA, Epstein JI. Florid hyperplasia of mesonephric remnants involving prostate and periprostatic tissue. Possible confusion with adenocarcinoma. *Am J Surg Pathol.* 1993;17:454–460.

53. Chen YB, Fine SW, Epstein JI. Mesonephric remnant hyperplasia involving prostate and periprostatic tissue: findings at radical prostatectomy. *Am J Surg Pathol.* 2011;35:1054–1061.

54. Jensen KM, Sonneland P, Madsen PO. Seminal vesicle tissue in "resectate" of transurethral resection of prostate. *Urology.* 1983;22:20–23.

55. Tsuang MT, Weiss MA, Evans AT. Transurethral resection of the prostate with partial resection of the seminal vesicle. *J Urol.* 1981;126:615–617.

56. Arias-Stella J, Takano-Moron J. Atypical epithelial changes in the seminal vesicle. *AMA Arch Pathol*. 1958;66:761–766.

57. Brennick JB, O'Connell JX, Dickersin GR, et al. Lipofuscin pigmentation (so-called "melanosis") of the prostate. *Am J Surg Pathol*. 1994;18:446–454.

58. Leroy X, Ballereau C, Villers A, et al. MUC6 is a marker of seminal vesicle-ejaculatory duct epithelium and is useful for the differential diagnosis with prostate adenocarcinoma. *Am J Surg Pathol*. 2003;27:519–521.

59. Varma M, Morgan M, O'Rourke D, et al. Prostate specific antigen (PSA) and prostate specific acid phosphatase (PSAP) immunoreactivity in benign seminal vesicle\ejaculatory duct epithelium: a potential pitfall in the diagnosis of prostate cancer in needle biopsy specimens. *Histopathology*. 2004;44:405–406.

60. Gagucas RJ, Brown RW, Wheeler TM. Verumontanum mucosal gland hyperplasia. *Am J Surg Pathol*. 1995;19:30–36.

61. Gaudin PB, Wheeler TM, Epstein JI. Verumontanum mucosal gland hyperplasia in prostatic needle biopsy specimens. A mimic of low grade prostatic adenocarcinoma. *Am J Clin Pathol*. 1995;104:620–626.

62. Frauenhoffer EE, Ro JY, el-Naggar AK, et al. Clear cell cribriform hyperplasia of the prostate. Immunohistochemical and DNA flow cytometric study. *Am J Clin Pathol*. 1991;95:446–453.

63. Stillwell TJ, Engen DE, Farrow GM. The clinical spectrum of granulomatous prostatitis: a report of 200 cases. *J Urol*. 1987;138:320–323.

64. Oppenheimer JR, Kahane H, Epstein JI. Granulomatous prostatitis on needle biopsy. *Arch Pathol Lab Med*. 1997;121:724–729.

65. Blumenfeld W, Tucci S, Narayan P. Incidental lymphocytic prostatitis. Selective involvement with nonmalignant glands. *Am J Surg Pathol*. 1992;16:975–981.

66. Presti B, Weidner N. Granulomatous prostatitis and poorly differentiated prostate carcinoma. Their distinction with the use of immunohistochemical methods. *Am J Clin Pathol*. 1991;95:330–334.

67. Ostrowski ML, Wheeler TM. Paraganglia of the prostate. Location, frequency, and differentiation from prostatic adenocarcinoma. *Am J Surg Pathol*. 1994;18:412–420.

68. Kawabata K. Paraganglion of the prostate in a needle biopsy: a potential diagnostic pitfall. *Arch Pathol Lab Med*. 1997;121:515–516.

69. Chen KT, Schiff JJ. Adenomatoid prostatic tumor. *Urology*. 1983;21:88–89.

70. Grignon DJ, Ro JY, Srigley JR, et al. Sclerosing adenosis of the prostate gland. A lesion showing myoepithelial differentiation. *Am J Surg Pathol*. 1992;16:383–391.

71. Jones EC, Clement PB, Young RH. Sclerosing adenosis of the prostate gland. A clinicopathological and immunohistochemical study of 11 cases. *Am J Surg Pathol*. 1991; 15:1171–1180.

72. Sakamoto N, Tsuneyoshi M, Enjoji M. Sclerosing adenosis of the prostate. Histopathologic and immunohistochemical analysis. *Am J Surg Pathol*. 1991;15:660–667.

73. Luque RJ, Lopez-Beltran A, Perez-Seoane C, et al. Sclerosing adenosis of the prostate. Histologic features in needle biopsy specimens. *Arch Pathol Lab Med*. 2003;127: e14–e16.

74. Alguacil-Garcia A. Artifactual changes mimicking signet ring cell carcinoma in transurethral prostatectomy specimens. *Am J Surg Pathol*. 1986;10:795–800.

75. Sebo TJ, Bostwick DG, Farrow GM, et al. Prostatic xanthoma: a mimic of prostatic adenocarcinoma. *Hum Pathol*. 1994;25:386–389.

76. Chuang AY, Epstein JI. Xanthoma of the prostate: a mimicker of high-grade prostate adenocarcinoma. *Am J Surg Pathol*. 2007;31:1225–1230.

8

REPORTING CANCER: INFLUENCE ON PROGNOSIS AND TREATMENT

NEEDLE BIOPSY

Use of Macros (Canned Text)

We have made extensive use of abbreviations in our pathology reports concerning prostate specimens. The advantages of these macros are multiple: (a) shorten transcription time with reduction in typographical errors, (b) create uniform terminology for clinicians, (c) prevent omission of important points relating to treatment and prognosis, (d) save the pathologist's time by not having to "reinvent the wheel" each time he or she has to add a comment, and (e) allow one to search for prior diagnoses based on standard verbiage used. The macros that we use are listed in the appendix. The only potential disadvantage of using macros is if one relies on them too heavily. For the occasional case that does not fit a macro, it is necessary to abandon them for the use of free text or to add free text at the end of the macro.

Quantification of Amount of Cancer on Needle Biopsy

Multiple techniques of quantifying the amount of cancer found on needle biopsy have been developed and studied.[1,2] The most common measurements studied include the (a) number of positive cores, (b) total millimeters of cancer among all cores, (c) percentage of each core occupied by cancer, (d) total percent of cancer in the entire specimen, and (e) fraction of positive cores (# positive cores/# total cores). From the cited measurements, one can even develop more refined means of quantifying tumor. For example, after calculating the percentage of each core with cancer, one can assess the highest percentage of cancer at any core or percentage of cancer at the site with the highest Gleason score. All of the cited measurements of cancer volume on needle biopsy are tightly correlated with each other, such that it is difficult to demonstrate the superiority of one technique over the other.

PREDICTION OF PATHOLOGIC STAGE AND MARGINS. Earlier studies demonstrated that percent of cancer on biopsy and the number of positive cores correlated with pathologic stage and margins.[3–11] Subsequently, there has been a growing consensus on the importance of the fraction of positive cores (no. of positive cores/total cores) to predict radical prostatectomy stage and margins of resection.[12–19] An advantage of using fraction of positive cores is that the number of cores sampled by the urologist or radiologist can widely vary, which the fraction of positive cores accounts for. Whereas most studies demonstrate the correlation of fraction of positive cores with stage statistically but without showing raw data, Gancarczyk et al.[14] illustrates the power of this measurement broken down by various percentages of the cores with cancer (Table 8.1). The best approach to factoring in needle biopsy tumor volume is using nomograms to predict pathologic stage factoring in pretreatment prostate-specific antigen (PSA), biopsy Gleason score, and percentage of cores positive for tumor.[14] However, prostate cancer limited to even one or two needle biopsy cores offers no guarantee of favorable findings at final surgical staging. In a study that specifically developed a nomogram to predict seminal vesicle invasion, which evaluated numerous biopsy tumor volume measurements, the best model was the percent of cancer at the base, clinical stage, biopsy Gleason score, and PSA.[17] Although the incidence of lymph node metastases at radical prostatectomy has come down as a result of earlier detection of prostate cancer, Conrad et al.[20] was able to identify tumors with a 42% to 45% likelihood of nodal metastases when there were more than three sextant cores with any Gleason pattern 4 or 5.

Currently, there is no consensus as to the optimal method for measuring tumor length or percentage of cancer on a core when there are two or more foci of prostate cancer in a single core separated by benign intervening glands and stroma.[2] Some urologic pathologists, including our group,

TABLE 8.1 **Pathologic Stage Stratified by the Percent of Biopsy Cores Positive for Cancer**

Percent Biopsy Positive	OC	EPE	SV+	LN+	Total No.
<20	64.6%	29.1%	4.1%	2.2%	636
≥20 to <30	59.3%	29.2%	8%	3.5%	113
≥30 to <40	61.6%	32.5%	4.3%	1.7%	304
≥40 to <50	50.9%	36.8%	12.3%	0%	57
≥50 to <60	44%	40.4%	12.4%	3.2%	218
≥60 to <70	51.2%	38.1%	6%	4.8%	84
≥70 to <80	46.2%	30.8%	15.4%	7.7%	13
≥80 to <90	39.5%	44.7%	7.9%	7.9%	38
≥90 to 100	34.7%	36.8%	18.4%	10.2%	49

OC, organ confined; EPE, extraprostatic extension; SV+, seminal vesicle invasion; LN+, lymph node metastases.

measure discontinuous foci of cancer as if they were a single continuous focus. The rationale is that these discontinuous foci are undoubtedly the same cancer going in and out of the plane of section. Others choose to add the measurements of the individual separate foci of cancer, ignoring the extent of the intervening benign prostate tissue. In a recent study from our group, Karram et al.[21] demonstrated that for prostate cancer in which the needle biopsy grade is representative of the entire tumor, quantifying cancer extent on biopsy by measuring discontinuous cancer on biopsy from one end to the other as opposed to "collapsing" the cancer by subtracting out the intervening benign prostate tissue correlates better with organ-confined disease and risk of positive margins.

PREDICTION OF POSTTREATMENT PROGRESSION. Several studies have demonstrated that percent of positive cores factored in with biopsy Gleason score, PSA, and clinical stage predict progression following radical prostatectomy.[22–25] Other biopsy tumor measurements that have been reported in these studies to correlate with progression following surgery are (a) percent total needle biopsy specimen with cancer (total length of cancer/total length of cores), (b) greatest percentage of cancer on a given core, and (c) percent positive cores from the most involved side (i.e., left or right). Similarly, percent of positive cores have been shown to independently predict recurrence following either brachytherapy or external beam radiotherapy after factoring in PSA and biopsy Gleason score.[26–30]

PREDICTION OF PROSTATECTOMY TUMOR VOLUME AND POTENTIALLY INSIGNIFICANT TUMOR. Multiple studies have demonstrated that measurements of cancer on the needle biopsy correlate with radical prostatectomy tumor volume.[15,31–35] These include linear extent of cancer, percent of cancer, bilateral tumor, greatest percent of cancer, and number of positive cores. However, all of these studies emphasize that the correlation is very weak. The importance of preoperatively attempting to predict tumor volume is to predict which men harbor potentially insignificant cancers that could be treated expectantly with watchful waiting.[36] Typically, finding limited cancer on needle biopsy, by itself, is not sufficiently predictive of insignificant cancer without factoring in other clinical and other pathologic information (reviewed in Anast et al.).[37–39] For example, Guzzo et al.[40] reported that if there was less than 5% of Gleason score less than or equal to 6 cancer on sextant biopsy, only 37% of radical prostatectomies had less than 5% cancer. The same limited amount of cancer on more extended biopsy was more predictive with 73% having less than 5% cancer in the prostatectomy. Zackrisson et al.[41] found that on sextant biopsies, if the total cancer length on biopsy was less than 3 mm, only one-third of the corresponding radical prostatectomy specimens contained less than 0.5 cc of tumor. One could only predict with 95% confidence that there was more than 0.5 cc tumor if the total tumor length on biopsy was more than 10 mm. Multiple studies have demonstrated that a limited extent (<3 mm) of cancer on biopsy does not necessarily predict "insignificant" amounts of tumor in the entire prostate.[31,36,42 45] One feasible and rational approach would be to have pathologists report the number of cores containing cancer, as well as one other system quantifying tumor extent. This was formally studied by Bismar et al.,[12] where multiple measurements of tumor volume on needle biopsy were tested to predict radical prostatectomy tumor volume. They concluded that several measurements of needle biopsy tumor volume (as opposed to only one) provided maximal information on prostate cancer size.[12] In their study, they found that number of positive cores and total tumor length along with PSA best predicted whole gland tumor volume. At our institution, the number of cores containing cancer is reported along with the percentage of cancer present on each involved core. Calculating the percent of each core involved by cancer is based on a visual estimate of the length of the cancer involvement divided by the length of the core. An example of how we report our needle biopsy findings is as follows: "Adenocarcinoma of the prostate, Gleason score $3 + 3 = 6$, involving three cores (10%, 15%, 30%)." In cases where the cores are fragmented and difficult to assess, we state that the specimen is fragmented and give an estimate as to the percentage of the entire slide involved by cancer. Occasionally, there will be scattered small foci of cancer occupying, for example, 80% of the length of the core, yet only 5% of the total core volume. Merely reporting such a case as showing 80% involvement by cancer may be misleading, because one would expect to see extensive cancer on the biopsy. On the other hand, such a case should be distinguished from one with only a single minute focus of cancer involving 5% of the core. An example of how we report such a case is as follows: "Scattered small foci of adenocarcinoma, Gleason score $3 + 3 = 6$, discontinuously involving 80% of the length of one core." We would predict that such a tumor would not be insignificant and would need definitive therapy in contrast to some cases with only a single minute focus of cancer. A recent report demonstrated that quantifying discontinuous foci of cancer on needle biopsy by measuring from one end of the cancer to the other with inclusion of intervening benign tissue in the measurement correlated better with radical prostatectomy tumor volume, as opposed to "collapsing the cancer" and ignoring intervening benign prostate tissue.[46]

PREDICTION OF EXTRAPROSTATIC EXTENSION INTO NEUROVASCULAR BUNDLE: IMPLICATIONS FOR POTENCY-PRESERVING SURGERY. The critical decision the urologist must make either before or during radical prostatectomy is whether to spare the neurovascular bundle(s) (NVB[s]) to preserve potency or to resect the bundle(s) in cases where there is a high risk of extraprostatic extension (EPE) in the region of the NVB. How to select the right patients for nerve-sparing radical prostatectomy is still controversial. One option that might be more reliable than various preoperative algorithms would be to assess surgical margins in the region of the NVB by intraoperative frozen sections. There have been conflicting studies as to the utility of performing frozen sections for this purpose, because the technique has significant false-positive and false-negative rates.[47-49] Another method of predicting NVB invasion relies on intraoperative visual and tactile assessment at the time of surgery. We have demonstrated that a very experienced urologist can do so with excellent reliability.[50] However, such skills and subjective evaluations are not easily transferable to other less experienced urologists. Thus, the most widely used method in predicting EPE to decide whether to spare the NVB(s) relies on various preoperative algorithms. The most complete models utilize needle biopsy cancer tumor volume, grade, and PSA values. Most of these nomograms report the probability of EPE somewhere in the prostate, not specifically within the area of the NVB. Graefen et al.[51] reported the presence in a lobe of more than two positive cores containing Gleason grade 4/5 cancer or the presence of more than two positive cores in a lobe with a PSA value more than 10 ng/mL regardless of the Gleason score able to predict side-specific EPE. The Steuber et al.[52] model to predict side-specific EPE included PSA, clinical stage, and Gleason score and percent cancer in the ipsilateral biopsy specimen. Ohori et al.[53] developed a nomogram to predict side-specific EPE factoring in PSA and the following side-specific variables of digital rectal exam (DRE), maximum Gleason score, percent positive cores, and length of cancer/total length of cores. There have been two studies that specifically defined preoperative parameters to identify patients with a low likelihood of side-specific EPE in the region of the NVB who could safely undergo nerve-sparing prostatectomy without compromising cancer control. Shah et al.[54] showed that PSA, clinical stage, ipsilateral Gleason score, and tumor volume in the needle biopsies were statistically significant by multivariate analysis for predicting side-specific EPE in the NVB region. Our group at Hopkins found in a study of 2,660 cases that PSA of 10 or more, side-specific Gleason score of 7 or more, abnormal DRE, more than one-third of side-specific cores with tumor, and more than 20% average percent involvement of each positive core per side were independent predictors of NVB penetration.[55] If no more than one of the cited adverse features was present, urologists could predict with 90% or greater accuracy that a man would be an ideal candidate for nerve-sparing radical prostatectomy. Perineural invasion (PNI) on needle biopsy was not independently predictive of NVB EPE in the Hopkins study, although D'Amico[56] found that when the NVB was resected as a result of PNI on biopsy, the positive margin rate was decreased as opposed to if the NVB was spared and left within the patient. Rubin et al.[57] reported that only 24% of urologists use the presence of PNI on biopsy to determine whether to resect the NVB, although surgeons who do more radical prostatectomies were more likely to consider PNI important.[57]

LOCATION OF POSITIVE BIOPSY CORES

Some urologists hesitate to submit routine sextant needle biopsies as six separate cores in six separate containers and instead submit them as left- and right-sided cores. There are several advantages to submitting cores by

TABLE 8.2	Advantages of Submitting Cores by Separate Sextant Site

- Distribution of cancer for planning RT (e.g., brachytherapy)
- Location of cancer helps target additional tissue or block sampling in cases with no apparent cancer in radical prostatectomy.
- Biopsy site helps recognize potential diagnostic pitfalls (e.g., seminal vesicle or central zone, seen at base and Cowper glands at apex).
- In "atypical" cases, directs more focused repeat biopsies
- 1–2 cores per slide helps block/slide preparation with complete visualization of cores and detection of small foci of cancer.
- 1–2 cores reduces fragmentation to determine number of cores involved.

RT, radiation therapy.

separate sextant site (Table 8.2). Evidence to support lumping the cores together is provided by a study reporting that the positive predictive value of an individual positive core for the location of EPE was not sufficient to guide the surgical decision to spare or excise an NVB.[58] However, biopsy core location is of potentially critical importance in the 5% to 10% of biopsies diagnosed as atypical and suspicious for cancer. We advocate the precise labeling of the initial biopsies to localize the sites of an initial atypical diagnosis and to direct the location of repeat biopsies, because increased sampling of the initial atypical site and adjacent ipsilateral and adjacent contralateral sites will increase the yield of cancer detection on repeat biopsy.[59]

Several studies have demonstrated that the location of a positive biopsy core is predictive of adverse findings at radical prostatectomy. Badalament et al.[3] reported that the percentage of cancer in the biopsies from the base and apex correlated with EPE and positive margins, respectively. Similarly, Koh et al.[17] reported that percent of cancer at the base on biopsy along with clinical stage, Gleason score, and PSA predicted seminal vesicle invasion. The presence of cancer in multiple sextant sites is predictive of the presence of multifocal rather than solitary cancer at radical prostatectomy; however, these differences do not correlate with pathologic stage or margin positivity.[60] Bilateral cancer in most studies correlates with EPE and total tumor volume.[15,33]

The submission of needle biopsy specimens in separate containers may lead to much larger pathology charges, although the payments for the pathologist's services are less than the charges. If this is an issue, it is important for urologists and pathologists to come up with alternative strategies that result in agreeable charges while preserving the maximum possible predictive value for biopsy specimens. One option is to put the biopsies from the left gland and the biopsies from the right gland in separate containers. Biopsy cores from the mid and basal areas can be marked with different colors of dye, with the apex unstained, such that the specimens could be submitted together with their sextant origin preserved. A third option would be to dye only biopsies from one side of the gland (i.e., left), with three separate containers (apex, mid, base) submitted to the pathologist. With these options, the pathologist would still be able to identify the site of the atypical focus, and the patient would only be charged for either two or three parts to a case. It has also been demonstrated that with increased numbers of cores per part, there is increased core fragmentation, which can impact in some cases accurate Gleason grading and quantification of number of positive cores, such that a maximum of two cores per cassette is recommended.[61]

NEEDLE BIOPSY PERINEURAL INVASION

PNI is defined as the presence of prostate cancer tracking along or around a nerve (eFigs. 8.1 and 8.2). The role of prostate needle biopsy PNI in treatment planning has been a source of considerable debate. PNI has been demonstrated to be one of the major mechanisms of extension of prostate cancer from the prostatic parenchyma to the periprostatic soft tissue.[62] Whether PNI extensive enough to be sampled on needle biopsy signals an increased risk of EPE of cancer is controversial (reviewed in Bismar et al.).[12] In many studies of PNI, assessment of EPE was performed on only partially submitted prostates such that it was most likely underrecognized. Most studies show PNI on needle biopsy to be predictive of EPE on univariate analysis but not independently predictive once other preoperative clinical and pathologic features are factored in. Other studies show PNI to be predictive of EPE also in multivariate analyses, whereas an equal number finds PNI not be predictive even in univariate analysis (Table 8.3).

TABLE 8.3 Perineural Invasion on Needle Biopsy: Risk of Extraprostatic Extension		
Author	% EPE	Independent[a]
Vargas	38	Yes
Egan	49	No
Taille	52	Yes
Ukimura	61	Yes
Ravery	74	Not assessed
Holmes	78	Not assessed
Bastacky	93	Not assessed

[a]Independently significant in multivariate analysis.
EPE, extraprostatic extension.
Modified from Bismar TA, Lewis JS Jr, Vollmer RT, et al. Multiple measures of carcinoma extent versus perineural invasion in prostate needle biopsy tissue in prediction of pathologic stage in a screening population. *Am J Surg Pathol.* 2003;27:432–440.

The data as to whether PNI on needle biopsy predicts progression after radiotherapy and surgery is also contradictory and experienced surgeons are almost equally divided as to whether PNI on biopsies influence their treatment decisions.[57] In a recent study from our institution, Loeb et al.[63] evaluated the relationship of PNI on prostate biopsy and radical prostatectomy outcomes in a contemporary series of 1,256 radical prostatectomies performed by one urologist. On multivariate analysis, PNI was significantly associated with EPE and seminal vesicle invasion. Biochemical progression was more likely in patients with PNI; however, PNI was not a significant independent predictor of biochemical progression on multivariate analysis. Furthermore, the study found that bilateral nerve-sparing surgery did not compromise the oncologic outcomes for patients with PNI on biopsy.[63] Harnden et al.[64] in a systematic review of the importance of PNI on needle biopsy following radiotherapy or surgery concluded that the weight of the evidence in 21 studies is that this finding is a significant prognostic indicator, particularly in specific patient subgroups defined by serum PSA and Gleason scores. Over two-thirds of the studies using external beam radiotherapy but none using brachytherapy showed prognostic significance for PNI. Difficulty with interpreting studies included (a) varying biopsy techniques (needle angle, location of sampling, number of cores) can affect the type and amount of prostatic tissue sampled and the number of nerves present; (b) number of levels histologically examined can vary; (c) in some studies, data taken from reports where recording of PNI may not be uniformly performed; (d) whether any nerves are present in the specimen is often not taken into account; (e) different pathologists can have interobserver variation in diagnosis of PNI; and (f) pathologists are not blinded to outcome. As some studies have found PNI prognostically useful, some radiotherapists favor the use of external beam radiotherapy over brachytherapy (interstitial seed therapy) in order to treat cases with PNI and a potentially higher risk of cancer being exterior to the prostate. Given that PNI is readily identifiable in most cases, that it is prognostic in some studies although the data is conflicting, and that it is uncertain what factors an individual clinician may consider in treatment decisions, it is the opinion of these authors that it is reasonable for pathologists to note its presence on the biopsy pathology report.

The role of PNI in prostate cancer patients who are candidates for active surveillance has been recently evaluated by our group. Assessing a large cohort (313 cases) of patients who met the biopsy criteria for active surveillance, and elected to undergo immediate radical prostatectomy, the study found that despite a greater extent of cancer on biopsy, cases with and those without PNI on biopsy showed no significant difference in surgical margin involvement or organ-confined disease. Based on the latter findings, in our institution, patients with PNI who meet criteria for active surveillance are not excluded from this treatment option.[65]

Vascular invasion is rarely seen on needle biopsy and its significance on biopsy has not been studied, although typically, it is seen in the setting of other adverse histopathologic features (eFigs. 8.3 and 8.4). As vascular invasion at radical prostatectomy is an independent predictor of progression, its finding on needle biopsy is likely to be associated with a relatively poor prognosis.

USE OF NOMOGRAMS

Various nomograms have been developed to predict pathologic stage and postradical prostatectomy progression.[66–71] These nomograms use preoperative variables such as Gleason score; clinical stage; serum PSA; and in a more recent study, the extent of cancer on biopsy to predict the risk of extraprostatic disease, seminal vesicle invasion, and lymph node metastases. Nomograms using the same preoperative variables have also been formulated to predict the risk and the outcome after radiotherapy.[72] The most widely used of these are the Partin tables and Kattan nomograms, which are used by urologists, radiotherapists, oncologists, and patients to predict pathologic stage.[71] The validity of these tables in part rests on accurate Gleason scoring, which is dealt with in the next chapter.

DIRECT STAGING ON NEEDLE BIOPSY

Skeletal muscle fibers admix within the normal prostate, especially distally (apically) and anteriorly. Recognition of this finding is important for two reasons. First, nonneoplastic prostate glands may be seen admixed with skeletal muscle fibers occasionally in both transurethral resection (TUR) material as well as on needle biopsy (Fig. 3.5) and should not be diagnosed

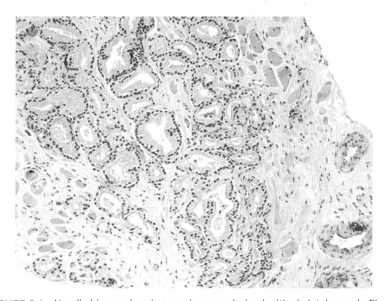

FIGURE 8.1   Needle biopsy showing carcinoma admixed with skeletal muscle fibers.

as prostate carcinoma. Also, the finding of adenocarcinoma of the prostate admixed with skeletal muscle fibers is not diagnostic of EPE by carcinoma (Fig. 8.1, eFig. 8.5).[73] Most patients with limited Gleason score 6 cancer involvement of skeletal muscle on biopsy have organ-confined disease and negative margins.[73]

In order to diagnose EPE on needle biopsy, it is necessary to demonstrate adenocarcinoma infiltrating periprostatic adipose tissue, which is not a common finding (Fig. 8.2, eFigs. 8.6 and 8.7). A study from our group revealed that the presence of EPE, as defined earlier, on needle core biopsy is associated with extensive, high-grade tumors with very poor prognosis. At a mean follow-up of only 2.9 years, 40% of the patients had metastases and 14% died from cancer, regardless of treatment.[74]

Cancer can sometimes be identified infiltrating thick, well-formed smooth muscle bundles, which is suggestive of bladder neck muscle (eFigs. 8.8 to 8.10). As ganglion cells are sometimes located within the prostate, cancer invading ganglion cells are not diagnostic of EPE.[75] On occasion, the urologist may purposely biopsy the seminal vesicle to detect whether there is invasion. Those who recommend this procedure restrict this procedure to patients with abnormal seminal vesicles on ultrasound, markedly elevated PSA levels, or abnormal seminal vesicles on DRE.[76,77] In some cases, carcinoma may be identified invading the seminal vesicle (Fig. 8.3, eFigs. 8.11 to 8.15). If the urologist does not specify that he or she is biopsying the seminal vesicles, one has to be cautious in the interpretation of what appears to be seminal vesicle invasion by cancer.

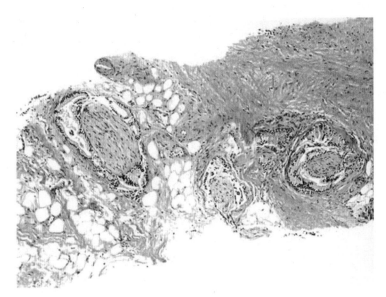

FIGURE 8.2 Adenocarcinoma infiltrating adipose tissue on needle biopsy diagnostic of capsular penetration.

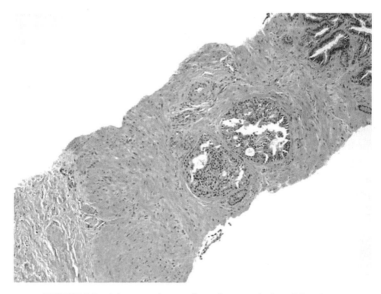

FIGURE 8.3   Adenocarcinoma invading seminal vesicles *(left)*.

Cancer invading the ejaculatory ducts will appear identical on biopsy yet does not indicate that the tumor is surgically incurable, as is the case with seminal vesicle invasion.

TRANSURETHRAL RESECTION

Currently, fewer cancers are incidentally detected on TUR as compared to a few years ago. This phenomenon results from a combination of factors. First, urologists are employing various medical therapies for the treatment of benign prostatic hyperplasia in an increasing number of men. Secondly, alternative surgical treatment options, such as lasers, cryosurgery, balloon dilatation, stents, and microwave therapy, may not provide tissue for histologic examination. Finally, in the workup of men with urinary obstructive symptoms, serum PSA tests and ultrasound studies may lead to a needle biopsy diagnosis of cancer. Nonetheless, TURs will continue to be performed either as an initial line of therapy in some men or in men who fail alternative treatment options.

Carcinoma that is unsuspected clinically and incidentally discovered in TUR specimens usually removed for benign prostatic hyperplasia is referred to as stage T1a and T1b disease. This situation occurs when either (a) the amount of carcinoma within the gland is very focal and not detectable by rectal exam, (b) when the tumor diffusely infiltrates the prostate without resulting in induration or a clinically detectable nodule, or (c) when the tumor is predominantly anteriorly or centrally located and not detectable on rectal examination even though there may be significant amount of tumor present. As one would expect, the behavior of the tumor in these various situations differs considerably. In fact, patients with a significant amount of clinically unsuspected tumor on transurethral resection of the prostate (TURP) tend to have higher pathologic stage in terms of EPE, seminal vesicle involvement, and pelvic lymph node metastases than patients with unilateral palpable carcinoma.[78] Because the tumor is not recognized clinically, the entire staging system used to evaluate these tumors is based on a histologic examination of the tumor. It is therefore the pathologists' responsibility to determine which system for classification of stage T1a and T1b disease is to be utilized and to advise the clinicians on the prognosis of incidental carcinomas of varying grades and quantities.

Subclassification

Approximately 16% (range 13% to 22%) of TURs performed for presumed benign prostatic hyperplasia reveal incidental adenocarcinoma of the prostate.[79] Incidental adenocarcinoma of the prostate is divided into those tumors that are relatively low-volume and low-grade (stage T1a) and those that are high-volume or high-grade (stage T1b). The definition of stage T1a disease is tumor occupying less than 5% of the specimen and not high-grade (Gleason sum <7), and stage T1b was originally defined as higher volume or high-grade tumor but is currently defined as tumors that are more than 5% volume regardless of their grade. There have been several articles published on the long-term progression rate of untreated stage T1a disease (reviewed in Matzkin et al.).[79] The progression rates in these studies ranged from 8% to 27% with the minimum follow-up ranging from 5 to 10 years. Data from these long-term studies shed some light on the question of whether low-volume, intermediate-grade tumor should be considered stage T1a or T1b. As long as the tumor occupies less than 5% of the specimen, there is no difference in the progression rate at 8 years following diagnosis whether the Gleason sum is less than 4 or 5 to 6. Newer techniques, such as DNA ploidy and nuclear morphometry, have in some studies enhanced our ability to predict progression in stage T1a and T1b tumors, although these tests have not been adopted for clinical use.[80,81]

It is important for the pathologist to accurately stage T1a or T1b disease when incidental adenocarcinoma is found on TURP. Depending on the age of the patient, stage T1b patients are treated definitively with surgery or radiotherapy, whereas most stage T1a patients are followed expectantly. There are two situations where subclassification is not as critical, because both T1a and T1b disease are treated definitively. Some young men with stage T1a disease may be offered radical prostatectomy as a treatment option because of their increased long-term risk of progression. The other situation where a man with stage T1a cancer might undergo radical prostatectomy is if his post-TURP serum PSA level is high, suggesting significant residual tumor.[82]

Calculating the percent of the TUR involved by cancer is not always straightforward unless the amount of cancer is at the extremes (i.e., >30% or <1%). To assess the percentage of cancer, first, only the cancer is circled on the glass slide, not the entire chip that contains the cancer (eFig. 8.16). Second, choose the size of a chip that you are going to consider as a "typical chip." Then add on all the slides how many typical chips of cancer there are; two small areas of circled cancer on two chips may equal one typical chip of cancer. Next, calculate the total number of typical chips there are in the entire specimen by estimating the number of typical chips there are on one slide and multiplying it by the total number of slides (assuming an approximately equal amount of tissue per slide). The percentage of the specimen involved by cancer is the number of typical chips with cancer divided by the total number of typical chips.

REFERENCES

1. Fine SW, Amin MB, Berney DM, et al. A contemporary update on pathology reporting for prostate cancer: biopsy and radical prostatectomy specimens. *Eur Urol.* 2012;62: 20–39.
2. Epstein JI. Prognostic significance of tumor volume in radical prostatectomy and needle biopsy specimens. *J Urol.* 2011;186:790–797.
3. Badalament RA, Miller MC, Peller PA, et al. An algorithm for predicting nonorgan confined prostate cancer using the results obtained from sextant core biopsies with prostate specific antigen level. *J Urol.* 1996;156:1375–1380.
4. Huland H, Hammerer P, Henke RP, et al. Preoperative prediction of tumor heterogeneity and recurrence after radical prostatectomy for localized prostatic carcinoma with digital rectal, examination prostate specific antigen and the results of 6 systematic biopsies. *J Urol.* 1996;155:1344–1347.
5. Peller PA, Young DC, Marmaduke DP, et al. Sextant prostate biopsies. A histopathologic correlation with radical prostatectomy specimens. *Cancer.* 1995;75:530–538.
6. Ravery V, Boccon-Gibod LA, Dauge-Geffroy MC, et al. Systematic biopsies accurately predict extracapsular extension of prostate cancer and persistent/recurrent detectable PSA after radical prostatectomy. *Urology.* 1994;44:371–376.
7. Ravery V, Chastang C, Toublanc M, et al. Percentage of cancer on biopsy cores accurately predicts extracapsular extension and biochemical relapse after radical prostatectomy for T1-T2 prostate cancer. *Eur Urol.* 2000;37:449–455.
8. Rubin MA, Bassily N, Sanda M, et al. Relationship and significance of greatest percentage of tumor and perineural invasion on needle biopsy in prostatic adenocarcinoma. *Am J Surg Pathol.* 2000;24:183–189.
9. Tigrani VS, Bhargava V, Shinohara K, et al. Number of positive systematic sextant biopsies predicts surgical margin status at radical prostatectomy. *Urology.* 1999;54: 689–693.
10. Ukimura O, Troncoso P, Ramirez EI, et al. Prostate cancer staging: correlation between ultrasound determined tumor contact length and pathologically confirmed extraprostatic extension. *J Urol.* 1998;159:1251–1259.
11. Wills ML, Sauvageot J, Partin AW, et al. Ability of sextant biopsies to predict radical prostatectomy stage. *Urology.* 1998;51:759–764.
12. Bismar TA, Lewis JS Jr, Vollmer RT, et al. Multiple measures of carcinoma extent versus perineural invasion in prostate needle biopsy tissue in prediction of pathologic stage in a screening population. *Am J Surg Pathol.* 2003;27:432–440.

13. Freedland SJ, Csathy GS, Dorey F, et al. Percent prostate needle biopsy tissue with cancer is more predictive of biochemical failure or adverse pathology after radical prostatectomy than prostate specific antigen or Gleason score. *J Urol.* 2002;167:516–520.

14. Gancarczyk KJ, Wu H, McLeod DG, et al. Using the percentage of biopsy cores positive for cancer, pretreatment PSA, and highest biopsy Gleason sum to predict pathologic stage after radical prostatectomy: the Center for Prostate Disease Research nomograms. *Urology.* 2003;61:589–595.

15. Grossklaus DJ, Coffey CS, Shappell SB, et al. Percent of cancer in the biopsy set predicts pathological findings after prostatectomy. *J Urol.* 2002;167:2032–2035; discussion 2036.

16. Guzzo TJ, Vira M, Wang Y, et al. Preoperative parameters, including percent positive biopsy, in predicting seminal vesicle involvement in patients with prostate cancer. *J Urol.* 2006;175:518–521; discussion 521–522.

17. Koh H, Kattan MW, Scardino PT, et al. A nomogram to predict seminal vesicle invasion by the extent and location of cancer in systematic biopsy results. *J Urol.* 2003;170:1203–1208.

18. Lotan Y, Shariat SF, Khoddami SM, et al. The percent of biopsy cores positive for cancer is a predictor of advanced pathological stage and poor clinical outcomes in patients treated with radical prostatectomy. *J Urol.* 2004;171:2209–2214.

19. Sebo TJ, Bock BJ, Cheville JC, et al. The percent of cores positive for cancer in prostate needle biopsy specimens is strongly predictive of tumor stage and volume at radical prostatectomy. *J Urol.* 2000;163:174–178.

20. Conrad S, Graefen M, Pichlmeier U, et al. Prospective validation of an algorithm with systematic sextant biopsy to predict pelvic lymph node metastasis in patients with clinically localized prostatic carcinoma. *J Urol.* 2002;167:521–525.

21. Karram S, Trock BJ, Netto GJ, et al. Should intervening benign tissue be included in the measurement of discontinuous foci of cancer on prostate needle biopsy? Correlation with radical prostatectomy findings. *Am J Surg Pathol.* 2011;35:1351–1355.

22. Freedland SJ, Terris MK, Csathy GS, et al. Preoperative model for predicting prostate specific antigen recurrence after radical prostatectomy using percent of biopsy tissue with cancer, biopsy Gleason grade and serum prostate specific antigen. *J Urol.* 2004;171: 2215–2220.

23. Grossfeld GD, Latini DM, Lubeck DP, et al. Predicting disease recurrence in intermediate and high-risk patients undergoing radical prostatectomy using percent positive biopsies: results from CaPSURE. *Urology.* 2002;59:560–565.

24. Nelson CP, Rubin MA, Strawderman M, et al. Preoperative parameters for predicting early prostate cancer recurrence after radical prostatectomy. *Urology.* 2002;59:740–745.

25. Quinn DI, Henshall SM, Brenner PC, et al. Prognostic significance of preoperative factors in localized prostate carcinoma treated with radical prostatectomy: importance of percentage of biopsies that contain tumor and the presence of biopsy perineural invasion. *Cancer.* 2003;97:1884–1893.

26. Merrick GS, Butler WM, Wallner KE, et al. Prognostic significance of perineural invasion on biochemical progression-free survival after prostate brachytherapy. *Urology.* 2005;66:1048–1053.

27. Kestin LL, Goldstein NS, Vicini FA, et al. Percentage of positive biopsy cores as predictor of clinical outcome in prostate cancer treated with radiotherapy. *J Urol.* 2002;168: 1994–1999.

28. Rossi PJ, Clark PE, Papagikos MA, et al. Percentage of positive biopsies associated with freedom from biochemical recurrence after low-dose-rate prostate brachytherapy alone for clinically localized prostate cancer. *Urology.* 2006;67:349–353.

29. Lieberfarb ME, Schultz D, Whittington R, et al. Using PSA, biopsy Gleason score, clinical stage, and the percentage of positive biopsies to identify optimal candidates for prostate-only radiation therapy. *Int J Radiat Oncol Biol Phys.* 2002;53:898–903.

30. Wong WW, Schild SE, Vora SA, et al. Association of percent positive prostate biopsies and perineural invasion with biochemical outcome after external beam radiotherapy for localized prostate cancer. *Int J Radiat Oncol Biol Phys.* 2004;60:24–29.

31. Cupp MR, Bostwick DG, Myers RP, et al. The volume of prostate cancer in the biopsy specimen cannot reliably predict the quantity of cancer in the radical prostatectomy specimen on an individual basis. *J Urol.* 1995;153:1543–1548.

32. Lewis JS Jr, Vollmer RT, Humphrey PA. Carcinoma extent in prostate needle biopsy tissue in the prediction of whole gland tumor volume in a screening population. *Am J Clin Pathol.* 2002;118:442–450.

33. Poulos CK, Daggy JK, Cheng L. Prostate needle biopsies: multiple variables are predictive of final tumor volume in radical prostatectomy specimens. *Cancer.* 2004;101:527–532.

34. Noguchi M, Stamey TA, McNeal JE, et al. Relationship between systematic biopsies and histological features of 222 radical prostatectomy specimens: lack of prediction of tumor significance for men with nonpalpable prostate cancer. *J Urol.* 2001;166:104–109.

35. Terris MK, Haney DJ, Johnstone IM, et al. Prediction of prostate cancer volume using prostate-specific antigen levels, transrectal ultrasound, and systematic sextant biopsies. *Urology.* 1995;45:75–80.

36. Epstein JI, Walsh PC, Carmichael M, et al. Pathologic and clinical findings to predict tumor extent of nonpalpable (stage T1c) prostate cancer. *JAMA.* 1994;271:368–374.

37. Anast JW, Andriole GL, Bismar TA, et al. Relating biopsy and clinical variables to radical prostatectomy findings: can insignificant and advanced prostate cancer be predicted in a screening population? *Urology.* 2004;64:544–550.

38. Allan RW, Sanderson H, Epstein JI. Correlation of minute (0.5 MM or less) focus of prostate adenocarcinoma on needle biopsy with radical prostatectomy specimen: role of prostate specific antigen density. *J Urol.* 2003;170:370–372.

39. Ochiai A, Troncoso P, Chen ME, et al. The relationship between tumor volume and the number of positive cores in men undergoing multisite extended biopsy: implication for expectant management. *J Urol.* 2005;174:2164–2168.

40. Guzzo TJ, Vira M, Hwang WT, et al. Impact of multiple biopsy cores on predicting final tumor volume in prostate cancer detected by a single microscopic focus of cancer on biopsy. *Urology.* 2005;66:361–365.

41. Zackrisson B, Aus G, Bergdahl S, et al. The risk of finding focal cancer (less than 3 mm) remains high on re-biopsy of patients with persistently increased prostate specific antigen but the clinical significance is questionable. *J Urol.* 2004;171:1500–1503.

42. Bruce RG, Rankin WR, Cibull ML, et al. Single focus of adenocarcinoma in the prostate biopsy specimen is not predictive of the pathologic stage of disease. *Urology.* 1996;48:75–79.

43. Dietrick DD, McNeal JE, Stamey TA. Core cancer length in ultrasound-guided systematic sextant biopsies: a preoperative evaluation of prostate cancer volume. *Urology.* 1995;45:987–992.

44. Wang X, Brannigan RE, Rademaker AW, et al. One core positive prostate biopsy is a poor predictor of cancer volume in the radical prostatectomy specimen. *J Urol.* 1997;158:1431–1435.

45. Weldon VE, Tavel FR, Neuwirth H, et al. Failure of focal prostate cancer on biopsy to predict focal prostate cancer: the importance of prevalence. *J Urol.* 1995;154:1074–1077.

46. Schultz L, Maluf CE, da Silva RC, et al. Discontinuous foci of cancer in a single core of prostatic biopsy: when it occurs and performance of quantification methods in a private-practice setting. *Am J Surg Pathol.* 2013;37:1831–1836.

47. Fromont G, Baumert H, Cathelineau X, et al. Intraoperative frozen section analysis during nerve sparing laparoscopic radical prostatectomy: feasibility study. *J Urol.* 2003;170:1843–1846.

48. Goharderakhshan RZ, Sudilovsky D, Carroll LA, et al. Utility of intraoperative frozen section analysis of surgical margins in region of neurovascular bundles at radical prostatectomy. *Urology*. 2002;59:709–714.

49. Vaidya A, Hawke C, Tiguert R, et al. Intraoperative T staging in radical retropubic prostatectomy: is it reliable? *Urology*. 2001;57:949–954.

50. Hernandez DJ, Epstein JI, Trock BJ, et al. Radical retropubic prostatectomy. How often do experienced surgeons have positive surgical margins when there is extraprostatic extension in the region of the neurovascular bundle? *J Urol*. 2005;173:446–449.

51. Graefen M, Haese A, Pichlmeier U, et al. A validated strategy for side specific prediction of organ confined prostate cancer: a tool to select for nerve sparing radical prostatectomy. *J Urol*. 2001;165:857–863.

52. Steuber T, Graefen M, Haese A, et al. Validation of a nomogram for prediction of side specific extracapsular extension at radical prostatectomy. *J Urol*. 2006;175:939–944.

53. Ohori M, Kattan MW, Koh H, et al. Predicting the presence and side of extracapsular extension: a nomogram for staging prostate cancer. *J Urol*. 2004;171:1844–1849.

54. Shah O, Robbins DA, Melamed J, et al. The New York University nerve sparing algorithm decreases the rate of positive surgical margins following radical retropubic prostatectomy. *J Urol*. 2003;169:2147–2152.

55. Tsuzuki T, Hernandez DJ, Aydin H, et al. Prediction of extraprostatic extension in the neurovascular bundle based on prostate needle biopsy pathology, serum prostate specific antigen and digital rectal examination. *J Urol*. 2005;173:450–453.

56. D'Amico AV. Perineural invasion as a predictor of PSA outcome following local therapy for patients with clinically localized prostate cancer. *Cancer J*. 2001;7:375–376.

57. Rubin MA, Bismar TA, Curtis S, et al. Prostate needle biopsy reporting: how are the surgical members of the Society of Urologic Oncology using pathology reports to guide treatment of prostate cancer patients? *Am J Surg Pathol*. 2004;28:946–952.

58. Taneja SS, Penson DF, Epelbaum A, et al. Does site specific labeling of sextant biopsy cores predict the site of extracapsular extension in radical prostatectomy surgical specimen. *J Urol*. 1999;162:1352–1357.

59. Allen EA, Kahane H, Epstein JI. Repeat biopsy strategies for men with atypical diagnoses on initial prostate needle biopsy. *Urology*. 1998;52:803–807.

60. Epstein JI, Lecksell K, Carter HB. Prostate cancer sampled on sextant needle biopsy: significance of cancer on multiple cores from different areas of the prostate. *Urology*. 1999;54:291–294.

61. Fajardo DA, Epstein JI. Fragmentation of prostatic needle biopsy cores containing adenocarcinoma: the role of specimen submission. *BJU Int*. 2010;105:172–175.

62. Villers A, McNeal JE, Redwine EA, et al. The role of perineural space invasion in the local spread of prostatic adenocarcinoma. *J Urol*. 1989;142:763–768.

63. Loeb S, Epstein JI, Humphreys EB, et al. Does perineural invasion on prostate biopsy predict adverse prostatectomy outcomes? *BJU Int*. 2010;105:1510–1513.

64. Harnden P, Shelley MD, Clements H, et al. The prognostic significance of perineural invasion in prostatic cancer biopsies: a systematic review. *Cancer*. 2007;109:13–24.

65. Al-Hussain T, Carter HB, Epstein JI. Significance of prostate adenocarcinoma perineural invasion on biopsy in patients who are otherwise candidates for active surveillance. *J Urol*. 2011;186:470–473.

66. Ross PL, Scardino PT, Kattan MW. A catalog of prostate cancer nomograms. *J Urol*. 2001;165:1562–1568.

67. Partin AW, Kattan MW, Subong EN, et al. Combination of prostate-specific antigen, clinical stage, and Gleason score to predict pathological stage of localized prostate cancer. A multi-institutional update. *JAMA*. 1997;277:1445–1451.

68. Kattan MW, Eastham JA, Stapleton AM, et al. A preoperative nomogram for disease recurrence following radical prostatectomy for prostate cancer. *J Natl Cancer Inst.* 1998;90:766–771.

69. D'Amico AV, Whittington R, Malkowicz SB, et al. Combination of the preoperative PSA level, biopsy Gleason score, percentage of positive biopsies, and MRI T-stage to predict early PSA failure in men with clinically localized prostate cancer. *Urology.* 2000;55: 572–577.

70. Han M, Partin AW, Zahurak M, et al. Biochemical (prostate specific antigen) recurrence probability following radical prostatectomy for clinically localized prostate cancer. *J Urol.* 2003;169:517–523.

71. Han M, Partin AW. Nomograms for clinically localized prostate cancer. Part I: radical prostatectomy. *Semin Urol Oncol.* 2002;20:123–130.

72. Kattan MW, Zelefsky MJ, Kupelian PA, et al. Pretreatment nomogram for predicting the outcome of three-dimensional conformal radiotherapy in prostate cancer. *J Clin Oncol.* 2000;18:3352–3359.

73. Ye H, Walsh PC, Epstein JI. Skeletal muscle involvement by limited Gleason score 6 adenocarcinoma of the prostate on needle biopsy is not associated with adverse findings at radical prostatectomy. *J Urol.* 2010;184:2308–2312.

74. Miller JS, Chen Y, Ye H, et al. Extraprostatic extension of prostatic adenocarcinoma on needle core biopsy: report of 72 cases with clinical follow-up. *BJU Int.* 2010;106: 330–333.

75. Yorukoglu K, Tuna B, Kirkali Z. Ganglion cells in the human prostate. *Prostate Cancer Prostatic Dis.* 2000;3:34–36.

76. Vallancien G, Bochereau G, Wetzel O, et al. Influence of preoperative positive seminal vesicle biopsy on the staging of prostatic cancer. *J Urol.* 1994;152:1152–1156.

77. Terris MK, McNeal JE, Freiha FS, et al. Efficacy of transrectal ultrasound-guided seminal vesicle biopsies in the detection of seminal vesicle invasion by prostate cancer. *J Urol.* 1993;149:1035–1039.

78. Christensen WN, Partin AW, Walsh PC, et al. Pathologic findings in clinical stage A2 prostate cancer. Relation of tumor volume, grade, and location to pathologic stage. *Cancer.* 1990;65:1021–1027.

79. Matzkin H, Patel JP, Altwein JE, et al. Stage T1A carcinoma of prostate. *Urology.* 1994;43:11–21.

80. McIntire TL, Murphy WM, Coon JS, et al. The prognostic value of DNA ploidy combined with histologic substaging for incidental carcinoma of the prostate gland. *Am J Clin Pathol.* 1988;89:370–373.

81. Epstein JI, Berry SJ, Eggleston JC. Nuclear roundness factor. A predictor of progression in untreated Stage A2 prostate cancer. *Cancer.* 1984;54:1666–1671.

82. Carter HB, Partin AW, Epstein JI, et al. The relationship of prostate specific antigen levels and residual tumor volume in stage A prostate cancer. *J Urol.* 1990;144:1167–1170.

9

GRADING OF PROSTATIC ADENOCARCINOMAS

HISTORICAL BACKGROUND

Donald F. Gleason in 1966 created a unique grading system for prostatic carcinoma based solely on the architectural pattern of the tumor.[1-4] Five patterns were described (Tables 9.1 and 9.2; Fig. 9.1, eFig. 9.1). Initially, some of the patterns were subdivided to denote different morphologies within the same Gleason grade pattern. For example, pattern 3A denoted medium-sized single glands; 3B, small to very small glands; and 3C, papillary and cribriform epithelium in smooth, rounded cylinders and masses. Over time, these subdivisions within a given pattern were dropped. Another innovative aspect of this system was, rather than assigning the worst grade as the grade of the carcinoma, which was the norm, the grade was defined as the sum of the two most common grade patterns, reported as the Gleason score. Synonyms for "Gleason score" are "combined Gleason grade" and "Gleason sum." Both the primary (predominant) and the secondary (second most prevalent) architectural patterns are identified and assigned a number from 1 to 5, with 1 the most differentiated and 5 the least differentiated. If a tumor has only one histologic pattern, then the primary and secondary patterns are given the same number. Gleason scores range from 2 ($1 + 1 = 2$), which represents tumors uniformly composed of Gleason pattern 1 tumor, to 10 ($5 + 5 = 10$), which represents totally undifferentiated tumors (eFigs. 9.2 to 9.6). A tumor that is predominantly Gleason pattern 3 with a lesser amount of Gleason pattern 4 has a Gleason score of 7 ($3 + 4 = 7$), as does a tumor that is predominantly Gleason pattern 4 with a lesser amount of Gleason pattern 3 tumor ($4 + 3 = 7$). Gleason score $4 + 3 = 7$ on needle biopsy is associated with increased pathologic stage and progression after radical prostatectomy, even when the number of positive cores, maximum percent of cancer per core, and serum prostate-specific antigen (PSA) are accounted for.[5] To distinguish between these two scores, which has prognostic significance, Gleason scores $3 + 4 = 7$ and $4 + 3 = 7$ are occasionally referred to as Gleason scores 7a and 7b, respectively. In describing the breakdown of Gleason patterns among 2,911 cases, Gleason pattern 1 was seen in 3.5%, pattern 2 in 24.4%, pattern 3 in 87.7%, pattern 4 in 12.1%, and pattern 5 in 22.6%. These percentages added up to approximately 150% because 50%

TABLE 9.1	Original Gleason System: 1966 and 1967

Pattern 1:

Very well differentiated, small, closely packed, uniform glands

Essentially circumscribed masses

Pattern 2:

Similar (to pattern 1) but with moderate variation in size and shape of glands

Cribriform pattern may be present, still essentially circumscribed, but more loosely arranged.

Pattern 3:

Similar to pattern 2 but marked irregularity in size and shape of glands

Tiny glands or individual cells invading stroma away from circumscribed mass

Solid cords and masses with easily identifiable glandular differentiation

Includes poorly formed individual glands

Pattern 4:

Large, clear cells growing in a diffuse pattern resembling hypernephroma

May show gland formation

Pattern 5:

Very poorly differentiated tumors

Usually solid masses or diffuse growth with little or no differentiation into glands

TABLE 9.2	Gleason's Modifications: 1974 and 1977

Patterns 1 and 2:

Unchanged

Pattern 3:

Adds to earlier description: may be papillary or cribriform (1974), which vary in size and may be quite large, but the essential feature is the smooth and usually rounded edge around all the circumscribed masses of tumor (1977).

Pattern 4:

Adds to earlier description: raggedly infiltrating, fused-glandular tumor (1974). Glands are not single and separate but coalesce and branch (1977).

Pattern 5:

Adds to earlier description: can resemble comedocarcinoma of the breast (1977). Almost absent gland pattern with few tiny glands or signet cells (1977).

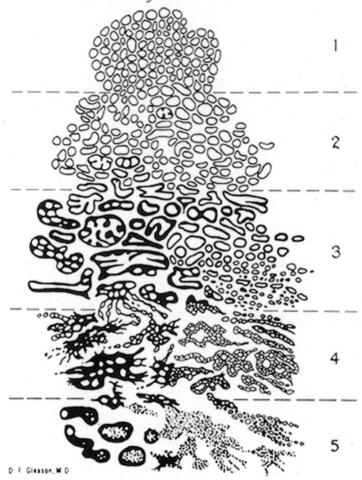

FIGURE 9.1   Original Gleason grading diagram.

of the tumors showed at least two different patterns. The only comment relating to tertiary patterns was "occasionally, small areas of a third pattern were observed."

THE 2005 INTERNATIONAL SOCIETY OF UROLOGICAL PATHOLOGY MODIFICATIONS TO THE GLEASON GRADE

Why the Need for a Consensus on Gleason Grading?

Since the late 1960s when the Gleason grading system was derived, the field of prostate carcinoma has changed dramatically. In the 1960s, there was no screening for prostate cancer other than by digital rectal examination, as serum PSA had not yet been discovered. In Gleason's 1974 study, the vast majority (86%) of men had advanced disease with either local extension out of the prostate on clinical exam or distant metastases. Only 6% of patients had nonpalpable tumor diagnosed by transurethral resection and only 8% of patients were diagnosed with a localized nodule on rectal examination.[1] The method of obtaining prostate tissue was also very different from today's practice. Typically, only a couple of thick-gauge needle biopsies were directed into an area of palpable abnormality. The use of 18-gauge thin biopsy needles and the concept of sextant needle biopsies to more extensively sample the prostate were not developed until the late 1980s.[6] Consequently, the grading of prostate cancer in thin cores and in multiple cores from different sites of the prostate were not issues in Gleason's era.

The Gleason system also predated the use of immunohistochemistry. It is likely that with immunostaining for basal cells that many of Gleason's original 1 + 1 = 2 adenocarcinomas of the prostate would today be regarded as adenosis (atypical adenomatous hyperplasia), a mimicker of cancer.[7] Similarly, many of the cases in 1967 diagnosed as cribriform Gleason pattern 3 carcinoma would probably be currently referred to as cribriform high-grade prostatic intraepithelial neoplasia (PIN) or intraductal carcinoma of the prostate, if labeled with basal cell markers.[8,9]

Another issue that was not dealt with in the original Gleason grading system is how to grade newly described variants of adenocarcinoma of the prostate. Some of the more common variants where grading issues arise include mucinous carcinoma (see Chapter 13), ductal adenocarcinoma (see Chapter 11), foamy gland carcinoma, and pseudohyperplastic adenocarcinoma of the prostate. In addition, there are certain patterns of adenocarcinoma of the prostate such as those with glomeruloid features and mucinous fibroplasia (collagenous micronodules) where the use of Gleason grading was not defined. The application of the Gleason system for all of the reasons noted earlier varies considerably in contemporary surgical pathology practice compared to Gleason's era, and there arose a need for a formal updating of the Gleason grading system.

2005 International Society of Urological Pathology Consensus Conference

A group of urologic pathologists convened at the 2005 United States and Canadian Academy of Pathology (USCAP) meeting in an attempt to achieve consensus in controversial areas relating to the Gleason grading system.[10] Over 70 urologic pathologists from around the world were invited to attend, with most attending. A schematic diagram was developed to reflect the modified Gleason grading system, which was subsequently slightly further modified to reflect changes in grading cribriform cancer (Table 9.3; Fig. 9.2, eFig. 9.1).

TABLE 9.3 Current International Society of Urological Pathology Modified Gleason System

Pattern 1:
- Circumscribed nodule of closely packed but separate, uniform, rounded to oval, medium-sized acini (larger glands than pattern 3).

Pattern 2:
- Like pattern 1, fairly circumscribed, yet at the edge of the tumor nodule, there may be minimal infiltration.
- Glands are more loosely arranged and not quite as uniform as Gleason pattern 1.

Pattern 3:
- Discrete glandular units
- Typically smaller glands than seen in Gleason pattern 1 or 2
- Infiltrates in and among nonneoplastic prostate acini
- Marked variation in size and shape

Pattern 4:
- Fused microacinar glands
- Ill-defined glands with poorly formed glandular lumina
- Cribriform glands
- Hypernephromatoid

Pattern 5:
- Essentially no glandular differentiation, composed of solid sheets, cords, or single cells
- Comedocarcinoma with central necrosis surrounded by papillary, cribriform, or solid masses

It is remarkable that nearly 40 years after the inception of the Gleason grading system, it remains one of the most powerful prognostic predictors in prostate cancer. In part, this system has remained timely by adaptations of the system to accommodate the changing practice of medicine. The Gleason grading consensus conference resulted in a modified updated Gleason grading system that is more relevant to today's practice.

GENERAL APPLICATIONS OF THE GLEASON GRADING SYSTEM

The initial grading of prostate carcinoma should be performed at low magnification using the 4× and 10× objective.[1,10] After one assesses the case at scanning magnification, one may proceed to use the 20× objective to verify the grade. For example, at low magnification, one may have the impression of fused glands or necrosis but may require higher magnification

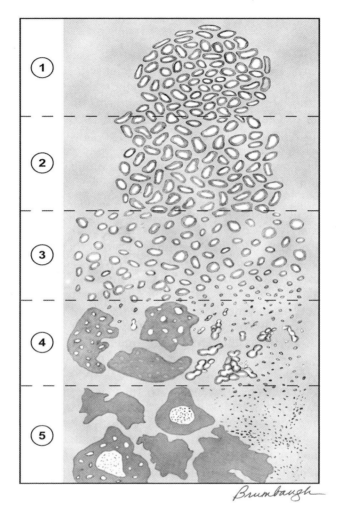

FIGURE 9.2 Modified Gleason grading diagram.

at 20× to confirm its presence. One should not initially use the 20× or 40× objectives to look for rare fused glands or a few individual cells seen only at higher power, which would lead to an overdiagnosis of Gleason pattern 4 or 5, respectively (eFig. 9.7).

The best way to report the Gleason grades in a pathology report is in a mathematical equation (i.e., Gleason score 3 + 3 = 6). Alternative methods in use may be misconstrued. For example, reports of "Gleason 3/5" could be interpreted as either Gleason score 3 + 5 = 8 or the tumor is Gleason pattern 3 out of a maximum of 5 patterns (i.e., Gleason score 3 + 3 = 6). Cases diagnosed as "Gleason grade 4" can be considered as either Gleason score 2 + 2 = 4 or Gleason score 4 + 4 = 8.

GLEASON PATTERNS

Gleason Patterns 1 and 2

Gleason patterns 1 and 2 consist of fairly circumscribed nodules of closely packed glands (eFigs. 9.8 to 9.14). The glands are uniform in their size and shape with slightly more variation in pattern 2 than pattern 1. Smaller glands typical of Gleason pattern 3 are absent. It is now accepted that Gleason score 2 to 4 should not be assigned to cancer on needle biopsy for several reasons including poor reproducibility even among experts. Several studies have demonstrated that tumors on needle biopsy assigned a Gleason score of 2 to 4 are not infrequently associated with higher grade and high-stage disease at radical prostatectomy.[11–13] The major limitation of rendering a diagnosis of Gleason score 4 on needle biopsy is that one cannot see the entire edge of the lesion to determine if it is completely circumscribed. Consequently, most of the lesions that appear to be very low-grade on needle biopsies are diagnosed by urologic pathologists as Gleason score 3 + 2 = 5 or 3 + 3 = 6. Studies have shown a dramatic decrease in the incidence of diagnosing Gleason score 2 to 4 on needle biopsy over the last decade. In one study, 24% of pathologists rendered a diagnosis of Gleason score of 2 to 4 on biopsy in 1991, which decreased to 2.4% in 2001.[14] In another study analyzing biopsies from 2002 to 2003, only 1.6% were graded as Gleason score 2 to 4 compared to 22.3% of the biopsies in 1994.[12,15]

Low-grade cancers are rarely seen on needle biopsy because low-grade cancers are predominantly located anteriorly in the prostate within the transition zone and they tend to be small. Low-grade prostate cancer does exist and Gleason score 3 and 4 adenocarcinomas may be uncommonly diagnosed on transurethral resection of the prostate (TURP) (Fig. 9.3). Typically, both Gleason pattern 1 and Gleason pattern 2 carcinomas have abundant pale eosinophilic cytoplasm. It has been proposed that transition zone cancers be termed *clear cell carcinomas*.[16,17] These tumors do not have a unique histology but rather reflect the finding that transition zone cancers are frequently low grade. Carcinomas with pale cytoplasm may also be found in the peripheral zone.

Gleason Pattern 3

Gleason pattern 3 cancer consists of variably sized individual glands that are well formed (Fig. 9.4, eFigs. 9.15 to 9.27). In contrast to Gleason pattern 4, the glands in Gleason pattern 3 are discrete units. If one can mentally draw a circle around well-formed individual glands, then it is Gleason pattern 3. One should assign a Gleason grade at relatively low power (i.e., 2.5× or 4× objective). The presence of a few poorly formed glands at high power, which could represent a tangential section off of small well-formed glands, is still consistent with Gleason pattern 3 tumor. Gleason pattern 3 glands are either (a) infiltrative between benign glands, (b) more variably sized, or (c) smaller than Gleason patterns 1 and 2.

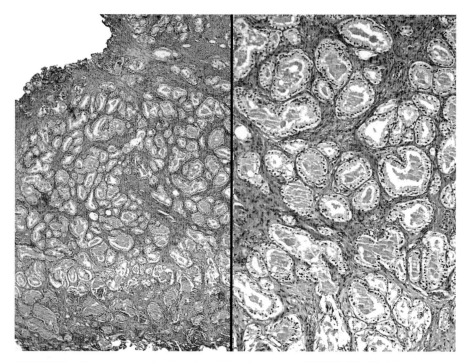

FIGURE 9.3   Gleason score 2 + 2 = 4 nodule of cancer on TURP **(left)** with higher magnification **(right)** showing relatively uniformly sized and shaped larger glands than Gleason pattern 3.

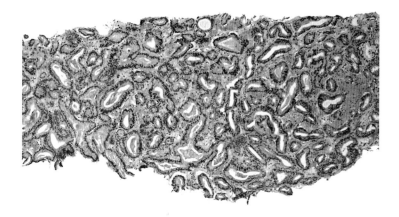

FIGURE 9.4   Gleason score 3 + 3 = 6 prostate carcinoma composed of small discrete glands.

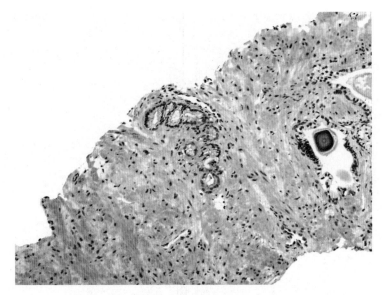

FIGURE 9.5   Small focus of Gleason score 3 + 3 = 6.

Some pathologists may not feel comfortable assigning both a primary and secondary pattern 3 to very small foci of carcinoma on biopsy. However, small foci of Gleason score 3 + 3 = 6 cancer on biopsy is more often associated with Gleason score 3 + 3 = 6 at radical prostatectomy compared to cases with more extensive Gleason score 3 + 3 = 6 on biopsy (Fig. 9.5).[12] The reason is that greater amounts of cancer on needle biopsy correlate with larger tumors that are more likely to have areas of pattern 4 at radical prostatectomy.

A major point of divergence from the original Gleason system is with assignment of grade to cribriform glands. Within Gleason's[18] original illustrations of his cribriform pattern 3, he depicts large, cribriform glands. At the time of the 2005 International Society of Urological Pathology (ISUP) grading consensus meeting, expert uropathologists uniformly had been diagnosing these lesions as cribriform pattern 4 (Figure 3D in [19]). The consensus conference proposed extremely stringent criteria for cribriform Gleason pattern 3.[10] Subsequently, a study showed that even in a highly selected set of images thought to be the best candidates for cribriform pattern 3, most experts interpreted the cribriform patterns as pattern 4.[20] In a subsequent study specifically addressing the prognosis of cribriform prostate cancer glands, both small and large cribriform glands were equally linked to progression after radical prostatectomy.[21] These findings fit conceptually, because one would expect the change in grade from pattern 3 to pattern 4 to be reflected in a distinct architectural paradigm shift where cribriform as opposed to individual glands are formed rather than merely a subjective continuum of differences in size, shape, and contour of cribriform glands. The only reason why cribriform pattern 3 even exists is because of the original Gleason schematic diagram. However, Gleason never specifically published the prognostic difference between what he called cribriform Gleason pattern 3 compared to cribriform Gleason pattern 4. Many of Gleason's cribriform Gleason pattern 3 cancers may not even have been infiltrating carcinomas due to the lack of availability of immunohistochemistry for basal cell markers. Today, we might have diagnosed them either as cribriform high-grade PIN or intraductal carcinoma of the prostate (concepts not present in Gleason's era).[8,9] Based on all the given data, all cribriform cancer should be interpreted as Gleason pattern 4.

There are certain situations that lead to overgrading of Gleason pattern 3 as pattern 4. Crowded glands at low magnification can have the appearance of fused glands, mimicking Gleason pattern 4 cancer (Fig. 9.6). Small glands are acceptable for Gleason pattern 3 as long as they are well formed and not fused with other glands. Probably, the most common scenario where Gleason pattern 3 is overgraded as Gleason pattern 4 is when a few tangentially sectioned small glands of pattern 3 are present and seen at higher magnification. Given the presence of small glands in Gleason pattern 3, a few glands will invariably be tangentially sectioned, resulting in a gland that appears not well formed (Fig. 9.7). Consequently, only when there is a cluster of poorly formed glands seen at 10× where it is unlikely that they all represent tangentially sectioned glands should Gleason pattern 4 be diagnosed. Branching glands appear more complex than simple round glands, yet as long as they are not fused or cribriform, branching glands are still consistent with Gleason pattern 3. Glands that artifactually appear poorly formed as a result of crush artifact must be distinguished from Gleason pattern 4. Thick, poorly

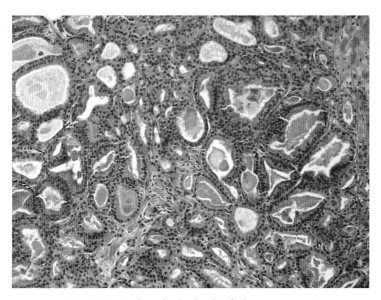

FIGURE 9.6 Back-to-back glands of Gleason pattern 3.

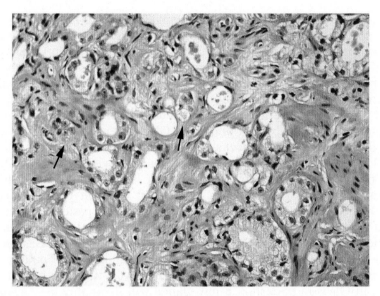

FIGURE 9.7 Gleason pattern 3 with occasional glands without visible lumina *(arrows)* representing tangential sections off of adjacent well-formed glands.

sectioned tissue can result in multilayering and the appearance of poorly formed glands or solid nests of cells, mimicking higher grade carcinoma.

When glands surround a nerve (perineural invasion), the glands often develop a more complex papillary, crowded appearance (Fig. 9.8). Consequently, one should be cautious in diagnosing Gleason pattern 4

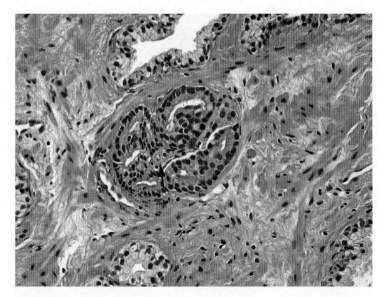

FIGURE 9.8 Perineural invasion with small nerve *(arrow)* surrounded by crowded, well-formed glands of Gleason pattern 3.

based on glands within perineural invasion in the absence of Gleason pattern 4 elsewhere. Similarly, the delicate ingrowth of fibrous tissue seen with mucinous fibroplasia (collagenous micronodules) can result in glands appearing to be fused resembling cribriform structures, although the underlying architecture is really that of individual discrete rounded glands invested by loose collagen. The tumor should be graded on the underlying glandular architecture, whereby the majority are graded as Gleason score 3 + 3 = 6 (Fig. 9.9).[22] Only when there are distinct cribriform glands in areas of mucinous fibroplasia should Gleason pattern 4 be diagnosed (Fig. 9.10).

Gleason Pattern 4

The 2005 ISUP consensus conference agreed with the original Gleason system that fused glands, irregular cribriform glands, and the hypernephroma pattern were designated as Gleason pattern 4.[10] As described earlier, subsequent studies support the inclusion of any cribriform glands as pattern 4 (eFigs. 9.28 to 9.93). In addition, the consensus conference reported that ill-defined glands with poorly formed glandular lumina also warrant the diagnosis of Gleason pattern 4. In contrast, Gleason's original description of pattern 4 included only the hypernephromatoid pattern and in subsequent years, fused glandular masses.[19,23] Gleason pattern 4 closely resembling renal cell carcinoma (hypernephromatoid pattern) is rare, despite occupying a prominent role in the original Gleason grading system. Cribriform glands in one study were associated with a higher risk of postradical prostatectomy failure as compared to fused glands.[21] The

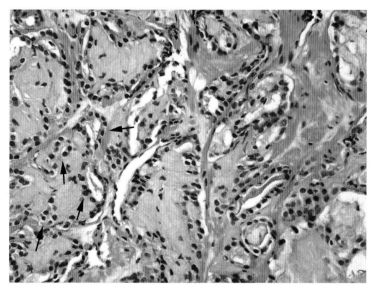

FIGURE 9.9 Well-formed glands of Gleason pattern 3 (arrows) distorted by mucinous fibroplasia.

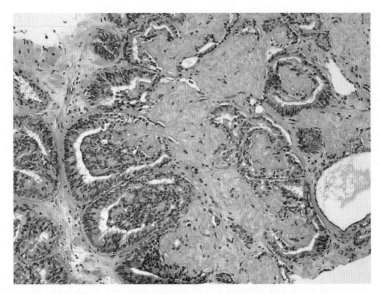

FIGURE 9.10   Mucinous fibroplasia involving cribriform glands of Gleason pattern 4.

current spectrum of morphology in Gleason pattern 4 is depicted schematically in Figure 9.2.

There are some difficulties in distinguishing better developed cribriform glands of pattern 4 from poorly formed cribriform glands with barely identifiable acini that are best characterized as pattern 5 (see Gleason pattern 5 in the following discussion). Despite being high grade based on the architectural pattern, cribriform Gleason pattern 4 can be cytologically bland (Fig. 9.11). Cribriform pattern 4 glands on biopsy can appear rounded irregularly and shaped with ragged borders (Fig. 9.12). On needle biopsy, cribriform Gleason pattern 4 tumor often manifests as fragments of cribriform tumor because there is little supporting stroma in larger cribriform glands (Fig. 9.13).

Cribriform prostate cancer glands span a broad spectrum in terms of their differentiation. At one end, there are well-developed cribriform glands with well-formed lumina (Fig. 9.14). In some less differentiated examples, cribriform glands have lumina that are not as open, yet they are still readily recognizable as cribriform structures and hence are still considered Gleason pattern 4 (Fig. 9.15). These cases are better differentiated than some cases of Gleason pattern 5 where the cribriform structures are so poorly developed that they are barely recognizable (see Gleason pattern 5 in the following section).

A variant morphology of cribriform prostatic adenocarcinoma glands are glomeruloid glands (Fig. 9.16, eFigs. 9.94 to 9.96). They are characterized by dilated glands containing intraluminal cribriform structures with a single point of attachment, resembling a renal glomerulus.[22]

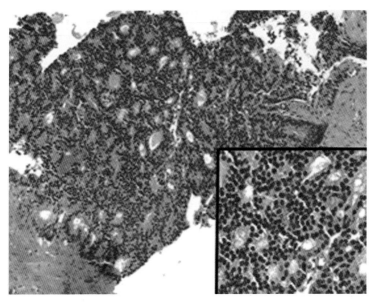

FIGURE 9.11   Circumscribed cribriform Gleason pattern 4 on needle biopsy. *Inset* shows bland cytology.

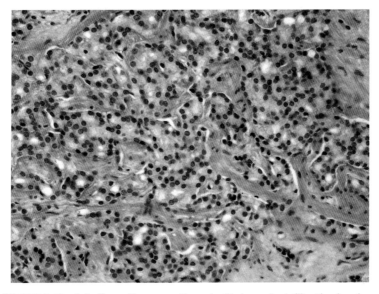

FIGURE 9.12   Cribriform Gleason pattern 4 with irregular infiltrative borders.

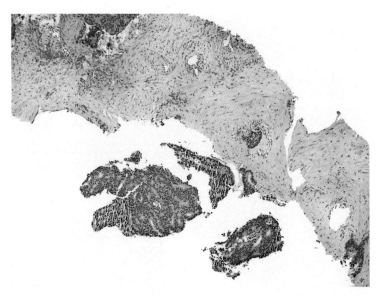

FIGURE 9.13   Detached cribriform Gleason pattern 4 on needle biopsy.

On prostate biopsy, glomeruloid glands are exclusively associated with carcinoma and not associated with benign mimickers. A study from Hopkins subsequent to the consensus conference indicated that glomerulations were overwhelmingly associated with concurrent Gleason pattern 4 or higher grade carcinoma.[24] In several cases, transition could

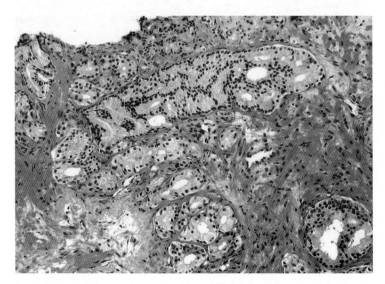

FIGURE 9.14   Gleason score 3 + 4 = 7 with small glands of Gleason pattern 4 and small well-circumscribed cribriform Gleason pattern 4.

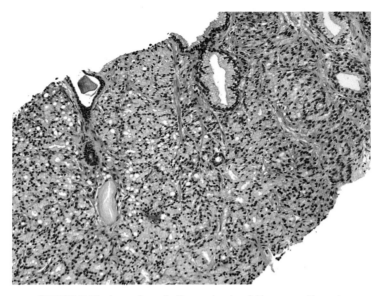

FIGURE 9.15 Irregular cribriform glands of Gleason pattern 4.

be seen between small glomerulations, large glomeruloid structures, and cribriform pattern 4 cancer. These data suggest that glomerulations represent an early stage of cribriform pattern 4 cancer and are best graded as Gleason pattern 4. A mimicker of glomeruloid glands is telescoping of neoplastic glands within glands (Fig. 9.17). With telescoping glands,

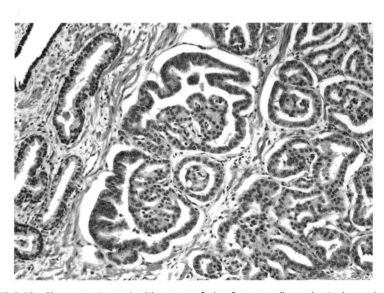

FIGURE 9.16 Gleason pattern 4 with range of size from small regular to larger irregular glomeruloid structures.

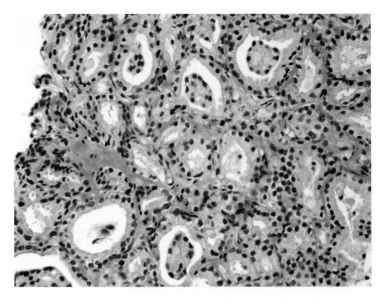

FIGURE 9.17 Gleason pattern 3 cancer with telescoping.

the intraluminal structure consists of a well-formed gland rather than a cribriform gland.

In addition to cribriform glands, the other major morphologies of Gleason pattern 4 are poorly formed and fused glands. Only when there is a cluster of poorly formed glands, where a tangential section of Gleason pattern 3 glands cannot account for the histology, should the focus be

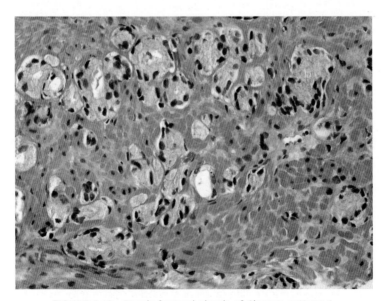

FIGURE 9.18 Poorly formed glands of Gleason pattern 4.

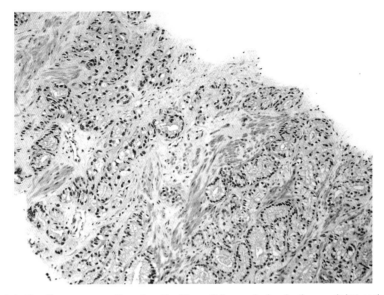

FIGURE 9.19 Gleason score 3 + 4 = 7 with well-formed glands *(lower right)* and poorly formed glands *(upper left)*.

graded as Gleason pattern 4 (Figs. 9.18 and 9.19). In other cases, the majority of glands are more well formed, yet rather than being discrete glands, they are fused to each other and are also graded Gleason pattern 4 (Fig. 9.20). In other cases, ill-defined glands with poorly formed glandular lumina are accompanied by fused glands.

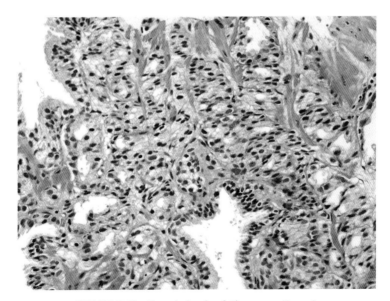

FIGURE 9.20 Fused glands of Gleason pattern 4.

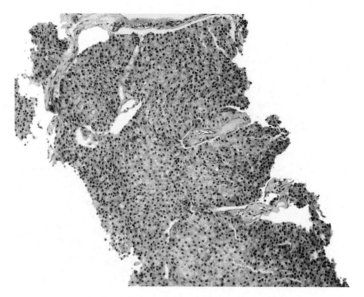

FIGURE 9.21   Sheets of Gleason pattern 5.

Gleason Pattern 5

Gleason pattern 5 consists of sheets of tumor, individual cells, and cords of cells (Figs. 9.21 and 9.22, eFigs. 9.97 to 9.117). Less commonly, there are nests of cells. There is a tendency for general pathologists to underdiagnose Gleason pattern 5 on needle biopsy. In two separate studies,

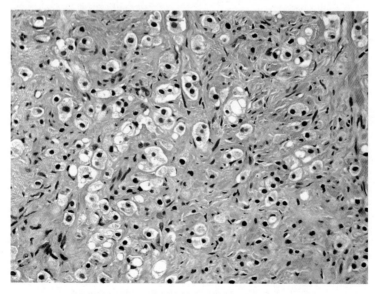

FIGURE 9.22   Individual cell of Gleason pattern 5.

Gleason pattern 5 was not reported by general pathologists in 50% of needle biopsy specimens compared to an expert review. Of the various morphologies of Gleason pattern 5, the only situation where it was more routinely recognized was with solid sheets as the primary pattern.[25,26]

Solid nests of cells with vague microacinar or only occasional gland space formation are still consistent with Gleason pattern 5 (Figs. 9.23 and 9.24). Single cells are another frequent morphology of Gleason pattern 5. It is not uncommon to see poorly formed glands along with single cells, resulting in a Gleason score of 4 + 5 = 9 or 5 + 4 = 9. Whether a tumor is Gleason score 4 + 5 = 9, 5 + 4 = 9, or 5 + 5 = 10 is not that critical, because together, they are considered relatively undifferentiated tumor with typically a poor prognosis. Most cases of Gleason score 9 and 10 are fairly extensive on needle biopsy, although uncommonly, only a small focus of such high-grade cancer is present on biopsy. Although the majority of cases with Gleason pattern 5 are either Gleason score 9 or 10, some cases are Gleason score 3 + 5 = 8 or 5 + 3 = 8.

A relatively uncommon morphology is comedonecrosis with solid nests (Fig. 9.25). Occasionally, one can see necrosis with cribriform masses that by themselves might be cribriform pattern 4; the consensus is that these patterns should be regarded as Gleason pattern 5 (Fig. 9.26). One must be stringent as to the definition of comedonecrosis, requiring intraluminal necrotic cells and/or karyorrhexis, especially in the setting of cribriform glands. Occasionally, cribriform glands have eosinophilic material within their lumina that if unaccompanied by necrotic cells at the periphery should not be considered Gleason pattern 5.

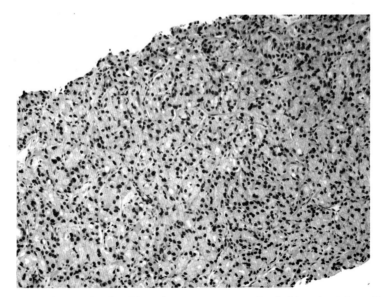

FIGURE 9.23 Sheets of cells with such vague attempt of primitive gland formation still consistent with Gleason pattern 5.

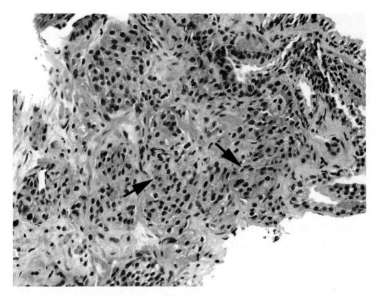

FIGURE 9.24   Nests of cells with such vague attempt of primitive gland formation *(arrows)* still consistent with Gleason pattern 5.

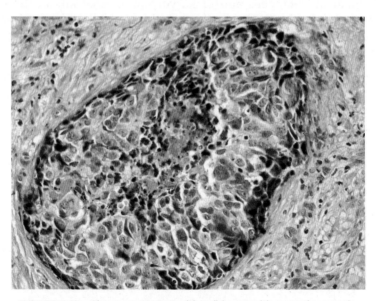

FIGURE 9.25   Gleason pattern 5 with solid nest with comedonecrosis.

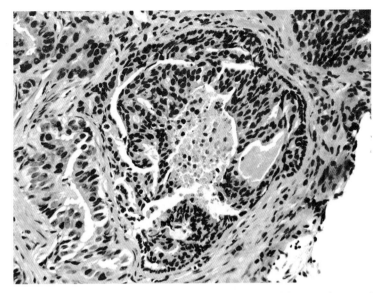

FIGURE 9.26   Gleason pattern 5 with cribriform gland with comedonecrosis.

Other less common morphologies seen with Gleason pattern 5 are small nests and cords of cells. The nested growth may be confused with urothelial carcinoma, whereas cords are patterns not seen in urothelial carcinoma.

GRADING VARIANTS OF PROSTATE CARCINOMA

Adenocarcinoma with Vacuoles

Adenocarcinomas of the prostate may contain clear vacuoles which differ from true signet-ring cell carcinomas that contain mucin.[2,27] In Gleason's[2] original description, vacuoles are described under pattern 5 tumor. Although vacuoles are typically seen within Gleason pattern 4 or 5 cancer (Fig. 9.27), they may also be seen within Gleason pattern 3 tumors (Fig. 9.28, eFig. 9.118). Tumors should be graded, as if the vacuoles are not present, by only evaluating the underlying architectural pattern.

Foamy Gland Carcinoma

One should ignore the foamy cytoplasm and grade the tumor solely based on the underlying architecture. Initially, foamy gland cancer was described as consisting of discrete well-formed glands.[28] A subsequent study demonstrated that the full range of architectural patterns seen in usual prostate cancer can also be seen in foamy gland cancer.[29] Foamy gland cancer with poorly formed/fused/cribriform glands and those lacking gland formation should be graded as Gleason patterns 4 and 5, respectively (Fig. 9.29).

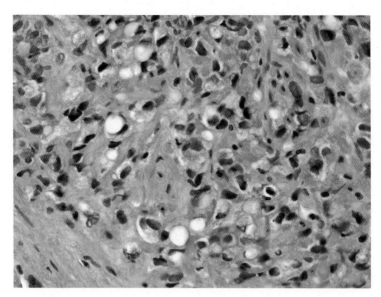

FIGURE 9.27   Gleason pattern 5 with individual cells containing signet ring cell–like vacuoles.

Foamy gland carcinoma is most commonly seen with Gleason score 7 tumor. An unusual variant of foamy gland consists of widely separated foamy glands associated with a very prominent desmoplastic stroma. These tumors tend to be extensive, aggressive cancers and typically are high grade despite the relative paucity of malignant glands.[29]

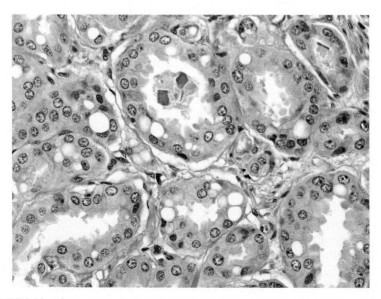

FIGURE 9.28   Gleason pattern 3 with glands containing signet ring cell–like vacuoles.

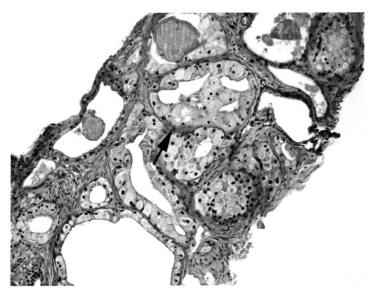

FIGURE 9.29   Gleason score 3 + 4 = 7 foamy gland adenocarcinoma with discrete glands and cribriform glands *(arrow)*.

Pseudohyperplastic Adenocarcinoma

These cancers should be graded as Gleason score 3 + 3 = 6 with pseudohyperplastic features (eFig. 9.119).[30,31] This convention is in large part based on the recognition that they are most often accompanied by more ordinary Gleason score 3 + 3 = 6 adenocarcinoma. In the uncommon case where some of the glands with pseudohyperplastic features have cribriform morphology, a Gleason pattern 4 should be assigned.

REPORTING GLEASON GRADE ON BIOPSY

Different Cores with Different Grades

This issue assumes its greatest importance when one or more of the cores shows pure high-grade cancer (i.e., Gleason score 4 + 4 = 8) and the other cores show pattern 3 cancer. Assume a case with Gleason score 4 + 4 = 8 on one core with pattern 3 (3 + 3 = 6, 3 + 4 = 7, or 4 + 3 = 7) on other cores. The "global" score for the entire case, averaging all involved needle biopsies together as if they were one long positive core, would be 4 + 3 = 7 or 3 + 4 = 7, depending on whether pattern 4 or 3 predominated. Several studies have demonstrated that in cases with different cores having different grades, the highest Gleason score on a given core correlates better with stage and Gleason score at radical prostatectomy than the average or most frequent grade among the cores.[32–35] Additional support for giving cores a separate grade rather than an overall score for the entire case is that all of the various tables (i.e., Partin tables) and nomograms that have been validated and proven to be prognostically useful have used the highest core grade in cases where there are multiple cores of different grades. Whether the highest grade per core or the overall score is used impacts a significant number of cases.[36]

It is therefore incumbent on pathologists to report the grades of each core separately as long as the cores are submitted in separate containers or the cores are in the same container yet specified by the urologist as to their location (i.e., by different color inks). As a consequence, the core with the highest grade tumor can be selected by the clinician as the grade of the entire case to determine treatment.[37,38] In addition to giving separate cores individual Gleason scores, it is an option for pathologists to also give an overall score at the end of the case.

There is no consensus how to grade different cores with different grades when the different cores are present within the same specimen container without a designation as to site.[10] For example, there may be two cores of tissue from the left base in one jar without further designation or multiple cores divided into containers from the left and right side of the gland. In the setting of multiple undesignated cores with cancer per container, some urologic pathologists still grade each core separately with the remaining experts in the field giving an overall grade for the specimen container. A rationale for the latter approach is that it is implicit that clinicians submitting multiple cores together in one container do not value the specific information derived from the cores within a given container. On the other hand, assigning a Gleason score to each core even when there are multiple positive cores in a given jar provides the most accurate information for patient care.[35]

In cases with multiple fragmented cores in a jar, only an overall Gleason score for that jar can be assigned. For example, diagnosing Gleason score $4 + 4 = 8$ on a tiny tissue fragment where there are other fragments with a greater amount of Gleason pattern 3 could be in error; if the cores were intact and the tumor was all on one core, it would be assigned a Gleason score $3 + 4 = 7$.

Tertiary Gleason Patterns

On needle biopsies with patterns 3, 4, and 5, both the primary pattern and the highest grade should be recorded, which is a departure from the original Gleason grading system.[10] For example, needle biopsies with predominantly Gleason pattern 3, lesser amount of Gleason pattern 4, and an even lesser amount of pattern 5 would be recorded as Gleason score $3 + 5 = 8$. Men with biopsy Gleason score 7 with focal pattern 5 have a higher risk of PSA failure whether treated with radical prostatectomy or radiation therapy when compared to men with biopsy Gleason score 7 without focal pattern 5 and have a comparable risk with men with biopsy Gleason scores 8 to 10.[39,40] In cases where there are three patterns consisting of patterns 2, 3, and 4, pattern 2 is ignored and the biopsy is graded as Gleason score $3 + 4 = 7$ or Gleason score $4 + 3 = 7$, depending on whether pattern 3 or pattern 4 is more prevalent.

Reporting Secondary Patterns of Higher Grade When Present to a Limited Extent

High-grade tumor of any quantity on needle biopsy should be included within the Gleason score.[10] Consequently, a needle biopsy with 98% Gleason pattern 3 and 2% Gleason pattern 4 should be graded as Gleason score 3 + 4 = 7.

Reporting Secondary Patterns of Lower Grade When Present to a Limited Extent

In all specimens, in the setting of high-grade cancer, one should ignore lower grade patterns if they occupy less than 5% of the area of the tumor. For example, tumor composed of 98% Gleason pattern 4 and 2% Gleason pattern 3 should be graded as Gleason score 4 + 4 = 8.[10] The only setting where very limited Gleason pattern 3 on needle biopsy is factored into the Gleason score is with a millimeter or less focus of otherwise Gleason pattern 4 cancer. In the setting of very limited cancer on needle biopsy, the few glands of pattern 3 typically occupy over 5% of the area of the tumor focus, resulting in a Gleason score 4 + 3 = 7.

CORRELATION NEEDLE BIOPSY AND RADICAL PROSTATECTOMY GRADE

It is most accurate to group Gleason scores into the following five prognostically homogeneous categories: 2 to 6, 3 + 4 = 7, 4 + 3 = 7, 8, and 9 and 10.[41] As seen in Table 9.4, representing data from Hopkins, 36.3% of cases were upgraded from a needle biopsy Gleason score 6 to a higher grade at radical prostatectomy. Within the literature, upgrading from Gleason score 6 on needle biopsy to radical prostatectomy was seen in 4,614 out of 13,163 (35%) of the cases, virtually the same as with our own experience. The relation of other biopsy grades to the grades at resection can be seen in Table 9.4.

Explanations for Grading Discrepancies

One source of grading discrepancy between needle and radical prostatectomy grade is that the differences between different Gleason patterns are on a continuum. For example, it can be subjective whether there are small glands of pattern 3 or poorly formed glands of pattern 4. Similarly, it may be a judgment call whether there are very poorly formed glands of pattern 4 as opposed to pattern 5 with barely appreciable glandular differentiation.

Another source of discrepancy is needle biopsy sampling error. The most common sampling error occurs when a higher grade component present in the radical prostatectomy is missed on the needle biopsy, resulting in undergrading of the needle biopsy. Alternatively, a very focal high-grade component may not be identified in the radical prostatectomy report when the high-grade component remains deeper within a paraffin block and not sectioned onto glass slides.

TABLE 9.4 Radical Prostatectomy Grades Stratified by Biopsy Gleason Scores

RPGS	No.	%	RPGS	No.	%
Biopsy Gleason score (GS) 3 + 3 = 6			**Biopsy Gleason score (GS) 8**		
3 + 3 = 6	3,230	(63.7)	3 + 3 = 6	3	(1.1)
3 + 3 + T	567	(11.2)	3 + 3 + T	3	(1.1)
3 + 4 = 7	946	(18.7)	3 + 4 = 7	32	(12.3)
3 + 4 + T	70	(1.4)	3 + 4 + T	16	(6.1)
4 + 3 = 7	152	(3.0)	4 + 3 = 7	49	(18.8)
4 + 3 + T	47	(0.9)	4 + 3 + T	31	(11.9)
GS 8	26	(0.5)	GS 8	56	(21.5)
GS 8 + T	11	(0.2)	GS 8 + T	24	(9.2)
GS 9–10	22	(0.4)	GS 9–10	47	(18.0)
Total	5,071	(100)	Total	261	(100)
Biopsy Gleason score (GS) 3 + 4 = 7			**Biopsy Gleason score (GS) 9–10**		
3 + 3 = 6	190	(12.0)	3 + 3 = 6	4	(3.4)
3 + 3 + T	196	(12.4)	3 + 3 + T	1	(0.8)
3 + 4 = 7	784	(49.7)	3 + 4 = 7	4	(3.4)
3 + 4 + T	74	(4.7)	3 + 4 + T	5	(4.2)
4 + 3 = 7	201	(12.8)	4 + 3 = 7	6	(5.0)
4 + 3 + T	84	(5.3)	4 + 3 + T	17	(14.3)
GS 8	25	(1.6)	GS 8	6	(5.0)
GS 8 + T	4	(0.3)	GS 8 + T	7	(5.9)
GS 9–10	19	(1.2)	GS 9–10	69	(58.0)
Total	1,577	(100)	Total	119	(100)
Biopsy Gleason score 4 + 3 = 7					
3 + 3 = 6	33	(5.4)			
3 + 3 + T	22	(3.6)			
3 + 4 = 7	172	(28.0)			
3 + 4 + T	26	(4.2)			
4 + 3 = 7	174	(28.3)			
4 + 3 + T	105	(17.1)			
GS 8	25	(4.0)			
GS 8 + T	25	(4.0)			
GS 9–10	33	(5.4)			
Total	615	(100)			

RP, radical prostatectomy; T, tertiary higher grade pattern.

A third explanation of grade discrepancy between biopsy and radical prostatectomy is that a needle biopsy can sample a tertiary higher grade component in the radical prostatectomy, which is then not recorded in the standard Gleason score reporting, resulting in apparent overgrading on the needle biopsy. At Johns Hopkins, 17.5% of radical prostatectomies have a tertiary grade component.[41] This is a critical issue that other articles analyzing the relationship between biopsy and radical prostatectomy Gleason score do not account for.[42] For example, 16.0% of our biopsies had Gleason score 7, where the corresponding radical prostatectomy was Gleason score 6 with a tertiary higher grade component. If the tertiary patterns were not recorded, the erroneous explanation would have been overgrading of the biopsy as opposed to what happened where the biopsy sampled a small component of Gleason pattern 4.

Factors Associated with Increased Upgrading from Biopsy to Prostatectomy

Sampling error is a well-established predictor of upgrading.[43–45] Numerous studies have demonstrated that extended biopsies, whether more than 10, or 12 cores, are associated with less upgrading than sextant biopsies. More cancers on biopsy or those seen with higher serum PSA values are more likely to be upgraded because these findings are associated with larger, higher grade tumors at radical prostatectomy.

INTEROBSERVER REPRODUCIBILITY

The typical method of reporting levels of agreement is by a kappa score. Kappa scores of 0.00 to 0.20 reflect slight agreement; 0.21 to 0.40, fair agreement; 0.41 to 0.60, moderate agreement; 0.61 to 0.80, substantial agreement; and 0.81 to 1.00, almost perfect agreement. The latter is virtually never seen in clinical practice regardless of the issue being studied. The mean kappa among the needle biopsy studies with general pathologists was at the lowest end of moderate agreement (0.41), whereas it was at the highest end of moderate agreement (0.59) for urologic pathologists. Among urologic and general pathologists, major problem areas of nonconsensus are (a) cases borderline between two grades, (b) differentiating tangential sections of Gleason pattern 3 glands versus poorly formed glands of Gleason pattern 4, and (c) cases with cancer present on multiple cores.

PROGNOSTIC GLEASON GRADE GROUPING

A problem with the current grading system is that Gleason score 6 is typically the lowest grade assigned on biopsy material. However, the Gleason scale ranges from 2 to 10, so consequently, patients are unduly concerned when told they have Gleason score 6 cancer on biopsy, logically but incorrectly assuming that their tumor is in the midrange of aggressiveness. Another consequence of the modified grading system is that there is an expanded definition of Gleason pattern 4 to include a broader range of histologic patterns, as discussed and illustrated earlier in this chapter. There are several prognostic consequences of the reclassification of many former Gleason score 6 tumors to Gleason score 7 in the modified system. Gleason score 6 tumors are currently more homogeneous and have a uniformly better prognosis. For example, virtually no organ-confined Gleason score 6 tumor is associated with progression after radical prostatectomy, whereas using the original Gleason system, this occasionally occurred.[46]

Using the modified Gleason system, a study from Hopkins correlated biopsy and radical prostatectomy Gleason score with pathologic stage and biochemical recurrence in 6,462 men (Fig. 9.30).[47] In this study, almost 95%

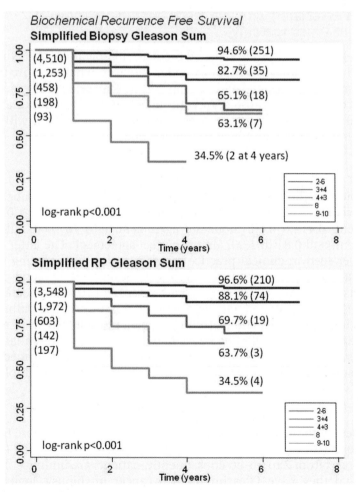

FIGURE 9.30 Biochemical recurrence–free survival stratified by Gleason Prognostic Grade Groups on biopsy (top) and radical prostatectomy (bottom).

TABLE 9.5	Prognostic Grade Grouping
Gleason score 2–6, Prognostic Grade Group I/V	
Gleason score 3 + 4 = 7, Prognostic Grade Group II/V	
Gleason score 4 + 3 = 7, Prognostic Grade Group III/V	
Gleason score 8, Prognostic Grade Group IV/V	
Gleason score 9–10, Prognostic Grade Group V/V	

and 97% of patients with Gleason score 6 cancer at biopsy and radical prostatectomy (no tertiary pattern 4 at radical prostatectomy), respectively, were predicted to be cured of disease at 5 years following radical prostatectomy. Using the modified Gleason system, this study showed that Gleason score 3 + 4 = 7 tumor has a very favorable prognosis with an estimated 5-year biochemical free survival of 83% and 88% for biopsy and radical prostatectomy, respectively. Gleason scores 9 and 10 tumor had almost twice the risk of progression compared to Gleason score 8. An accurate grouping of Gleason scores can be accomplished with five Prognostic Grade Groups, as opposed to the individual nine Gleason scores (Table 9.5). Oversimplification of the Gleason grade classification, such as combining Gleason scores 8 to 10 or classifying patients into low-, intermediate-, and high-risk categories based on Gleason scores less than 7, 7, and greater than 7, loses critical prognostic information. In reporting grades on biopsy and radical prostatectomy, in addition to reporting the individual Gleason score, Prognostic Grade Groups could be added. One would still report a case as "Gleason score 9" or as "Gleason score 10" (rather than as "Gleason score 9–10") along with the Prognostic Grade Group V. Patients will, for example, be reassured that when diagnosed with a Gleason score 6, their Prognostic Grade Group is I out of V, not Gleason score 6 out of 10. The same would apply for Gleason score 3 + 4 = 7 tumor where the Prognostic Grade Group (II) is in line with their tumor's relatively less aggressive behavior. The use of biopsy grade to drive clinical therapy is beyond the scope of this book but has been covered in detail elsewhere by one of the authors.

CHANGE OF GRADE OVER TIME

There is limited data as to whether the grade of prostate cancer changes over time. In two studies addressing this issue, men who had two TURPs over time, each containing cancer, were compared.[48,49] The second TURP tended to have higher grade cancer, with the conclusion that grade worsened over time. However, the reason why a second TURP was performed in these men was that the tumor progressed. The majority of men with cancer on the initial TURP who did not progress and whose grade may have not changed did not get a second TURP and were not factored in.

In men who are being followed with active surveillance and yearly repeat biopsies, within the first 3 years after diagnosis of Gleason score 6 prostate cancer, there is a relatively low risk of grade progression (19%). In most cases with repeat biopsies showing higher grade within the first 3 years, it is likely that the tumor grade did not progress, but rather the higher grade component was initially not sampled, because most grade changes occurred relatively soon after biopsy. There are some cases showing an increase in grade after 3 years, which may represent true dedifferentiation, but the emergence of a separate focus of high-grade carcinoma is also possible.[50]

REFERENCES

1. Gleason DF, Mellinger GT. Prediction of prognosis for prostatic adenocarcinoma by combined histological grading and clinical staging. *J Urol.* 1974;111:58–64.

2. Gleason DF. Histological grading and staging of prostatic carcinoma. In: Tannenbaum M, ed. *The Prostate.* Philadelphia: Lea and Feibiger; 1977:171.

3. Mellinger GT, Gleason D, Bailar J 3rd. The histology and prognosis of prostatic cancer. *J Urol.* 1967;97:331–337.

4. Bailar JC 3rd, Mellinger GT, Gleason DF. Survival rates of patients with prostatic cancer, tumor stage, and differentiation—preliminary report. *Cancer Chemother Rep.* 1966;50:129–136.

5. Amin A, Partin A, Epstein JI. Gleason score 7 prostate cancer on needle biopsy: relation of primary pattern 3 or 4 to pathological stage and progression after radical prostatectomy. *J Urol.* 2011;186:1286–1290.

6. Hodge KK, McNeal JE, Terris MK, et al. Random systematic versus directed ultrasound guided transrectal core biopsies of the prostate. *J Urol.* 1989;142:71–74.

7. Gaudin PB, Epstein JI. Adenosis of the prostate. Histologic features in transurethral resection specimens. *Am J Surg Pathol.* 1994;18:863–870.

8. Amin MB, Schultz DS, Zarbo RJ. Analysis of cribriform morphology in prostatic neoplasia using antibody to high-molecular-weight cytokeratins. *Arch Pathol Lab Med.* 1994;118:260–264.

9. Robinson BD, Epstein JI. Intraductal carcinoma of the prostate without invasive carcinoma on needle biopsy: emphasis on radical prostatectomy findings. *J Urol.* 2010;184:1328–1333.

10. Epstein JI, Allsbrook WC Jr, Amin MB, et al. The 2005 International Society of Urological Pathology (ISUP) Consensus Conference on Gleason Grading of Prostatic Carcinoma. *Am J Surg Pathol.* 2005;29:1228–1242.

11. Epstein JI. Gleason score 2-4 adenocarcinoma of the prostate on needle biopsy: a diagnosis that should not be made. *Am J Surg Pathol.* 2000;24:477–478.

12. Steinberg DM, Sauvageot J, Piantadosi S, et al. Correlation of prostate needle biopsy and radical prostatectomy Gleason grade in academic and community settings. *Am J Surg Pathol.* 1997;21:566–576.

13. Cury J, Coelho RF, Srougi M. Well-differentiated prostate cancer in core biopsy specimens may be associated with extraprostatic disease. *Sao Paulo Med J.* 2008;126:119–122.

14. Ghani KR, Grigor K, Tulloch DN, et al. Trends in reporting Gleason score 1991 to 2001: changes in the pathologist's practice. *Eur Urol.* 2005;47:196–201.

15. Fine SW, Epstein JI. A contemporary study correlating prostate needle biopsy and radical prostatectomy Gleason score. *J Urol.* 2008;179:1335–1338; discussion 1338–1339.

16. McNeal JE, Redwine EA, Freiha FS, et al. Zonal distribution of prostatic adenocarcinoma. Correlation with histologic pattern and direction of spread. *Am J Surg Pathol*. 1988;12: 897–906.

17. Garcia JJ, Al-Ahmadie HA, Gopalan A, et al. Do prostatic transition zone tumors have a distinct morphology? *Am J Surg Pathol*. 2008;32:1709–1714.

18. Gleason DF. Histologic grading of prostate cancer: a perspective. *Hum Pathol*. 1992;23: 273–279.

19. Mellinger GT. Prognosis of prostatic carcinoma. *Recent Results Cancer Res*. 1977;(60): 61–72.

20. Latour M, Amin MB, Billis A, et al. Grading of invasive cribriform carcinoma on prostate needle biopsy: an interobserver study among experts in genitourinary pathology. *Am J Surg Pathol*. 2008;32:1532–1539.

21. Iczkowski KA, Torkko KC, Kotnis GR, et al. Digital quantification of five high-grade prostate cancer patterns, including the cribriform pattern, and their association with adverse outcome. *Am J Clin Pathol*. 2011;136:98–107.

22. Baisden BL, Kahane H, Epstein JI. Perineural invasion, mucinous fibroplasia, and glomerulations: diagnostic features of limited cancer on prostate needle biopsy. *Am J Surg Pathol*. 1999;23:918–924.

23. Gleason DF. Classification of prostatic carcinomas. *Cancer Chemother Rep*. 1966;50: 125–128.

24. Lotan TL, Epstein JI. Gleason grading of prostatic adenocarcinoma with glomeruloid features on needle biopsy. *Hum Pathol*. 2009;40:471–477.

25. Al-Hussain TO, Nagar MS, Epstein JI. Gleason pattern 5 is frequently underdiagnosed on prostate needle-core biopsy. *Urology*. 2012; 79:178–181.

26. Fajardo DA, Miyamoto H, Miller JS, et al. Identification of Gleason pattern 5 on prostatic needle core biopsy: frequency of underdiagnosis and relation to morphology. *Am J Surg Pathol*. 2011;35:1706–1711.

27. Ro JY, el-Naggar A, Ayala AG, et al. Signet-ring-cell carcinoma of the prostate. Electronmicroscopic and immunohistochemical studies of eight cases. *Am J Surg Pathol*. 1988;12: 453–460.

28. Nelson RS, Epstein JI. Prostatic carcinoma with abundant xanthomatous cytoplasm. Foamy gland carcinoma. *Am J Surg Pathol*. 1996;20:419–426.

29. Zhao J, Epstein JI. High-grade foamy gland prostatic adenocarcinoma on biopsy or transurethral resection: a morphologic study of 55 cases. *Am J Surg Pathol*. 2009;33: 583–590.

30. Humphrey PA, Kaleem Z, Swanson PE, et al. Pseudohyperplastic prostatic adenocarcinoma. *Am J Surg Pathol*. 1998;22:1239–1246.

31. Levi AW, Epstein JI. Pseudohyperplastic prostatic adenocarcinoma on needle biopsy and simple prostatectomy. *Am J Surg Pathol*. 2000;24:1039–1046.

32. Kunz GM Jr, Epstein JI. Should each core with prostate cancer be assigned a separate Gleason score? *Hum Pathol*. 2003;34:911–914.

33. Park HK, Choe G, Byun SS, et al. Evaluation of concordance of Gleason score between prostatectomy and biopsies that show more than two different Gleason scores in positive cores. *Urology*. 2006;67:110–114.

34. Poulos CK, Daggy JK, Cheng L. Preoperative prediction of Gleason grade in radical prostatectomy specimens: the influence of different Gleason grades from multiple positive biopsy sites. *Mod Pathol*. 2005;18:228–234.

35. Kunju LP, Daignault S, Wei JT, et al. Multiple prostate cancer cores with different Gleason grades submitted in the same specimen container without specific site designation: should each core be assigned an individual Gleason score? *Hum Pathol*. 2009;40:558–564.

36. Kuroiwa K, Uchino H, Yokomizo A, et al. Impact of reporting rules of biopsy Gleason score for prostate cancer. *J Clin Pathol*. 2009;62:260–263.

37. Rubin MA, Bismar TA, Curtis S, et al. Prostate needle biopsy reporting: how are the surgical members of the Society of Urologic Oncology using pathology reports to guide treatment of prostate cancer patients? *Am J Surg Pathol*. 2004;28:946–952.

38. Descazeaud A, Rubin MA, Allory Y, et al. What information are urologists extracting from prostate needle biopsy reports and what do they need for clinical management of prostate cancer? *Eur Urol*. 2005;48:911–915.

39. Trpkov K, Zhang J, Chan M, et al. Prostate cancer with tertiary Gleason pattern 5 in prostate needle biopsy: clinicopathologic findings and disease progression. *Am J Surg Pathol*. 2009;33:233–240.

40. Patel AA, Chen MH, Renshaw AA, et al. PSA failure following definitive treatment of prostate cancer having biopsy Gleason score 7 with tertiary grade 5. *JAMA*. 2007;298: 1533–1538.

41. Epstein JI, Feng Z, Trock BJ, et al. Upgrading/downgrading of prostate cancer from biopsy to radical prostatectomy: incidence and predictive factors. *Eur Urol*. 2012;61: 1019–1024.

42. Trock BJ, Guo CC, Gonzalgo ML, et al. Tertiary Gleason patterns and biochemical recurrence after prostatectomy: proposal for a modified Gleason scoring system. *J Urol*. 2009;182:1364–1370.

43. Capitanio U, Karakiewicz PI, Valiquette L, et al. Biopsy core number represents one of foremost predictors of clinically significant Gleason sum upgrading in patients with low-risk prostate cancer. *Urology*. 2009;73:1087–1091.

44. Freedland SJ, Kane CJ, Amling CL, et al. Upgrading and downgrading of prostate needle biopsy specimens: risk factors and clinical implications. *Urology*. 2007;69:495–499.

45. Richstone L, Bianco FJ, Shah HH, et al. Radical prostatectomy in men aged > or = 70 years: effect of age on upgrading, upstaging, and the accuracy of a preoperative nomogram. *BJU Int*. 2008;101:541–546.

46. Hernandez DJ, Nielsen ME, Han M, et al. Natural history of pathologically organ-confined (pT2), Gleason score 6 or less, prostate cancer after radical prostatectomy. *Urology*. 2008;72:172–176.

47. Pierorazio PM, Walsh PC, Partin AW, et al. Prognostic Gleason grade grouping: data based on the modified Gleason scoring system. *BJU Int*. 2013;111:753–760.

48. Brawn PN. The dedifferentiation of prostate carcinoma. *Cancer*. 1983;52:246–251.

49. Cumming JA, Ritchie AW, Goodman CM, et al. De-differentiation with time in prostate cancer and the influence of treatment on the course of the disease. *Br J Urol*. 1990;65: 271–274.

50. Sheridan TB, Carter HB, Wang W, et al. Change in prostate cancer grade over time in men followed expectantly for stage T1c disease. *J Urol*. 2008;179:901–904.

10

FINDINGS OF ATYPICAL GLANDS SUSPICIOUS FOR CANCER

TERMINOLOGY

The term *atypical hyperplasia* is nonspecific and has been used to denote such diverse entities as prostatic intraepithelial neoplasia (PIN), adenosis (a benign mimicker of cancer), and foci suspicious for infiltrating carcinoma. As the term atypical hyperplasia is nonspecific, it should not be used.

The term *atypical small acinar proliferation* (ASAP) has been proposed.[1] Needle biopsies signed out as ASAP encompass such lesions as high-grade PIN, benign mimickers of cancer, reactive atypia, as well as many cases that in retrospect demonstrate focal carcinoma but contain insufficient cytologic or architectural atypia to establish a definitive diagnosis of cancer. Urologists frequently equate ASAP with high-grade PIN.[2,3] In a study by Park et al.,[4] men with high-grade PIN underwent repeat biopsy at 10.6 months as opposed to those with an atypical diagnosis who were rebiopsied at 23.8 months, suggesting that urologists are often more worried about a high-grade PIN diagnosis than an atypical diagnosis.[4] However, ASAP in contrast to high-grade PIN is not a specific entity but rather a broad group of lesions of varying clinical significance. It is important not to equate ASAP with high-grade PIN, because the likelihood of finding cancer on repeat biopsy is higher with a diagnosis of ASAP than with a finding of high-grade PIN.[5] The potential risk with using the diagnostic term atypical small acinar proliferation is that although many of these lesions are in fact infiltrating carcinomas, the term does not fully convey this risk and patients with this diagnosis may thus not receive repeat biopsy. Repeat biopsy is performed on average in only 56% of the cases with an atypical diagnosis.[1,6–9] Even when the term *repeat biopsy is recommended* was explicitly added to the pathology report, in one study, only 63% of atypical cases had a repeat biopsy, and in another study, the recommendation did not influence the likelihood of repeat biopsy.[6,7] Cases of an atypical diagnosis where a rebiopsy is not performed may reflect patient issues (i.e., patients lost to follow-up, patients refuse rebiopsy, medical complications prevent rebiopsy, change of health care providers, etc.) or reflect a lack of understanding by the urologist as to the significance of an atypical diagnosis in the pathology report. Nevertheless, approximately one-half of urologic pathologists use the term atypical small acinar proliferation.[10]

The remaining urologic pathologists and we favor the use of descriptive terminology in pathology reports.[10] At our institution, atypical biopsies are conveyed as "prostate tissue with small focus of atypical glands." We routinely note in needle biopsy reports that "while these findings are atypical and suspicious for adenocarcinoma, there is insufficient cytologic and/or architectural atypia to establish a definitive diagnosis" (see the Appendix for macros). Pathologists may add further information detailing why a diagnosis is atypical but not diagnostic of cancer, such that PIN or atrophy or adenosis cannot be excluded with certainty. A recommendation for repeat biopsy is made in the pathology report if the patient is younger than 75 years of age. In older men, we leave it up to the judgment of the urologist as to whether a repeat biopsy is justified.

INCIDENCE OF ATYPICAL DIAGNOSIS ON NEEDLE BIOPSY

On average, 5% of needle biopsy pathology reports have a diagnosis of atypical glands suspicious for carcinoma.[5] The median value is 4.4% with a wide range from 0.7% to 23.4%. There appears to be a trend over time in the reported incidence of atypical diagnoses on needle biopsy, with a decrease in more recent years.[5] In another study that addressed the issue of the changing incidence of atypical diagnoses over time, it was demonstrated that pathologists are becoming more skilled at diagnosing small foci of prostate cancer on needle biopsy and are referring for consultation predominantly cases with fewer cancer glands.[11] Correspondingly, many cases in the past that would have been sent to the expert as atypical would now be recognized as carcinoma by practicing pathologists and not sent to an expert for consultation.

INTEROBSERVER REPRODUCIBILITY

An atypical diagnosis reflects that a given acinar proliferation lacks the diagnostic criteria for a definitive diagnosis of carcinoma. Cancer may not be diagnosable as a result of the pathologist being unable to exclude mimickers of cancer, due to the presence of associated inflammation, or because of mechanical distortion from the needle biopsy procedure. One would therefore expect that there would be interpretive variability in cases diagnosed as atypical depending on the experience and skill of the pathologist. In three studies, cases signed out as atypical by general pathologists were diagnosed as benign in 5% to 17% of cases, and as carcinoma in 2% to 20% of cases when reviewed by a genitourinary pathologist.[1,9,12] Chan et al.[13] analyzed cases that were diagnosed as atypical in outside institutions and if not for the request of the patient and/or urologist for a second opinion of a urologic pathology expert, the atypical diagnosis would have remained the diagnosis on record. Of the 204 cases signed out as atypical by the outside pathologist, 45% were definitively diagnosed as cancer upon expert review with 16% diagnosed as benign.

PROSTATE CANCER RISK FOLLOWING A DIAGNOSIS OF ATYPIA

The average risk of cancer following an atypical diagnosis is 40.2% with a median of 38.5% (range: 17% to 70%).[5] More recent studies have reported similar findings.[14–17] There does not appear to be a trend over time in the reported risk of cancer following a repeat biopsy for an atypical diagnosis. Only three studies report the median time to rebiopsy with an average of approximately 9 months.[3,7,18] We recommend performing a repeat biopsy within 6 months of the initial atypical diagnosis, as the purpose of the repeat biopsy is to rule out carcinoma in an individual at high risk of harboring malignancy and no specific rationale exists for delaying repeat biopsy.

Of the 10 studies that have examined whether serum prostate-specific antigen (PSA) levels predict cancer following an atypical needle biopsy diagnosis, 9 showed no correlation.[5] In addition to serum PSA levels, percent free PSA levels as a predictor of cancer on repeat biopsy was examined in 4 studies with only 1 correlating.[15] Two studies have examined PSA velocity as a predictor and both found it to be significantly correlated with cancer on repeat biopsy.[19] Studies have shown no correlation with cancer based on the results of digital rectal exam and transrectal ultrasound findings.[5]

Several investigators have demonstrated that a diagnosis of "atypical, favor carcinoma" has a higher likelihood of having cancer on rebiopsy as opposed to a diagnosis of "atypical, favor benign."[1,11] Similarly, a markedly atypical biopsy is associated with an increased risk of cancer compared to a moderately atypical biopsy.[14] However, even an atypical, favor benign diagnosis has an appreciable risk of cancer, such that most urologic pathologists do not further specify an atypical diagnosis.[10] Occasionally, we subclassify an atypical diagnosis as being highly suspicious for cancer for a case that we strongly favor that carcinoma is present, yet the findings are not absolutely diagnostic. Similarly, there is a minority of cases that we will diagnose as mildly atypical, where we have a low suspicion for cancer, yet we cannot entirely exclude the possibility of malignancy.

Approximately 90% of cancers will be found on the initial repeat biopsy after an atypical diagnosis.[12,20] However, in the other 10% of cases, the first biopsy may be atypical and a repeat biopsy entirely benign. We have seen such cases where upon review of the initial biopsy, it was diagnostic of cancer. It is therefore incumbent upon the pathologist in these cases to have the initial biopsy sent off for consultation or try to re-solve the initial biopsy. If the pathologist is sufficiently worried with the initial biopsy to subject the patient to a surgical procedure (i.e., second needle biopsy), then there is an obligation to try to resolve the initial biopsy. If both the initial atypical biopsy and benign rebiopsy is performed using an extended technique ($\geq$10 cores), there is no data on the ultimate risk of cancer. It remains to be studied whether and how many times these men need additional tissue sampling.

REBIOPSY TECHNIQUES FOLLOWING A DIAGNOSIS OF ATYPIA

In most cases where cancer is found on rebiopsy following an atypical diagnosis, the atypical focus represents carcinoma, which on the initial sample was not diagnostic of malignancy. It is therefore logical that in order to maximize the detection of cancer following an atypical diag-nosis, one would want to concentrate the repeat biopsy sampling in the area of the atypical focus. Five studies have reported that following an atypical diagnosis, the likelihood of cancer being present in same sextant site as the initial atypical focus is 48% to 76%.[4,12,14,19,21] The likelihood of cancer being found either at the same sextant site or in the adjacent sextant sites is even higher, with two studies reporting rates of 71% and 85%.[4,21] The probability of cancer following an atypical diagnosis being located only on the contralateral side of the initial atypical biopsy has been reported in studies to be 17% to 27%.[7,12,14,19,21] It is recommended that urologists use the following rebiopsy strategy following an atypical diagnosis: (a) increased sampling of the initial atypical site, (b) increased sampling of the adjacent ipsilateral and adjacent contralateral sites, and (c) routine sampling of all the sextant sites. It is critical for urologists to submit needle biopsy specimens in a manner where the sextant location of each core can be determined so that pathologists can specify the sextant site containing the atypical focus.

RADICAL PROSTATECTOMY AFTER CANCER DIAGNOSED POSTATYPICAL BIOPSY

There have been two series addressing this issue. One from the Cleve-land Clinic found that at radical prostatectomy (RP), 49% had Gleason score 6; 37%, Gleason score 7; and 10%, Gleason score more than 8. Extraprostatic extension was seen in 15% with seminal vesicle invasion in 6%.[22] We have also studied this issue comparing cancer at RP follow-ing an atypical biopsy to RP in a control group which did not have a prior atypical biopsy.[23] Gleason score was 6 in 74.5%, Gleason score 7 in 24.9%, and Gleason score 8 in 0.6%. Extraprostatic extension was present in 17% with 1.2% seminal vesicle invasion. Cancer diagnosed following a prior atypical biopsy was associated with lower Gleason score and lower

TABLE 10.1 Features Arguing Against the Diagnosis of Adenocarcinoma
Atrophic cytoplasm
Merging in with benign glands (r/o adenosis)
Corpora amylacea
Inflammation
Adjacent PIN (r/o PINATYP)

r/o, rule out; PIN, prostatic intraepithelial neoplasia; PINATYP, (see Chapter 5).

pathologic stage compared to the control group without a prior atypical biopsy. The number of cores with atypical glands was not predictive of grade or stage at RP.

HISTOLOGY–ATYPICAL SMALL GLANDS

A diagnosis of "atypical, suspicious for cancer" results when there are some features of cancer, yet the features are limited quantitatively or qualitatively (Table 10.1). In some cases, cancer cannot be definitively diagnosed either due to atrophic features, where it is difficult to distinguish between benign atrophy and atrophic cancer (Figs. 10.1 to 10.3, eFigs. 10.1 to 10.83). In other

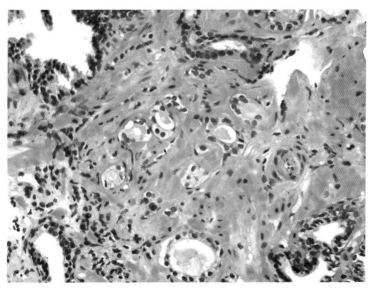

FIGURE 10.1 Crowded focus of atypical glands. Atrophic benign glands cannot be ruled out with certainty.

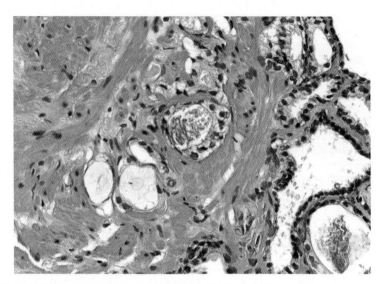

FIGURE 10.2 Small crowded glands *(left)* with slightly enlarged nuclei compared to more benign–appearing glands *(right)*.

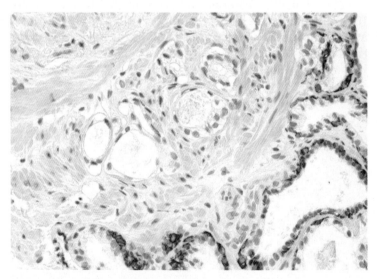

FIGURE 10.3 Same case as Figure 10.2 with negative stains for high molecular weight cytokeratin *(red chromogen)*. Despite negative stains, there are a limited number of negative glands and partial atrophy cannot be excluded with certainty.

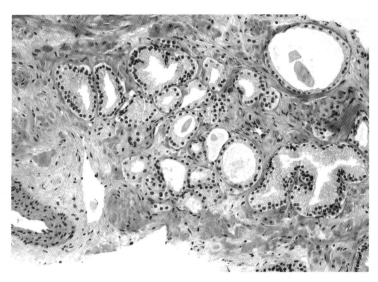

FIGURE 10.4 Crowded focus of atypical glands where adenosis cannot be ruled out. Small glands look similar to more recognizable benign glands.

examples, adenosis (Figs. 10.4 and 10.5) or high-grade PIN (Figs. 10.6 to 10.9) cannot be ruled out. Clusters of totally benign-appearing glands can also be negative for basal cell markers and positive for alpha-methylacyl-coenzyme A racemase (AMACR) (Figs. 10.10 and 10.11). If the morphology is definitively benign, where the stain was done to evaluate another focus,

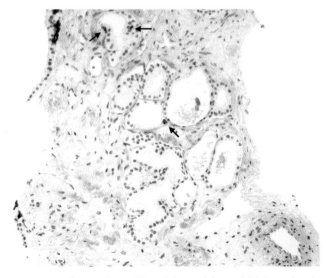

FIGURE 10.5 Same case as Figure 10.4 with patchy staining of high molecular weight cytokeratin (arrows).

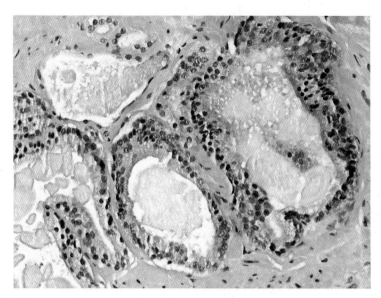

FIGURE 10.6 Several large atypical glands, some containing corpora amylacea. Differential diagnosis is high-grade PIN and carcinoma.

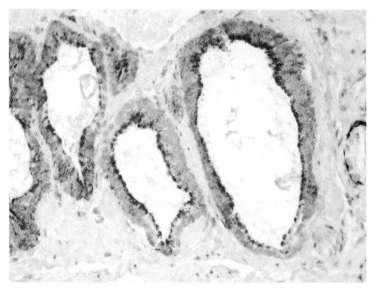

FIGURE 10.7 Same case as Figure 10.6. Despite negative basal cell markers *(brown)* and positive AMACR *(red)*, there are an insufficient number of atypical glands to rule out high-grade PIN. PIN may have such patchy basal cells that in a plane of section would appear negative for basal cell markers.

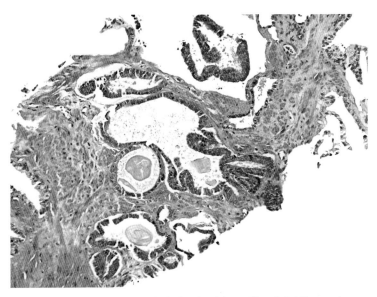

FIGURE 10.8 Large cytologically atypical glands with papillary infolding and corpora amy-lacea suggestive of high-grade PIN.

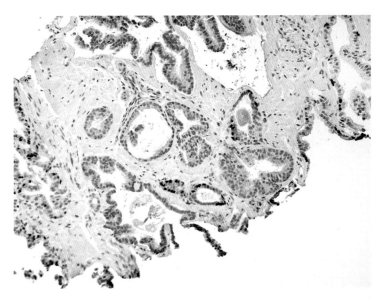

FIGURE 10.9 Same case as Figure 10.8 with all atypical glands negative for basal cell markers leading to a diagnosis of "atypical glands, cannot rule out high-grade PIN."

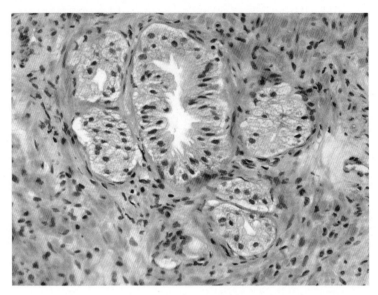

FIGURE 10.10 Glands with an entirely benign morphology.

the focus should still be considered benign. Cases where the atypical glands are at the edge of the core, where one cannot appreciate the infiltrative nature of the atypical glands among benign glands, are more likely to result in an atypical diagnosis (Figs. 10.12 and 10.13). Another situation where an atypical diagnosis may result is in the presence of crush artifact as a result of

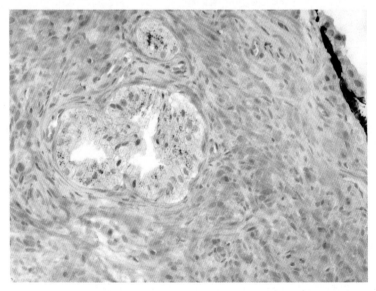

FIGURE 10.11 Same case as Figure 10.10 with negative stains for p63 and high molecular weight cytokeratin *(brown)* and positive for AMACR *(red)*. Case was sent in for consultation, whereby we diagnosed the focus as benign despite the immunohistochemical stains.

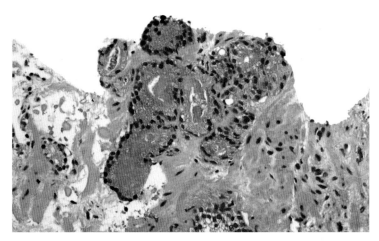

FIGURE 10.12 Cluster of small glands suspicious for carcinoma at the edge of the core. Despite focal intraluminal blue mucin and crowded small glands, there is insufficient cytologic atypia and the glands are at the edge of the core such that a definitive diagnosis of carcinoma should not be made.

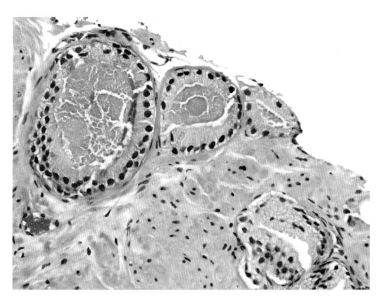

FIGURE 10.13 Atypical focus at the edge of the core with three glands with straight luminal borders, slightly amphophilic cytoplasm, and faint intraluminal blue mucin. There are only a few glands at the edge of the core and they lack prominent cytologic atypia, insufficient to definitively diagnose carcinoma.

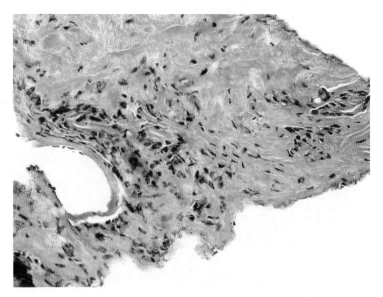

FIGURE 10.14   Crushed, poorly preserved glands suspicious for carcinoma.

mechanical distortion from the needle biopsy (Fig. 10.14), although a diagnosis of crushed cancer can sometimes be made (Fig. 10.15). When certain features more typical of cancer, such as blue-tinged or dense pink mucinous secretions, are present yet the atypical findings are minimal, a diagnosis of atypical glands suspicious for cancer is rendered.

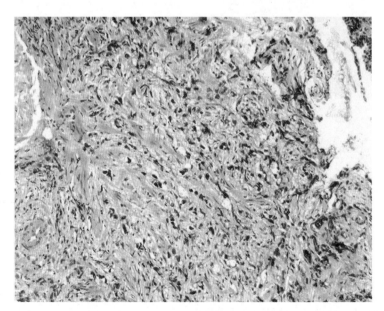

FIGURE 10.15   Numerous crushed individual cells that was positive for keratin and diagnostic of adenocarcinoma, Gleason score 5 + 5 = 10.

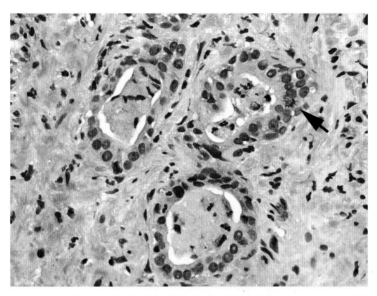

FIGURE 10.16 Atypical glands with mitotic figure *(arrow)*. Given the presence of intralumi-nal acute inflammation, reactive benign glands cannot be excluded.

In the presence of inflammation, one must be cautious in diagnosing cancer (Figs. 10.16 and 10.17). Rarely, one can establish a diagnosis of cancer associated with inflammation (Fig. 10.18). Figure 10.19 demonstrates a focus of crowded small glands infiltrating in between larger benign glands associated with extensive inflammation. This focus is diagnostic of cancer because

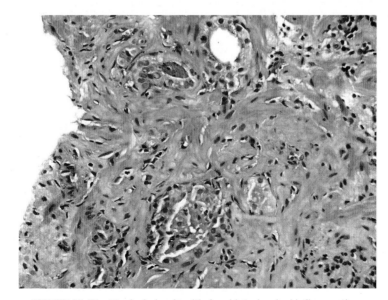

FIGURE 10.17 Atypical glands with focal intraluminal inflammation.

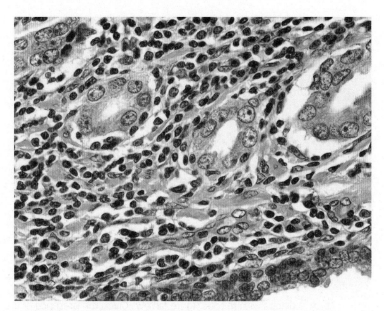

FIGURE 10.18 Adenocarcinoma with very prominent nucleoli compared to adjacent benign gland *(below)* in the setting of extensive chronic inflammation.

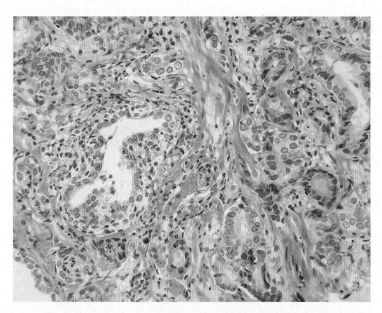

FIGURE 10.19 Adenocarcinoma with infiltrative patterns diagnostic of malignancy despite associated inflammation.

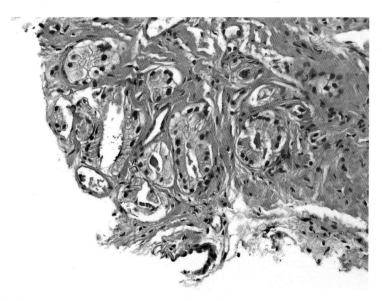

FIGURE 10.20 Focus of crowded glands with minimal atypia where adenosis cannot be ruled out.

the pattern of numerous small glands in between larger benign glands cannot be attributed to inflammation. Furthermore, the degree of cytologic atypia present in the small atypical glands is significantly greater than the adjacent benign glands even though both are exposed to the same inflammatory milieu.

In some cases where the number of atypical glands are so few or the glands have no other atypical features other than that they are crowded, adenosis cannot be excluded (Fig. 10.20). Even if the glands are negative for basal cell markers in a small focus, the lesion could still be adenosis because basal cell stains can be very patchy in adenosis. In a small focus of atypical glands on prostate biopsy, negative staining for basal cell markers should not necessarily lead to a definitive malignant diagnosis in all cases, because almost half of these biopsies on follow-up sampling are benign.[24]

In the setting of an inflamed prostate, one should also be cautious in the evaluation of isolated glands with abnormal architecture. Although rarely carcinomas may be inflamed, inflammation tends to preferentially localize away from malignant glands. In areas of intense chronic inflammation, prostatic acini appear atrophic with a high nuclear to cytoplasmic ratio. These basophilic glands may show some architectural abnormalities such as pseudocribriform formation with budding off of little glands (Fig. 10.21). Streaming of basophilic epithelium in areas of intense chronic inflammation resembles transitional cell metaplasia. The finding of occasional large nucleoli is not uncommon in areas of intense acute or chronic inflammation. The distinction of these inflammatory atypias from carcinoma first relies on the recognition that the atypical glands are located in an area of intense inflammation. In addition, the glands have a very

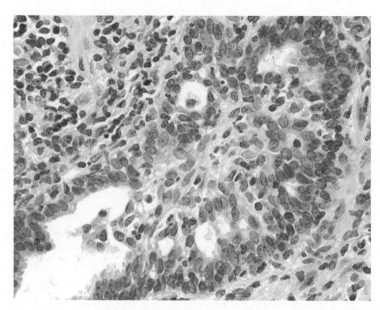

FIGURE 10.21   Pseudocribriform reactive gland with inflammation.

basophilic appearance in contrast to the usual gland-forming prostatic adenocarcinomas that have abundant, often pale-staining cytoplasm. The high nuclear to cytoplasmic ratio seen in inflamed glands is predominantly seen in only the more poorly differentiated prostatic carcinomas that lack good gland formation. Careful examination of these basophilic glands will also demonstrate the finding of a basal cell layer in most instances.

Many mimickers of prostate cancer illustrated in Chapter 7 are diagnosed as atypical. In addition, there are some other benign prostatic lesions that lack a specific name (i.e., crowded benign pale glands), which are often diagnosed as atypical. Another situation where benign glands are diagnosed as atypical is when their basal cells contain prominent nucleoli. We have also seen some men whose "normal" prostate looks abnormal throughout, containing small clusters of crowded glands with at most mild cytologic atypia, which we have termed *diffuse adenosis of the peripheral zone* (see Chapter 7).[25] Of the rebiopsied cases, 20 (57%) were subsequently diagnosed with carcinoma. Diffuse adenosis of the peripheral zone is a diagnostically challenging mimicker of prostate cancer seen in prostate needle biopsies from typically younger patients. It is a risk factor for prostate cancer and patients with this finding should be followed closely and rebiopsied.

One of the most frequent situations where one is left with an atypical diagnosis is when there are a few small atypical glands closely associated with a focus of high-grade PIN (see Chapter 5 for histologic description). We have termed this lesion *PINATYP*, where it cannot be determined whether the small atypical glands represent budding or tangentially sectioned glands from an adjacent high-grade PIN gland or invasive cancer next to the high-grade PIN. Studies have shown that PINATYP should be considered

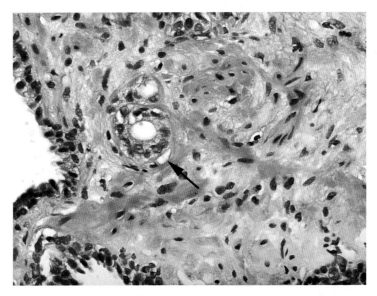

FIGURE 10.22 Single small atypical gland *(arrow)* highly suspicious for carcinoma.

in a similar fashion to those with atypical foci, suspicious for cancer as they have a higher risk of cancer on repeat biopsy compared to men with high-grade PIN alone.[26,27] When there are just a few small atypical glands that are not tightly packed between benign glands, one cannot exclude a section of an outpouching of high-grade PIN gland, where the majority of the PIN gland is not in the plane of section (Figs. 10.22 and 10.23).

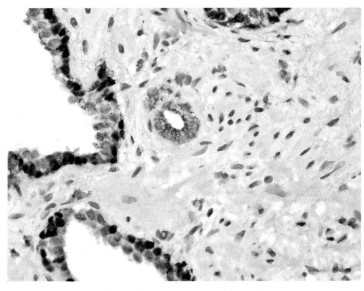

FIGURE 10.23 Same case as Figure 10.22 negative for basal cell markers *(brown)* and positive for AMACR *(red)* where an outpouching of high-grade PIN cannot be excluded with certainty.

REFERENCES

1. Iczkowski KA, MacLennan GT, Bostwick DG. Atypical small acinar proliferation suspicious for malignancy in prostate needle biopsies: clinical significance in 33 cases. *Am J Surg Pathol*. 1997;21:1489–1495.

2. Descazeaud A, Rubin MA, Allory Y, et al. What information are urologists extracting from prostate needle biopsy reports and what do they need for clinical management of prostate cancer? *Eur Urol*. 2005;48:911–915.

3. Rubin MA, Bismar TA, Curtis S, et al. Prostate needle biopsy reporting: how are the surgical members of the Society of Urologic Oncology using pathology reports to guide treatment of prostate cancer patients? *Am J Surg Pathol*. 2004;28:946–952.

4. Park S, Shinohara K, Grossfeld GD, et al. Prostate cancer detection in men with prior high grade prostatic intraepithelial neoplasia or atypical prostate biopsy. *J Urol*. 2001; 165:1409–1414.

5. Epstein JI, Herawi M. Prostate needle biopsies containing prostatic intraepithelial neoplasia or atypical foci suspicious for carcinoma: implications for patient care. *J Urol*. 2006;175:820–834.

6. Cheville JC, Reznicek MJ, Bostwick DG. The focus of "atypical glands, suspicious for malignancy" in prostatic needle biopsy specimens: incidence, histologic features, and clinical follow-up of cases diagnosed in a community practice. *Am J Clin Pathol*. 1997; 108:633–640.

7. Fadare O, Wang S, Mariappan MR. Practice patterns of clinicians following isolated diagnoses of atypical small acinar proliferation on prostate biopsy specimens. *Arch Pathol Lab Med*. 2004;128:557–560.

8. Iczkowski KA, Chen HM, Yang XJ, et al. Prostate cancer diagnosed after initial biopsy with atypical small acinar proliferation suspicious for malignancy is similar to cancer found on initial biopsy. *Urology*. 2002;60:851–854.

9. Renshaw AA, Santis WF, Richie JP. Clinicopathological characteristics of prostatic adenocarcinoma in men with atypical prostate needle biopsies. *J Urol*. 1998;159: 2018–2021.

10. Egevad L, Allsbrook WC Jr, Epstein JI. Current practice of diagnosis and reporting of prostate cancer on needle biopsy among genitourinary pathologists. *Hum Pathol*. 2006; 37:292–297.

11. Chan TY, Epstein JI. Follow-up of atypical prostate needle biopsies suspicious for cancer. *Urology*. 1999;53:351–355.

12. Iczkowski KA, Bassler TJ, Schwob VS, et al. Diagnosis of "suspicious for malignancy" in prostate biopsies: predictive value for cancer. *Urology*. 1998;51:749–757; discussion 757–758.

13. Chan TY, Epstein JI. Patient and urologist driven second opinion of prostate needle biopsies. *J Urol*. 2005;174:1390–1394; discussion 1394; author reply 1394.

14. Girasole CR, Cookson MS, Putzi MJ, et al. Significance of atypical and suspicious small acinar proliferations, and high grade prostatic intraepithelial neoplasia on prostate biopsy: implications for cancer detection and biopsy strategy. *J Urol*. 2006;175:929–933.

15. Mearini L, Costantini E, Bellezza G, et al. Is there any clinical parameter able to predict prostate cancer after initial diagnosis of atypical small acinar proliferation? *Urol Int*. 2008;81:29–35.

16. Lopez JI. Prostate adenocarcinoma detected after high-grade prostatic intraepithelial neoplasia or atypical small acinar proliferation. *BJU Int*. 2007;100:1272–1276.

17. Ploussard G, Plennevaux G, Allory Y, et al. High-grade prostatic intraepithelial neoplasia and atypical small acinar proliferation on initial 21-core extended biopsy scheme: incidence and implications for patient care and surveillance. *World J Urol*. 2009;27:587–592.

18. Postma R, Roobol M, Schroder FH, et al. Lesions predictive for prostate cancer in a screened population: first and second screening round findings. *Prostate.* 2004;61: 260–266.

19. Borboroglu PG, Sur RL, Roberts JL, et al. Repeat biopsy strategy in patients with atypical small acinar proliferation or high grade prostatic intraepithelial neoplasia on initial prostate needle biopsy. *J Urol.* 2001;166:866–870.

20. Moore CK, Karikehalli S, Nazeer T, et al. Prognostic significance of high grade prostatic intraepithelial neoplasia and atypical small acinar proliferation in the contemporary era. *J Urol.* 2005;173:70–72.

21. Allen EA, Kahane H, Epstein JI. Repeat biopsy strategies for men with atypical diagnoses on initial prostate needle biopsy. *Urology.* 1998;52:803–807.

22. Zhou M, Magi-Galluzzi C. Clinicopathological features of prostate cancers detected after an initial diagnosis of "atypical glands suspicious for cancer." *Pathology.* 2010;42: 334–338.

23. Chen YB, Pierorazio PM, Epstein JI. Initial atypical diagnosis with carcinoma on subsequent prostate needle biopsy: findings at radical prostatectomy. *J Urol.* 2010;184: 1953–1957.

24. Halushka MK, Kahane H, Epstein JI. Negative 34betaE12 staining in a small focus of atypical glands on prostate needle biopsy: a follow-up study of 332 cases. *Hum Pathol.* 2004;35:43–46.

25. Lotan TL, Epstein JI. Diffuse adenosis of the peripheral zone in prostate needle biopsy and prostatectomy specimens. *Am J Surg Pathol.* 2008;32:1360–1366.

26. Alsikafi NF, Brendler CB, Gerber GS, et al. High-grade prostatic intraepithelial neoplasia with adjacent atypia is associated with a higher incidence of cancer on subsequent needle biopsy than high-grade prostatic intraepithelial neoplasia alone. *Urology.* 2001;57:296–300.

27. Kronz JD, Shaikh AA, Epstein JI. High-grade prostatic intraepithelial neoplasia with adjacent small atypical glands on prostate biopsy. *Hum Pathol.* 2001;32:389–395.

11

PROSTATIC DUCT ADENOCARCINOMA

Although most adenocarcinomas of the prostate are composed of cuboidal cells arranged in acini, approximately 0.2% to 1.3% of prostate cancers show distinctive tall pseudostratified columnar cells and are classified as pure prostatic duct adenocarcinomas (eFigs. 11.1 to 11.54).[1–5] The initial impression in the pathology literature was that this was a truly "endometrial" tumor arising in a vestigial müllerian structure.[6,7] However, subsequent reports on favorable response to orchiectomy, ultrastructure of tumor cells, histochemistry, and immunohistochemistry have proven that this is a neoplasm of prostatic origin.[2,8–10] Consequently, the terms *endometrioid* and *endometrial* adenocarcinoma of the prostate are no longer justified.

Although prostatic duct adenocarcinoma can be the sole component, more frequently, it is found admixed with tumor showing acinar differentiation. The latter is encountered in about 8% to 13% of prostatic carcinoma.[5,11] The term *prostatic duct carcinoma* should not be used, because it also refers to prostatic duct urothelial carcinomas.

When prostatic duct adenocarcinomas arise in large primary periurethral prostatic ducts, they may grow as exophytic lesions into the urethra, most commonly in and around the verumontanum. These lesions cystoscopically closely resemble papillary urothelial carcinomas. Often in these cases, there are no abnormalities on rectal examination. Patients may present with either obstructive symptoms or gross or microscopic hematuria. Tumors arising in the more peripheral prostatic ducts may or may not have a urethral component and may be palpable on rectal examination. Although ductal adenocarcinomas strongly express prostate-specific antigen (PSA) immunohistochemically, they are associated with variable expression in the serum.[12,13]

Prostatic duct adenocarcinomas show a variety of architectural patterns (Table 11.1). Tumors that grow into the urethra as exophytic lesions are often papillary (Figs. 11.1 to 11.5). They are characterized by tall pseudostratified epithelial cells with abundant, usually amphophilic cytoplasm, in contrast to the cuboidal to columnar single cell layer of epithelium seen with acinar prostatic carcinomas. Occasionally, the papillary

TABLE 11.1   Architectural Patterns of Prostatic Ductal Adenocarcinoma
Papillary
Solid papillary
Solid nests
Cribriform
PIN-like
Individual glands—mimicking colonic adenocarcinoma

PIN, prostatic intraepithelial neoplasia.

fronds within prostatic duct adenocarcinoma may be composed of clear cells or mucinous epithelium yet have pseudostratification of the nuclei typical of prostatic duct adenocarcinomas. Although the papillary pattern of prostatic duct adenocarcinoma is most commonly seen on transurethral resection (TUR) material, occasionally, this papillary pattern may also be seen on needle biopsy material (Figs. 11.6 and 11.7). Uncommonly, benign glands can demonstrate papillary hyperplasia, which is distinguished from ductal adenocarcinoma by the presence of bland cuboidal epithelium.

The cribriform pattern of prostatic duct adenocarcinomas is more commonly seen deeper within the tissue, although it may also be noted

(text continues on p. 259)

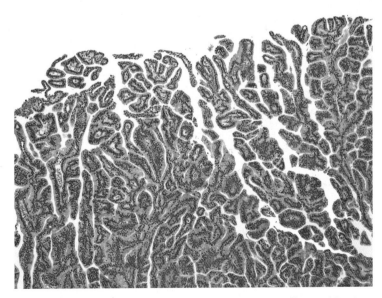

FIGURE 11.1   Prostatic ductal adenocarcinoma with papillary architecture.

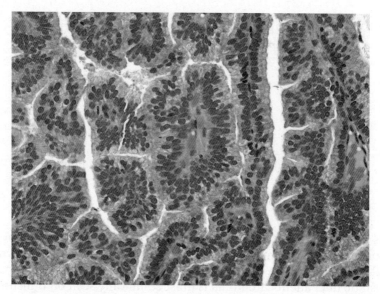

FIGURE 11.2   High magnification of Figure 11.1 with papillary fronds lined by pseudostratified columnar epithelium.

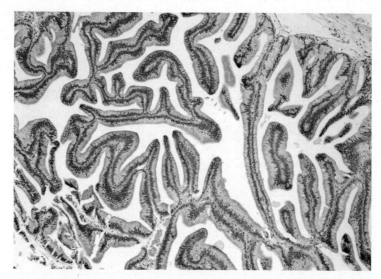

FIGURE 11.3   Papillary prostatic ductal adenocarcinoma.

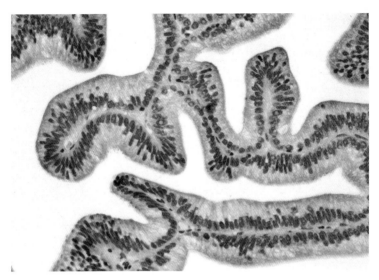

FIGURE 11.4   High magnification of Figure 11.3 with papillary fronds lined by pseudostratified columnar epithelium.

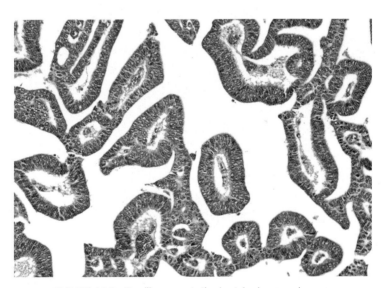

FIGURE 11.5   Papillary prostatic ductal adenocarcinoma.

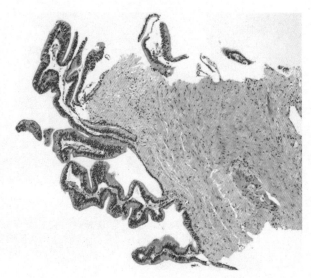

FIGURE 11.6   Papillary prostatic ductal adenocarcinoma at tip of needle biopsy core.

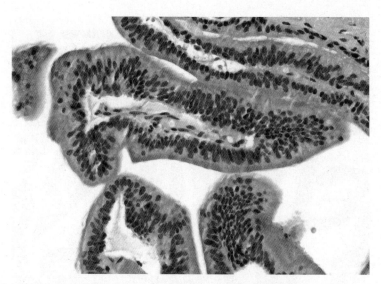

FIGURE 11.7   High magnification of Figure 11.6 with papillary fronds lined by pseudostratified relatively bland columnar epithelium.

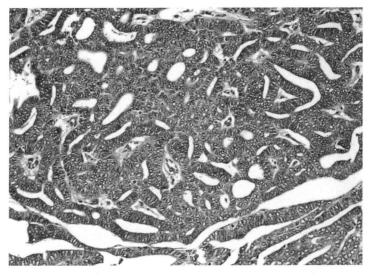

FIGURE 11.8   Cribriform prostatic duct adenocarcinoma.

in the exophytic urethral component of the lesion (Figs. 11.8 and 11.9). The cribriform pattern is formed by back-to-back large glands with intra-glandular epithelial bridging resulting in the formation of slit-like lumens. The epithelial lining is composed of pseudostratified tall columnar epithe-lium often with amphophilic cytoplasm. The pattern is somewhat remi-niscent of endometrial adenocarcinoma within the female. This pattern of prostatic adenocarcinoma differs from the cribriform pattern of prostatic

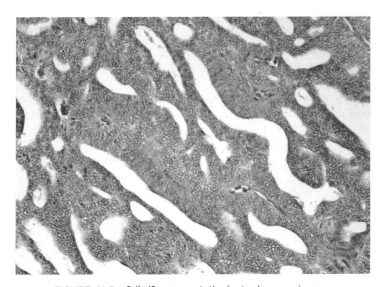

FIGURE 11.9   Cribriform prostatic duct adenocarcinoma.

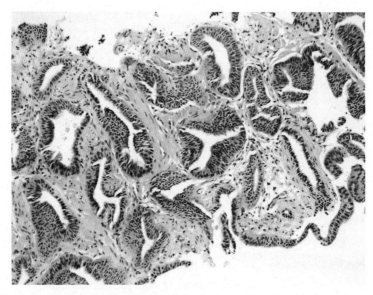

FIGURE 11.10 PIN-like ductal adenocarcinoma. Note strip of epithelium *(bottom)* that corresponds to a large dilated gland. Also note that most of the glands have a relatively flat architecture without the tufting typically seen in high-grade PIN.

acinar adenocarcinoma, which is composed of cuboidal epithelium and punched-out round lumina. It is not uncommon to find areas of papillary formation admixed with cribriform patterns.

The most recently described common pattern is prostatic intra-epithelial neoplasia (PIN)–like ductal adenocarcinoma (also see Chapter 5).[14,15] This variant consists of simple, often cystically dilated glands lined by pseudostratified columnar epithelium, definition of ductal adenocarcinoma (Figs. 11.10 to 11.12). On needle biopsy, the cystic nature of the glands can be discerned by strips of columnar epithelium lining the edge of the cores. The glandular lining is often flat, lacking the papillary or cribriform morphology initially described in ductal adenocarcinoma. As with other patterns of ductal adenocarcinoma, there can be a spectrum of cytologic atypia, although typically, PIN-like ductal adenocarcinoma lacks diffuse prominent nucleoli. Glands of PIN-like ductal adenocarcinoma can be more crowded than high-grade PIN or can be more spaced apart, more closely mimicking high-grade PIN. As a few glands of high-grade PIN can be negative for basal cell markers, one needs many negative glands in order to diagnose PIN-like ductal adenocarcinoma. Cases with only a few glands morphologically suggestive of PIN-like ductal adenocarcinoma are diagnosed as "atypical glands with the differential diagnosis of PIN-like ductal adenocarcinoma versus high-grade PIN. Repeat biopsy is recommended" (Figs. 11.13 and 11.14).

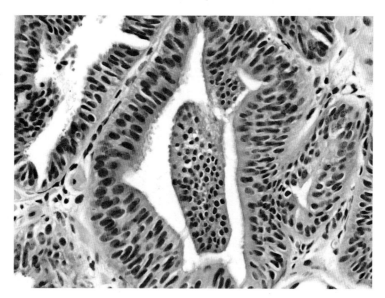

FIGURE 11.11 Same case as Figure 11.10 with relatively bland pseudostratified columnar epithelium.

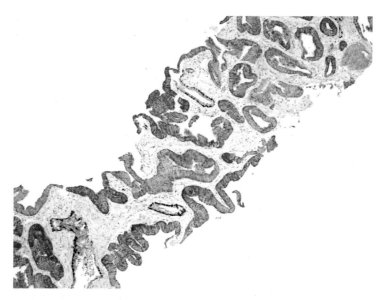

FIGURE 11.12 Same case as Figures 11.10 and 11.11 with triple stain showing PIN-like ductal adenocarcinoma lacking basal cells *(brown)* and positive for alpha-methylacyl-coenzyme A racemase (AMACR) *(red)*.

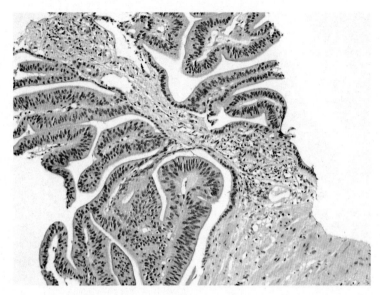

FIGURE 11.13 Atypical glands with the differential diagnosis of PIN-like ductal adenocarcinoma versus high-grade PIN.

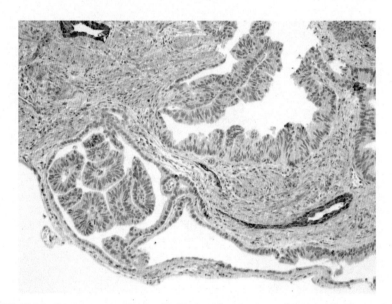

FIGURE 11.14 Same case as Figure 11.13. Despite absence of basal cells *(brown)*, there is an insufficient number of atypical negatively stained glands to rule out high-grade PIN.

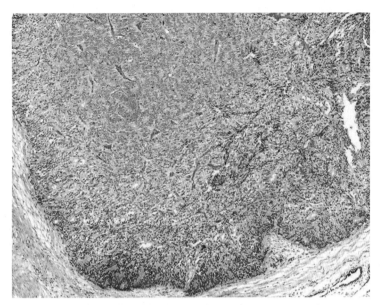

FIGURE 11.15   Solid papillary pattern of prostatic duct adenocarcinoma with evenly distributed thin capillaries.

Other patterns of prostatic duct adenocarcinoma, which by themselves may be difficult to identify as being of prostatic duct origin, may be seen in association with either the papillary or cribriform pattern. Occasionally, solid tumor masses with numerous thin-walled vessels distend prostatic ducts (Fig. 11.15). This pattern is a compact papillary form of prostatic duct adenocarcinoma, because areas can be seen where the solid pattern containing these thin fibrovascular cores open up into more recognizable papillary structures. Prostatic duct adenocarcinomas may also grow as solid nests of tumors with central necrosis. Without seeing this solid pattern in association with more recognizable prostatic duct adenocarcinoma, this pattern cannot be distinguished from poorly differentiated prostatic acinar adenocarcinoma. Prostatic duct adenocarcinomas may resemble infiltrating colonic adenocarcinoma. The differentiation between prostatic duct adenocarcinoma and secondary involvement of the prostate by colonic adenocarcinoma can be made by finding more typical prostatic duct adenocarcinoma elsewhere within the biopsy as well as by immunohistochemical demonstration of PSA and other prostate markers in ductal adenocarcinoma. Adding B-catenin, CDX-2, and villin for colon cancer to the immunohistochemistry panel can be of further use in such a differential.[16,17] However, one must be aware that rare cases of prostatic ductal adenocarcinoma can diffusely express CDX2.[18] *TMPRSS2-ERG* gene fusions are seen to a lesser frequency than with acinar carcinoma.[19] Prostatic duct adenocarcinoma on TUR specimens can also mimic papillary urothelial carcinoma. Nuclear features can be helpful in such differential; nuclei in urothelial carcinoma tend to be more pleomorphic and angulated. Immunohistochemical demonstration of PSA and other prostate markers and negative thrombomodulin and GATA3 staining in prostatic duct adenocarcinoma can also be of help.[17,20–22] Rarely, prostatic ductal adenocarcinoma can be focally lined by mucinous epithelium, although typically, this finding suggests extension from an intestinal primary (Fig. 11.16). Rare variations of ductal adenocarcinoma include those with goblet cells; foamy; and containing Paneth cell-like, micropapillary, and cystic features.[23]

In most cases with mixed acinar and ductal features, the two components are intimately comingled (Fig. 11.17). Other relationships seen between the two types include the coexistence of a centrally located duct carcinoma with a peripherally located acinar tumor. A prostatic duct adenocarcinoma can also express acinar differentiation in either prior or subsequent biopsies. Similarly, metastases from a ductal carcinoma may be purely ductal, acinar, or mixed.[2,24] Ductal adenocarcinoma on needle biopsy may be particularly difficult to diagnose in that there may be mild cytologic atypia without prominent nucleoli.[12] The other feature that can result in underdiagnosis of prostatic duct adenocarcinoma on needle biopsy is tumor fragmentation, resulting in small detached foci of carcinoma. One of the lesions most frequently confused with cytologically bland ductal adenocarcinoma is prostatic urethral polyp. Whereas ductal adenocarcinomas are composed of tall pseudostratified columnar cells, prostatic urethral polyps are polypoid nodules made up of entirely

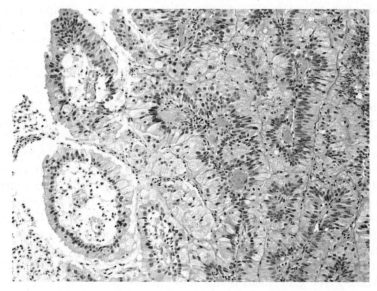

FIGURE 11.16 Prostatic duct adenocarcinoma lined by mucinous epithelium.

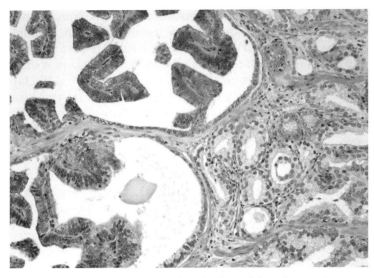

FIGURE 11.17 Mixed ductal *(left)* and acinar *(right)* adenocarcinoma.

benign-appearing prostate acini lined by prostatic glandular epithelium and urothelium (see Chapter 18).

We have found that the number of needle cores containing ductal adenocarcinoma correlate with positive margins at radical prostatectomy and with decreased time to progression. The proportion of ductal as opposed to acinar cancer on needle biopsy does not have predictive power, such that any ductal features on needle biopsy is an adverse prognostic feature.

Most studies consider ductal morphology to connote a more aggressive course than acinar prostate cancer.[1–3,10,25] Ductal adenocarcinomas overall are associated with increased extraprostatic extension, seminal vesicle invasion, and lower biochemical free survival following radical prostatectomy.[4,5,11–13,26,27] Most studies have shown that the percent of the ductal component is not prognostic.[5,11] Overall, the prognosis for usual ductal adenocarcinoma composed of cribriform or papillary architecture is similar to Gleason score 8 adenocarcinoma.[27] Variations of usual ductal adenocarcinoma are assigned different grades and discussed in Chapter 9. In cases with mixed acinar and ductal features, the ductal component is assigned either Gleason pattern 3, 4, or 5, depending on morphology of the ductal component (see Chapter 9).[28,29]

In cases where the urologist takes only a limited transurethral biopsy of the prostate, the entire specimen may consist of a small focus of prostatic duct adenocarcinoma. These tumor foci represent the "tip of the iceberg," where there is more extensive unsampled duct adenocarcinoma involving the underlying ductal system. Ductal adenocarcinomas, as they arise in ducts, may show residual staining for high molecular weight cytokeratin staining (see Chapter 5 for discussion on "intraductal carcinoma").

Regardless of whether the ductal adenocarcinomas consists of a small focus or there is basal cell staining, these tumors should be treated aggressively. The one exception to their treatment is the rare case when there is a good sampling of the prostate with a sizable TUR and there is only a small focus of ductal adenocarcinoma. These small periurethral ductal adenocarcinomas can be completely removed by transurethral resection of the prostate (TURP).[30] Our study of ductal adenocarcinoma on needle biopsy initially challenged the definition of ductal adenocarcinoma of the prostate as an entity unique to the transition zone.[12] We do not adhere to the belief that "clinical and pathologic evidence of involvement of large periurethral prostatic ducts or urethra is required for definitive diagnosis."[31] A large series of radical prostatectomies with ductal adenocarcinoma found that the majority of ductal adenocarcinomas involved the peripheral zone. The transition zone was purely or partly involved in only about 30% of cases with pure transition zone involvement in less than 5% of cases.[5]

REFERENCES

1. Bostwick DG, Kindrachuk RW, Rouse RV. Prostatic adenocarcinoma with endometrioid features. Clinical, pathologic, and ultrastructural findings. *Am J Surg Pathol.* 1985;9: 595–609.
2. Epstein JI, Woodruff JM. Adenocarcinoma of the prostate with endometrioid features. A light microscopic and immunohistochemical study of ten cases. *Cancer.* 1986;57: 111–119.
3. Greene LF, Farrow GM, Ravits JM, et al. Prostatic adenocarcinoma of ductal origin. *J Urol.* 1979;121:303–305.
4. Fine SW. Variants and unusual patterns of prostate cancer: clinicopathologic and differential diagnostic considerations. *Adv Anat Pathol.* 2012;19:204–216.
5. Seipel AH, Wiklund F, Wiklund NP, et al. Histopathological features of ductal adenocarcinoma of the prostate in 1,051 radical prostatectomy specimens. *Virchows Arch.* 2013;462:429–436.
6. Melicow MM, Pachter MR. Endometrial carcinoma of prostatic utricle (uterus masculinus). *Cancer.* 1967;20:1715–1722.
7. Melicow MM, Tannenbaum M. Endometrial carcinoma of uterus masculinus (prostatic utricle). Report of 6 cases. *J Urol.* 1971;106:892–902.
8. Young BW, Lagios MD. Endometrial (papillary) carcinoma of the prostatic utricle—response to orchiectomy. A case report. *Cancer.* 1973;32:1293–1300.
9. Zaloudek C, Williams JW, Kempson RL. "Endometrial" adenocarcinoma of the prostate: a distinctive tumor of probable prostatic duct origin. *Cancer.* 1976;37:2255–2262.
10. Ro JY, Ayala AG, Wishnow KI, et al. Prostatic duct adenocarcinoma with endometrioid features: immunohistochemical and electron microscopic study. *Semin Diagn Pathol.* 1988;5:301–311.
11. Samaratunga H, Duffy D, Yaxley J, et al. Any proportion of ductal adenocarcinoma in radical prostatectomy specimens predicts extraprostatic extension. *Hum Pathol.* 2010; 41:281–285.
12. Brinker DA, Potter SR, Epstein JI. Ductal adenocarcinoma of the prostate diagnosed on needle biopsy: correlation with clinical and radical prostatectomy findings and progression. *Am J Surg Pathol.* 1999;23:1471–1479.

13. Morgan TM, Welty CJ, Vakar-Lopez F, et al. Ductal adenocarcinoma of the prostate: increased mortality risk and decreased serum prostate specific antigen. *J Urol.* 2010; 184:2303–2307.

14. Tavora F, Epstein JI. High-grade prostatic intraepithelial neoplasialike ductal adenocarcinoma of the prostate: a clinicopathologic study of 28 cases. *Am J Surg Pathol.* 2008;32:1060–1067.

15. Hameed O, Humphrey PA. Stratified epithelium in prostatic adenocarcinoma: a mimic of high-grade prostatic intraepithelial neoplasia. *Mod Pathol.* 2006;19:899–906.

16. Owens CL, Epstein JI, Netto GJ. Distinguishing prostatic from colorectal adenocarcinoma on biopsy samples: the role of morphology and immunohistochemistry. *Arch Pathol Lab Med.* 2007;131:599–603.

17. Hameed O, Humphrey PA. Immunohistochemistry in diagnostic surgical pathology of the prostate. *Semin Diagn Pathol.* 2005;22:88–104.

18. Herawi M, De Marzo AM, Kristiansen G, et al. Expression of CDX2 in benign tissue and adenocarcinoma of the prostate. *Hum Pathol.* 2007;38:72–78.

19. Lotan TL, Toubaji A, Albadine R, et al. TMPRSS2-ERG gene fusions are infrequent in prostatic ductal adenocarcinomas. *Mod Pathol.* 2009;22:359–365.

20. Oxley J, Abbott C. Thrombomodulin immunostaining and ductal carcinoma of the prostate. *Histopathology.* 1998;33:391–392.

21. Chang A, Amin A, Gabrielson E, et al. Utility of GATA3 immunohistochemistry in differentiating urothelial carcinoma from prostate adenocarcinoma and squamous cell carcinomas of the uterine cervix, anus, and lung. *Am J Surg Pathol.* 2012;36:1472–1476.

22. Chuang AY, DeMarzo AM, Veltri RW, et al. Immunohistochemical differentiation of high-grade prostate carcinoma from urothelial carcinoma. *Am J Surg Pathol.* 2007; 31:1246–1255.

23. Lee TK, Miller JS, Epstein JI. Rare histological patterns of prostatic ductal adenocarcinoma. *Pathology.* 2010;42:319–324.

24. Gong Y, Caraway N, Stewart J, et al. Metastatic ductal adenocarcinoma of the prostate: cytologic features and clinical findings. *Am J Clin Pathol.* 2006;126:302–309.

25. Christensen WN, Steinberg G, Walsh PC, et al. Prostatic duct adenocarcinoma. Findings at radical prostatectomy. *Cancer.* 1991;67:2118–2124.

26. Amin A, Epstein JI. Pathologic stage of prostatic ductal adenocarcinoma at radical prostatectomy: effect of percentage of the ductal component and associated grade of acinar adenocarcinoma. *Am J Surg Pathol.* 2011;35:615–619.

27. Meeks JJ, Zhao LC, Cashy J, et al. Incidence and outcomes of ductal carcinoma of the prostate in the USA: analysis of data from the Surveillance, Epidemiology, and End Results program. *BJU Int.* 2012;109:831–834.

28. Epstein JI, Allsbrook WC Jr, Amin MB, et al. Update on the Gleason grading system for prostate cancer: results of an international consensus conference of urologic pathologists. *Adv Anat Pathol.* 2006;13:57–59.

29. Epstein JI, Allsbrook WC Jr, Amin MB, et al. The 2005 International Society of Urological Pathology (ISUP) Consensus Conference on Gleason Grading of Prostatic Carcinoma. *Am J Surg Pathol.* 2005;29:1228–1242.

30. Aydin H, Zhang J, Samaratunga H, et al. Ductal adenocarcinoma of the prostate diagnosed on transurethral biopsy or resection is not always indicative of aggressive disease: implications for clinical management. *BJU Int.* 2010;105:476–480.

31. Bostwick DG. Neoplasms of the prostate. In: Bostwick DG, Eble JN, eds. *Urologic Surgical Pathology.* St. Louis, MO: Mosby; 1997:366–368.

12

NEUROENDOCRINE DIFFERENTIATION IN THE BENIGN AND MALIGNANT PROSTATE

NEUROENDOCRINE CELLS IN NORMAL PROSTATE HISTOLOGY

The neuroendocrine (NE) component of the normal prostate consists of a small subset of cells, randomly scattered within the epithelium of the prostate glands in all anatomic zones. These cells contain a variety of peptide hormones, such as serotonin, histamine, chromogranin A, calcitonin, and other members of the calcitonin gene family, neuropeptide Y, vasoactive intestinal peptide, bombesin-/gastrin-releasing peptide, parathyroid hormone–related protein, neuron-specific enolase (NSE), thyroid-stimulating hormone–like peptide, somatostatin, vascular endothelial growth factor, and others.[1–3] These substances affect target cells by endocrine, paracrine, and autocrine mechanisms. By light microscopy, these cells rest on the basal cell layer between the secretory cells. They typically do not extend to the lumen but often have narrow apical and lateral dendritic extensions. They are not reliably recognizable by hematoxylin and eosin (H&E) examination but may contain granular eosinophilic cytoplasm distinct from Paneth cell-like change.[4,5] NE cells are more commonly present in the prostate than any other organ within the genitourinary tract.

NEUROENDOCRINE CELLS AND DIFFERENTIATION IN PROSTATE CANCER

NE cells are defined in current practice by immunohistochemical positivity for either synaptophysin, chromogranin, or CD56. NSE immunoreactivity is, despite its name, not sufficiently specific for the diagnosis of NE differentiation. NE cells have also been noted in neoplasms of the prostate, where they have generated recent interest in their relation to castration-resistant disease. NE cells lack androgen receptors (ARs) and NE differentiation increases after androgen deprivation and in castration-resistant prostate cancer (CRPC).[6] As a result of their secretory products, NE cells could stimulate the proliferation of prostate carcinoma cells and increase

TABLE 12.1 Classification of Neuroendocrine Differentiation in Prostate Carcinoma
Usual prostate adenocarcinoma with neuroendocrine differentiation
Adenocarcinoma with Paneth cell-like neuroendocrine differentiation
Carcinoid tumor
Small cell carcinoma
Large cell neuroendocrine carcinoma
Mixed neuroendocrine carcinoma—acinar adenocarcinoma
Prostate carcinoma with overlapping features of small cell and acinar adenocarcinoma
Castration-resistant prostate cancer (CRPC) with small cell carcinoma–like clinical presentation

their aggressiveness through the inhibition of apoptosis and stimulation of neoangiogenesis.[1,7–10] The amount of NE differentiation of prostate adenocarcinoma increases with disease progression and in response to androgen deprivation therapy (ADT).[6,11,12] There is also emerging evidence suggesting that transformation to a predominantly AR-negative prostate cancer with increasing NE differentiation by immunohistochemistry (IHC) may be an important resistance mechanism in castration-resistant disease and is likely more common than previously recognized. This may be related to patients living longer, more potent AR signaling inhibition with new approved therapies (i.e., abiraterone, enzalutamide), and/or increased awareness due to more common metastatic biopsy protocols in the setting of CRPC.[13,14]

The current World Health Organization (WHO) histologic classification of NE tumors of the prostate includes (a) focal NE differentiation in conventional prostate adenocarcinoma, (b) carcinoid tumor (WHO well-differentiated NE tumor), and (3) small cell NE carcinoma (WHO classification, poorly differentiated NE carcinoma).[15] Although this NE classification is analogous to other organs, it does not account for the unique aspects of NE differentiation in prostate cancer. The newly proposed classification of NE prostate carcinoma is outlined in Table 12.1.

USUAL PROSTATE ADENOCARCINOMA WITH NEUROENDOCRINE DIFFERENTIATION

In the early 1970s, Azzopardi and Evans[4] recognized the presence of argentaffin cells within normal prostatic adenocarcinoma. Immunohistochemically, usual adenocarcinoma of the prostate demonstrates scattered NE cells in 10% to 100% of cases, in part depending on the number of slides studied and the number of antibodies used (Fig. 12.1).[7,12,16,17]

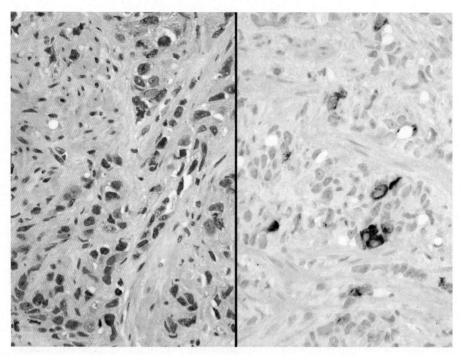

FIGURE 12.1   Gleason score 5 + 5 = 10 adenocarcinoma **(left)** with scattered synaptophysin positive cells **(right)**.

In these cases, prostate-specific antigen (PSA) is positive in the usual adenocarcinoma but variably positive in the NE cells.[18] It is controversial whether NE differentiation in typical adenocarcinomas worsens prognosis. In some studies suggesting a correlation, the prognostic relationship was weak and not sufficient to be useful clinically.[1,19–22] Most of the studies have shown no effect of NE differentiation on outcome, including one study each analyzing NE differentiation in prostate cancer on needle biopsy and transurethral resection of the prostate (TURP).[23–34]

Currently, as the clinical significance remains uncertain, it is not recommended to routinely employ immunohistochemical stains to detect any NE differentiation in an otherwise morphologically typical primary adenocarcinoma of the prostate.

ADENOCARCINOMA WITH PANETH CELL-LIKE NEUROENDOCRINE DIFFERENTIATION

The term *Paneth cell-like change* has been used to describe distinctive eosinophilic NE cells (eFig. 12.1).[35] Paneth cell-like NE differentiation in prostatic adenocarcinoma can be seen as either patchy isolated cells or diffusely involving glands or nests.[36,37] These Paneth cell-like cells may be present in well-formed glands of Gleason pattern 3 (Fig. 12.2) but also can

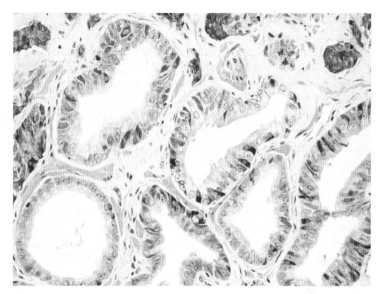

FIGURE 12.2   Gleason score 6 adenocarcinoma with Paneth cell-like NE granules.

be present in cords of cells with bland cytology, where strictly applying the Gleason grading system, one would assign a Gleason pattern 5 (Fig. 12.3, eFigs. 12.2 to 12.7). Although by the Gleason system areas of Paneth cell-like NE differentiation may be graded as pattern 5, their bland cytology, typically limited nature, and frequent association with lower grade conventional

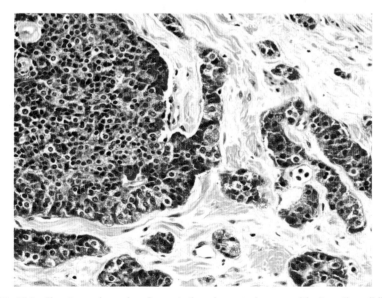

FIGURE 12.3   Sheets and cords of prostatic adenocarcinoma with Paneth cell-like NE granules.

adenocarcinoma raise questions as to whether this unique histology should not be diagnosed as high grade. Of 16 radical prostatectomy specimens with Paneth cell-like NE cells lacking glandular differentiation, there was organ-confined cancer in 62.5% of cases, only 4 cases with seminal vesicle invasion, and none with pelvic lymph node metastases. The postoperative course was also favorable with an over 90% actuarial PSA progression-free risk at 5 years. The prognosis seemed to be driven by conventional parameters independent of NE differentiation. The only two patients who progressed after radical prostatectomy had Gleason score 7 conventional cancer with extraprostatic extension and seminal vesicle invasion, with one also having ductal differentiation and positive margins. In cases in which the entire tumor is composed of Paneth cell-like cells and areas of the tumor lack glandular differentiation, it is questionable whether these tumors should be assigned a Gleason score. A comment could be provided as to the generally favorable prognosis of this morphologic variant of adenocarcinoma of the prostate based on the limited data available.[36] However, the data on the prognostic significance of Paneth cell-like differentiation is still limited, and we have seen anecdotal cases where such a tumor progressed to metastatic disease with small cell carcinoma.

In some cases, one can see a spectrum of Paneth cell-like cells with eosinophilic granules adjacent to identical cells with deeply amphophilic cytoplasm lacking granules, with both cell types labeling diffusely with NE markers (Figs. 12.4 and 12.5). Uncommonly, cancers may only consist of cords of cells with bland cytology and only amphophilic cytoplasm, either with rare or absence of the characteristic eosinophilic granules (Fig. 12.6).

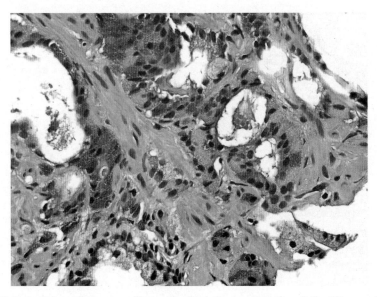

FIGURE 12.4 Adenocarcinoma with some glands having Paneth cell-like NE granules and other glands with deeply amphophilic cytoplasm.

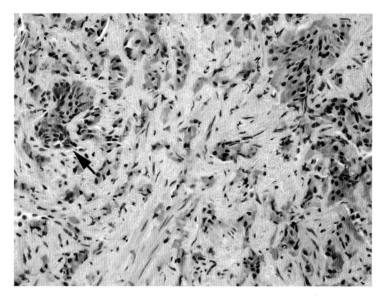

FIGURE 12.5   Cords of adenocarcinoma of the prostate with amphophilic cytoplasm and scattered cells with eosinophilic granules *(arrow)*.

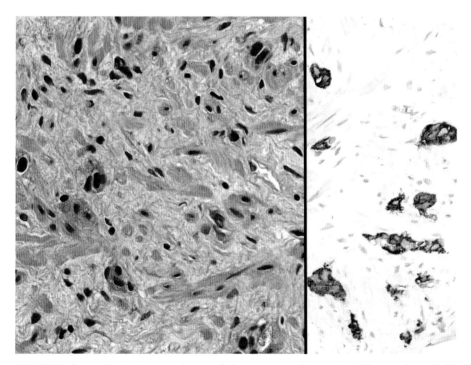

FIGURE 12.6   Cords of adenocarcinoma of the prostate with amphophilic cytoplasm **(left)** staining diffusely for synaptophysin **(right)**.

These cells are also diffusely positive for NE markers. These cells with amphophilic cytoplasm arranged in cords with bland cytology, typically in a very limited focus, are typically associated with other cells showing Paneth cell-like changes and should be considered a variant of Paneth cell-like change. Both the classic Paneth cell-like changes and this variant may not express prostate markers, possibly given that their cytoplasm is replaced by NE granules. The key to recognizing these cases is first to note the architectural pattern of nests and cords in a small focus. Secondly, these tumors have deeply amphophilic cytoplasm with careful search in most cases, revealing rare Paneth cell-like eosinophilic granules. Finally, the preceding finding in combination with either no prominent nucleoli or rare visible nucleoli may prompt immunohistochemical staining for NE markers.

Currently, as the clinical significance is incompletely understood, one may employ immunohistochemical stains to confirm NE differentiation in the eosinophilic (Paneth cell-like) and amphophilic cells. The term *adenocarcinoma with Paneth cell-like NE differentiation* should be used. Additionally, a comment may be made that in the absence of prior ADT, Gleason grading of areas showing Paneth cell-like or amphophilic NE change in areas without glandular differentiation may not be applicable.

CARCINOID TUMOR

True carcinoid tumors of the prostate are extremely rare. In order to diagnose a carcinoid of the prostate and distinguish it from a prostate adenocarcinoma with carcinoid-like features, the following features should be present: (a) not closely associated with concomitant adenocarcinoma of the prostate, (b) immunohistochemically positive for NE markers and negative for PSA, and (c) originating in the prostatic parenchyma. Of the cases in the literature, there are only five cases that satisfy this definition.[38-41] Some of the older reported cases of carcinoid tumor of the prostate predate the use of IHC and cannot be verified. One case based on the illustration provided is a urethral carcinoid as opposed to prostatic in origin.[42] The reports by Slater[43] in a 69-year-old and by Tash et al.[44] in a 38-year-old male may be carcinoids, yet immunohistochemical stains for PSA or any other prostatic marker were not reported. Similarly, in the study by Wasserstein and Goldman,[45] no IHC was performed. Murali et al.[46] illustrate images of two prostatic carcinoids in their review article, yet no details are provided about the cases. Turbat-Herrera et al.[47] reported a "prostatic carcinoid" that was negative for PSA, yet in contrast to carcinoids, only 2+ scattered synaptophysin-positive cells were present and the tumor had diffuse prominent nucleoli. The prostatic carcinoid reported by Egan et al.[48] had "intraductal carcinoid" and was admixed with usual prostate adenocarcinoma and most likely represents the recently described phenomenon of "small cell-like change in high-grade prostatic intraepithelial neoplasia, intraductal carcinoma, and invasive prostatic adenocarcinoma."[49] There are five bona fide cases of prostatic carcinoids. Two cases were in men in their 30s, younger than typically seen with adenocarcinoma of the prostate.[38,39] The remaining three cases were in even younger males with multiple endocrine neoplasia (MEN) IIB syndrome.[40,41] Patients were 7, 19, and 22 years of age. Although the data is limited, prostatic carcinoids tend to present with locally advanced disease, including some with regional lymph node metastases yet still have a favorable prognosis. It is reasonable for these true carcinoids to grade them in an analogous fashion to those of gastrointestinal tract based on mitotic rates and Ki67 proliferation rates.

Several cases have been reported where a "carcinoid-like" or "carcinoidal" appearance of the tumor with nested architecture and uniform nuclei has been present (eFigs. 12.8 and 12.9). These tumors may on occasion also exhibit immunohistochemical and/or ultrastructural evidence of NE differentiation. Some authors consider immunohistochemical staining with PSA a key discriminator where true prostatic carcinoids are negative and carcinoid-like carcinomas are positive. Most cases reported with carcinoid-like morphology have admixed usual prostate cancer or the carcinoid-like tumor expressed PSA.[50–56] Several carcinoid-like prostate cancers appear to be variants of Paneth cell-like NE differentiation with a paucity or absence of eosinophilic granules where PSA may be negative (Fig. 12.7).[57]

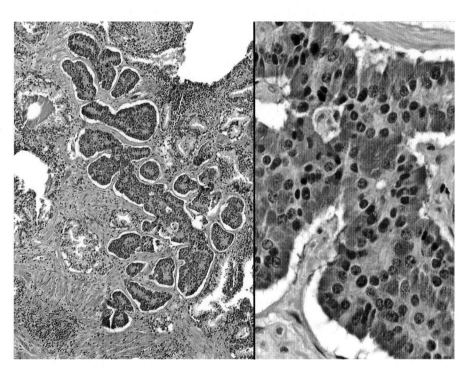

FIGURE 12.7 Carcinoid-like tumor with nests of cells **(left)**. Higher magnification **(right)** shows uniform round nuclei with "salt and pepper" chromatin and scattered Paneth cell-like granules. The tumor was positive for NE markers and negative for PSA. Adjacent was usual adenocarcinoma (not shown).

Clinically, carcinoid-like adenocarcinomas have behaved like ordinary pros-tate carcinomas and in none of these cases has a carcinoid syndrome been present. Prostate-specific acid phosphatase (PSAP) immunoreactivity is not discriminatory in the assessment of whether a tumor is a true carcinoid or adenocarcinoma with carcinoid-like features as even some nonprostatic carcinoid tumors express PSAP.[58] Although most carcinoid-like tumors have not produced clinical symptoms, several cases have produced adreno-corticotropic hormone (ACTH) in sufficient quantity to result in Cushing syndrome.[52]

The diagnosis of carcinoid tumor should be made very rarely and strictly, applying the criteria outlined earlier in the definition. In such cases, particularly in younger patients, investigation for stigmata of MEN syndrome should be initiated. Tumors with PSA-negative nests and cords of cells, which are admixed with usual prostate adenocarcinoma, should not be diagnosed as carcinoid tumor because such cases may represent adenocarcinoma with Paneth cell-like NE differentiation or its more subtle variant with cytoplasmic amphophilia.

SMALL CELL CARCINOMA

Small cell carcinoma is a high-grade tumor defined by characteristic nuclear features, including lack of prominent nucleoli, nuclear molding, fragility, and crush artifact. High nuclear to cytoplasmic ratio and indistinct cell borders are characteristic, as is a high mitotic rate and apoptotic bodies (Fig. 12.8, eFigs. 12.10 to 12.15). In resection specimens, as opposed to needle biopsy cores, geographic necrosis may be frequent.

Approximately 40% to 50% of small cell carcinomas have a history of usual prostatic adenocarcinoma. The interval between the diagnosis of small cell carcinoma and prior usual prostatic cancer ranges from 1 to 300 months (median: 25 months).[59] Historically, pure small cell carcinoma was seen at initial diagnosis in about 50% to 60% of cases, with the remaining cases admixed with prostate adenocarcinoma (as discussed later). Clinical recognition of the emergence of small cell carcinoma during the progres-sion of the disease is increasing and leading to more frequent biopsies of metastatic sites. Patients with this aggressive disease have frequent visceral metastases and less often paraneoplastic syndromes such as those associ-ated with ectopic ACTH, hypercalcemia, or inappropriate antidiuretic hormone (ADH) production. The diagnosis of small cell carcinoma of the prostate is reached based on morphologic features similar to those found in small cell carcinomas of the lung as defined in the 1999 WHO clas-sification criteria of pulmonary neoplasms.[60–62] Morphologic variations of small cell carcinoma include intermediate cell type with slightly more open chromatin and visible small nucleoli seen in about 30% to 40% of cases, which may be beyond that allowable in the strict diagnosis of small cell carcinoma of the lung (Fig. 12.9).[59] Less commonly, there is the presence of tumor giant cells and Indian filing.[59] Neurosecretory granules

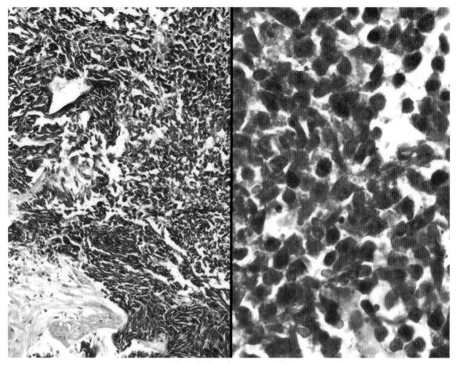

FIGURE 12.8   Low **(left)** and high **(right)** magnification of small cell carcinoma of the prostate.

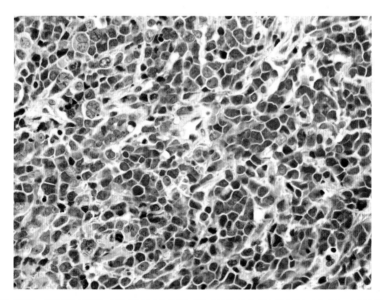

FIGURE 12.9   Intermediate cell type variant of small cell carcinoma of the prostate with slightly more open chromatin and occasional small nucleoli. Tumor was positive for NE markers (not shown).

have been demonstrated within several prostatic small cell carcinomas. Using immunohistochemical techniques, the small cell component is positive for one or more NE markers (synaptophysin, chromogranin, CD56) in almost 90% of cases.[59-61] PSA and other prostatic markers such as P501s are positive in about 17% to 25% of cases, although often very focally.[59-61] In 24% to 35% of cases, positivity is noted for p63 and high molecular weight cytokeratin, markers typically negative in prostatic carcinoma.[61] Studies have demonstrated TTF-1 expression in over 50% of small cell carcinomas of the prostate, limiting its use in distinguishing primary small cell carcinoma of the prostate from a metastasis from the lung.[59,61,63,64]

Because of the rarity of primary small cell carcinoma of the prostate, an important diagnostic consideration is exclusion of metastasis or local extension from other site such as bladder. A technique that can distinguish small cell carcinoma of the prostate from other small cell carcinomas is documentation by fluorescence in situ hybridization (FISH) or reverse transcriptase polymerase chain reaction (RT-PCR) of a gene fusion between members of the ETS family of genes, in particular *ERG* (ETS-related gene) and *TMPRSS2*, found in approximately one-half of usual prostatic adenocarcinoma.[65] In a similar percent of cases, small cell carcinoma of the prostate is positive for *TMPRSS2-ERG* gene fusion by FISH.[66-71] Importantly, it should be noted that compared to usual acinar carcinoma harboring *TMPRSS2-ERG* rearrangements, small cell carcinoma with *TMPRSS2-ERG* rearrangement is not reliably positive for ERG protein by IHC, presumably due to lack of AR expression in small cell carcinoma.[66] Additionally, in the setting of standard treatment for CRPC, ERG protein expression may not be present by IHC requiring the use of FISH. According to one study, there is strong and diffuse membrane staining for CD44 in all prostatic NE small cell carcinomas, whereas in usual prostatic adenocarcinomas, only rare positive scattered tumor cells are CD44 positive.[43] However, current work by one of the authors have not substantiated this finding and have concluded that this antibody is not useful in the distinction of high-grade adenocarcinoma of the prostate from small cell carcinoma.

The median cancer-specific survival of patients with small cell carcinoma of the prostate in 191 men according to the Surveillance, Epidemiology, and End Results (SEER) database from 1973 to 2004 was 19 months. Metastatic disease was presented by 60.5% of men, with a decreased survival related to stage. Two- and 5-year survival rates were 27.5% and 14.3%, respectively.[72] Given the high rate of occult metastases, clinically localized small cell prostate cancer is typically treated aggressively, often with multimodality therapy with chemotherapy and radiation similar to limited stage small cell lung cancer. Metastatic small cell carcinoma of the prostate is treated with platinum-based combination chemotherapy with regimens similar to those used to treat small cell lung carcinoma.[73-76] Some experts treat pure small cell carcinoma with chemotherapy alone, whereas others add ADT.

In summary, small cell carcinoma of the prostate is an aggressive malignancy recognized by relatively typical morphologic features although cases occurring in the prostate may exhibit a slightly wider spectrum of cytologic features than would be allowable at other tumor sites. In tumors showing classic morphology, IHC may not be necessary, although may be frequently useful for confirmation of the diagnosis in view of its important prognostic and therapeutic ramifications.

LARGE CELL NEUROENDOCRINE CARCINOMA

Large cell neuroendocrine carcinoma (LCNEC) of prostate is exceptionally rare, particularly its pure form. The largest series by Evans et al.[77] describes seven cases of LCNEC, only one pure and apparently de novo. Six other cases represented progression from prior typical prostate adenocarcinoma, following long-standing hormonal therapy. According to the authors, the large cell NE component was composed of sheets and ribbons of amphophilic cells with large nuclei, coarse chromatin, and prominent nucleoli (Fig. 12.10). Mitotic activity was high, and foci of necrosis were present. The LCNEC component was strongly positive for CD56, CD57, chromogranin A, synaptophysin, and P504S (Fig. 12.11). Ki67 proliferative index was greater than 50%. LCNEC has also been described in association with small cell carcinoma and adenocarcinoma.[78]

Importantly, in this series, a minor (<10%) component of conventional prostate adenocarcinoma showing hormonal deprivation effect was identified in all but the single de novo case. In the remainder of cases,

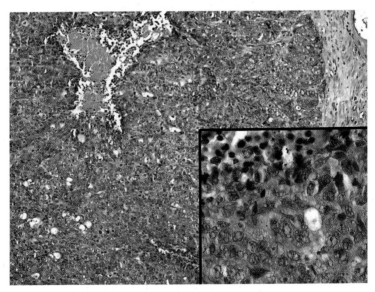

FIGURE 12.10 LCNEC sheets of cells and geographic necrosis *(left)* with prominent nucleoli *(inset)*.

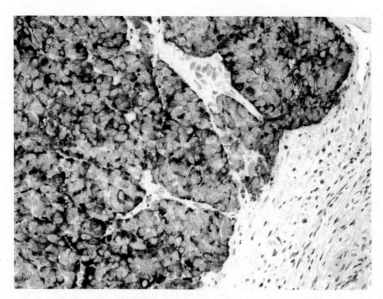

FIGURE 12.11 LCNEC (same case as Fig. 12.10) with diffuse chromogranin immuno-reactivity.

the authors describe "hybrid features of both LCNEC and conventional-type prostatic adenocarcinoma" with treatment effect. They describe PSA and PSAP expression in the conventional component that was focal or absent in the LCNEC areas. Although prostate markers are usually negative in LCNEC, we have noted cases with all the H&E and immunohistochemical features of LCNEC with PSA staining. Given that Gleason score 5 + 5 = 10 adenocarcinoma may on occasion diffusely express NE markers immunohistochemically, it is the consensus that the definition of LCNEC should be more restrictive than what was reported by Evans et al.[77] In addition to immunohistochemical expression of NE markers, there should also be evidence of morphologic NE differentiation consisting of large nests of cells with peripheral palisading. Diagnosed accordingly, LCNEC is extremely rare. Given its rarity and that usual high-grade prostate adenocarcinoma with immunohistochemical expression of NE markers have incorrectly been included in the past as LCNEC, additional studies are needed to categorize the treatment and prognosis of LCNEC. In the study by Evans et al.,[77] cases were associated with rapid dissemination and death with metastatic disease at a mean period of 7 months.

MIXED NEUROENDOCRINE CARCINOMA–ACINAR ADENOCARCINOMA

It is not infrequent that tumors are mixed small cell carcinoma and adenocarcinoma of the prostate.[59] In mixed cases, the transition between the small cell and acinar components is abrupt and each readily identifiable as distinctive (Figs. 12.12 and 12.13, eFigs. 12.16 to 12.18). Typically, the

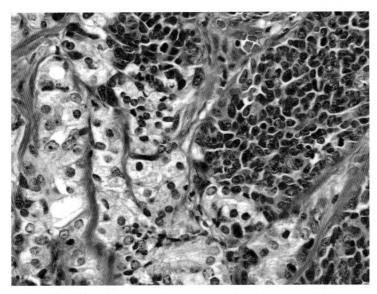

FIGURE 12.12 Mixed usual adenocarcinoma of the prostate *(left)* with small cell carcinoma *(right)*.

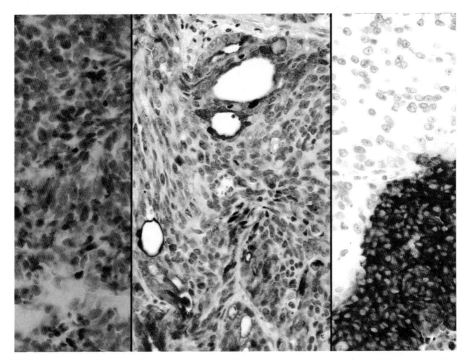

FIGURE 12.13 Same case as Figure 12.12 with small cell carcinoma component positive for TTF-1 **(left)**. Synaptophysin labeled the small cell carcinoma component **(right, bottom)** and not the adenocarcinoma component **(right, top)**. PSA **(center)** was positive in the adenocarcinoma component but not in the small cell carcinoma.

non–small cell component is usual conventional acinar adenocarcinoma, but rarely, the adenocarcinoma component may have ductal or other variant features. As with other unusual subtypes of prostate cancer, we do not assign a Gleason score to small cell carcinoma, but only to the conventional adenocarcinoma component if untreated. In reported mixed cases, small cell carcinoma predominated (median: 80% of the tumor); the Gleason score of the adenocarcinoma was 8 or higher in 85% of these cases.[59] According to the SEER database, in a study of 191 men with prostatic small cell carcinoma, the presence of concomitant high-grade adenocarcinoma as opposed to lower grade adenocarcinoma was an independent predictor of worse cancer-specific mortality.[72] In this study, the relative amount of small cell carcinoma was not recorded. Most patients with mixed small cell carcinoma and adenocarcinoma present with metastatic castration-resistant disease. In these cases, whether mixed small cell and adenocarcinoma are treated differently compared to pure small cell carcinoma depends on the clinical scenario. Patients with metastatic mixed tumors that are clinically aggressive are often treated with both ADT plus chemotherapy (platinum + etoposide or platinum + taxane).

In tumors showing classic morphology, IHC may not be necessary, although may be frequently useful for confirmation of the diagnosis in view of its important prognostic and therapeutic ramifications. Because the role of potent AR-targeted therapies such as abiraterone acetate and enzalutamide in cases of metastatic castration-resistant mixed NE-adenocarcinoma is uncertain, it is recommended that the percentage and grade of the acinar component be provided. This information may be valuable for individual case management and as data for further studies.

PROSTATE CARCINOMA WITH OVERLAPPING FEATURES OF SMALL CELL AND ACINAR ADENOCARCINOMA

Uncommonly, a significant component or the entire prostatic tumor shows overlap between small cell carcinoma and usual prostate adenocarcinoma without discrete classic small cell carcinoma or usual prostate adenocarcinoma components (Figs. 12.14 to 12.17) (eFig. 12.19). It should not be surprising that these cases exist as small cell carcinoma is currently thought to represent transdifferentiation from usual prostate adenocarcinoma.[79,80] These overlap cases are particularly difficult to determine whether they should be diagnosed as small cell carcinoma or Gleason pattern 5 adenocarcinoma. Tumor is typically arranged in sheets but lumen formation can be seen without the apical cytoplasm seen in gland-forming adenocarcinoma. Cells typically have scant cytoplasm with smaller nucleoli than seen in Gleason pattern 5 adenocarcinoma yet more prominent than seen in small cell carcinoma. Mitotic figures are common. Typically within the tumor, there is a continuum of morphologies present, with some areas showing more features of small cell carcinoma and

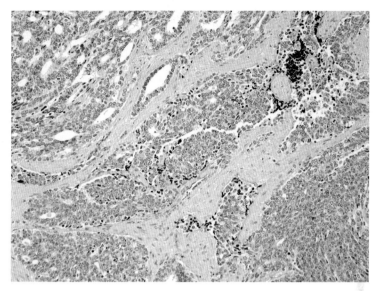

FIGURE 12.14   Case with overlapping features between small cell and usual adenocarcinoma with gland formation *(upper left)* and sheets of cells *(lower right)*.

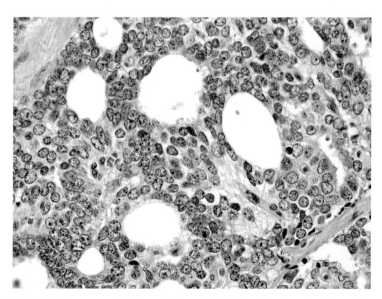

FIGURE 12.15   Higher magnification of Figure 12.14. Despite showing lumen formation, there is a lack of apical cytoplasm typical of usual adenocarcinoma of the prostate.

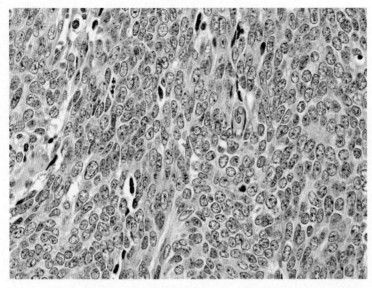

FIGURE 12.16 Higher magnification of Figure 12.14 with solid sheets of cells. Cells have a high nuclear to cytoplasmic ratio like small cell carcinoma yet lack its high mitotic/apoptotic rate. Nucleoli are intermediate between small cell and usual adenocarcinoma of the prostate.

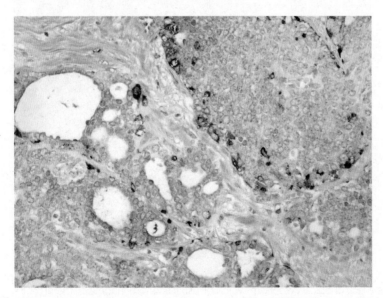

FIGURE 12.17 Same case as Figures 12.14 to 12.16 with positivity for synaptophysin in both solid and glandular areas.

others which more closely resemble high-grade adenocarcinoma. IHC for NE markers shows positivity as is the staining for prostate markers.

These tumors are best recognized when there is morphologic concern for NE carcinoma (sheetlike architecture and scant cytoplasm) but in which the morphologic features, particularly the cytology, are not typical for either small cell carcinoma or conventional acinar carcinoma. As there has not been a specific category for these lesions, there is no data on their prognosis and optimal treatment, and further studies are encouraged. Consequently, the issue of appropriateness of Gleason grading for these cases has not been addressed.

CASTRATION-RESISTANT PROSTATE CANCER WITH SMALL CELL CARCINOMA–LIKE CLINICAL PRESENTATION

Genitourinary oncologists have noted certain clinical features characteristic of small cell carcinoma of the prostate. These clinical features are distinct from what is typically seen in usual prostate adenocarcinoma and are present in a significant proportion of morphologically heterogeneous CRPCs. Some experts have hypothesized that prostate cancers that share clinical features with small cell prostate cancer (Table 12.2) also share its responsiveness to chemotherapy and underlying biology.[75] These cases have been termed *anaplastic prostate cancer* by clinicians. The term *anaplastic* is unsatisfactory because it has a more specific meaning for surgical pathologists denoting pleomorphic cytology and could lead to

---

TABLE 12.2 Clinical Manifestations Associated with Small Cell Carcinoma

- Visceral metastases
- Radiographically predominant lytic bone metastases by plain x-ray or CT scan
- Bulky (5 cm) lymphadenopathy or bulky (>5 cm) high-grade (Gleason >8) tumor mass in prostate/pelvis
- Low PSA at initial presentation (before ADT or at symptomatic progression in the castrate setting) plus high-volume tumor burden. High level of serum chromogranin can be detectable.
- Short interval (<6 months) to androgen-independent progression following the initiation of hormonal therapy with or without the presence of neuroendocrine markers.
- Any of the following in the absence of other causes: (a) elevated serum LDH (>2 × IULN), (b) malignant hypercalcemia, (c) elevated serum CEA (>2 × IULN)

CT, computed tomography; PSA, prostate-specific antigen; ADT, androgen deprivation therapy; LDH, lactate dehydrogenase; IULN, International units - limits of normal; CEA, carcinoembryonic antigen.

additional confusion. Morphologically, cases with these clinical findings could be pure or mixed small cell carcinoma, yet could also consist of the typical histology of high-grade usual prostatic adenocarcinoma or large cell NE carcinoma.[81] As there is greater understanding, acceptance, and refinement of CRPC, it is anticipated that tumors within this clinical category will be further classified into molecularly defined pathologic subsets. The understanding of their biology will facilitate the establishment of an optical nomenclature that encompasses the clinical and pathologic spectrum of these tumors. With the introduction of new potent hormonal agents into the clinic, its incidence is anticipated to escalate.

IMMUNOHISTOCHEMISTRY AND FLUORESCENCE IN SITU HYBRIDIZATION IN THE DIAGNOSIS AND CLASSIFICATION OF NEUROENDOCRINE DIFFERENTIATION IN PROSTATE CANCER

IHC plays a vital role and should be approached at two levels. For the issue of confirming NE differentiation, markers for NE differentiation include synaptophysin, chromogranin, and CD56. CD57 (Leu7) is expressed in a high percentage of acinar adenocarcinomas with and without NE differentiation and, along with NSE, are not recommended.

If there is any uncertainty about the histogenesis, that is, whether a tumor is primary to the prostate, markers for prostatic lineage—PSA, PSAP, prostate-specific membrane antigen (PSMA), prostein (p501s), NKX3.1, and ERG (by IHC or FISH)—may be used. In our opinion, PSA and ERG FISH detection would be the first line of approach.

Additional considerations for the role of IHC include for diagnosis, prognosis, and predictive purposes. The formal use of Ki67/MIB-1 IHC is not established, although Ki67 rates are typically higher than 50% and often higher than 80% in small cell carcinoma and LCNEC with much lower rates in usual high-grade adenocarcinoma of the prostate, carcinoid tumor, and adenocarcinoma with Paneth cell-like NE differentiation. Molecular studies of CRPC (which include cases showing NE differentiation) show alterations of AR signaling and loss of PSA expression by IHC. The IHC expression of AR across the proposed subtypes of NE carcinoma needs to be systematically evaluated such that its role in classification of these tumors may be determined. Promising new molecular targets that may be amenable to future IHC- or FISH-based classification and predictive strategies include Aurora A kinase and N-Myc, although these markers are not yet validated for clinical use.[80,81]

One final issue regarding the use of IHC in workup of these cases concerns the type of pathologic sample that is best for this analysis. In patients with multiple samples, including needle biopsies, radical prostatectomy, and sampling of a metastasis, the metastatic site and/or the histology of the sample most suspicious for NE differentiation should be evaluated.

REFERENCES

1. Abrahamsson PA. Neuroendocrine cells in tumour growth of the prostate. *Endocr Relat Cancer*. 1999;6:503–519.

2. Abrahamsson PA, Wadstrom LB, Alumets J, et al. Peptide-hormone- and serotonin-immunoreactive tumour cells in carcinoma of the prostate. *Pathol Res Pract*. 1987;182:298–307.

3. Bonkhoff H, Stein U, Remberger K. Androgen receptor status in endocrine-paracrine cell types of the normal, hyperplastic, and neoplastic human prostate. *Virchows Arch A Pathol Anat Histopathol*. 1993;423:291–294.

4. Azzopardi JG, Evans DJ. Argentaffin cells in prostatic carcinoma: differentiation from lipofuscin and melanin in prostatic epithelium. *J Pathol*. 1971;104:247–251.

5. Kazzaz BA. Argentaffin and argyrophil cells in the prostate. *J Pathol*. 1974;112:189–193.

6. Hirano D, Okada Y, Minei S, et al. Neuroendocrine differentiation in hormone refractory prostate cancer following androgen deprivation therapy. *Eur Urol*. 2004;45:586–592.

7. Abrahamsson PA. Neuroendocrine differentiation in prostatic carcinoma. *Prostate*. 1999;39:135–148.

8. Bonkhoff H. Neuroendocrine cells in benign and malignant prostate tissue: morphogenesis, proliferation, and androgen receptor status. *Prostate Suppl*. 1998;8:18–22.

9. Bonkhoff H, Wernert N, Dhom G, et al. Relation of endocrine-paracrine cells to cell proliferation in normal, hyperplastic, and neoplastic human prostate. *Prostate*. 1991;19:91–98.

10. Xing N, Qian J, Bostwick D, et al. Neuroendocrine cells in human prostate over-express the anti-apoptosis protein survivin. *Prostate*. 2001;48:7–15.

11. Berruti A, Mosca A, Porpiglia F, et al. Chromogranin A expression in patients with hormone naive prostate cancer predicts the development of hormone refractory disease. *J Urol*. 2007;178:838–843.

12. Mucci NR, Akdas G, Manely S, et al. Neuroendocrine expression in metastatic prostate cancer: evaluation of high throughput tissue microarrays to detect heterogeneous protein expression. *Hum Pathol*. 2000;31:406–414.

13. de Bono JS, Logothetis CJ, Molina A, et al. Abiraterone and increased survival in metastatic prostate cancer. *N Engl J Med*. 2011;364:1995–2005.

14. Scher HI, Fizazi K, Saad F, et al. Increased survival with enzalutamide in prostate cancer after chemotherapy. *N Engl J Med*. 2012;367:1187–1197.

15. Eble JN, Sauter G, Epstein JI, et al. *World Health Organization Classification of Tumours. Pathology and Genetics: Tumors of the Urinary System and Male Genital Organs*. Lyon, France: IARC Press; 2004.

16. Komiya A, Suzuki H, Imamoto T, et al. Neuroendocrine differentiation in the progression of prostate cancer. *Int J Urol*. 2009;16:37–44.

17. Vashchenko N, Abrahamsson PA. Neuroendocrine differentiation in prostate cancer: implications for new treatment modalities. *Eur Urol*. 2005;47:147–155.

18. Cohen RJ, Glezerson G, Haffejee Z. Prostate-specific antigen and prostate-specific acid phosphatase in neuroendocrine cells of prostate cancer. *Arch Pathol Lab Med*. 1992;116:65–66.

19. Berruti A, Mosca A, Tucci M, et al. Independent prognostic role of circulating chromogranin A in prostate cancer patients with hormone-refractory disease. *Endocr Relat Cancer*. 2005;12:109–117.

20. Bostwick DG, Qian J, Pacelli A, et al. Neuroendocrine expression in node positive prostate cancer: correlation with systemic progression and patient survival. *J Urol*. 2002;168:1204–1211.

21. Theodorescu D, Broder SR, Boyd JC, et al. Cathepsin D and chromogranin A as predictors of long term disease specific survival after radical prostatectomy for localized carcinoma of the prostate. *Cancer.* 1997;80:2109–2119.

22. Weinstein MH, Partin AW, Veltri RW, et al. Neuroendocrine differentiation in prostate cancer: enhanced prediction of progression after radical prostatectomy. *Hum Pathol.* 1996;27:683–687.

23. Cohen RJ, Glezerson G, Haffejee Z. Neuro-endocrine cells—a new prognostic parameter in prostate cancer. *Br J Urol.* 1991;68:258–262.

24. Shariff AH, Ather MH. Neuroendocrine differentiation in prostate cancer. *Urology.* 2006;68:2–8.

25. Casella R, Bubendorf L, Sauter G, et al. Focal neuroendocrine differentiation lacks prognostic significance in prostate core needle biopsies. *J Urol.* 1998;160:406–410.

26. Abrahamsson PA, Cockett AT, di Sant'Agnese PA. Prognostic significance of neuroendocrine differentiation in clinically localized prostatic carcinoma. *Prostate Suppl.* 1998;8:37–42.

27. Allen FJ, Van Velden DJ, Heyns CF. Are neuroendocrine cells of practical value as an independent prognostic parameter in prostate cancer? *Br J Urol.* 1995;75:751–754.

28. Ahlgren G, Pedersen K, Lundberg S, et al. Regressive changes and neuroendocrine differentiation in prostate cancer after neoadjuvant hormonal treatment. *Prostate.* 2000; 42:274–279.

29. Tan MO, Karaoglan U, Celik B, et al. Prostate cancer and neuroendocrine differentiation. *Int Urol Nephrol.* 1999;31:75–82.

30. Cohen MK, Arber DA, Coffield KS, et al. Neuroendocrine differentiation in prostatic adenocarcinoma and its relationship to tumor progression. *Cancer.* 1994;74:1899–1903.

31. Ishida E, Nakamura M, Shimada K, et al. Immunohistochemical analysis of neuroendocrine differentiation in prostate cancer. *Pathobiology.* 2009;76:30–38.

32. Jeetle SS, Fisher G, Yang ZH, et al. Neuroendocrine differentiation does not have independent prognostic value in conservatively treated prostate cancer. *Virchows Arch.* 2012;461:103–107.

33. Aprikian AG, Cordon-Cardo C, Fair WR, et al. Neuroendocrine differentiation in metastatic prostatic adenocarcinoma. *J Urol.* 1994;151:914–919.

34. Aprikian AG, Cordon-Cardo C, Fair WR, et al. Characterization of neuroendocrine differentiation in human benign prostate and prostatic adenocarcinoma. *Cancer.* 1993; 71:3952–3965.

35. Weaver MG, Abdul-Karim FW, Srigley J, et al. Paneth cell-like change of the prostate gland. A histological, immunohistochemical, and electron microscopic study. *Am J Surg Pathol.* 1992;16:62–68.

36. Tamas EF, Epstein JI. Prognostic significance of Paneth cell-like neuroendocrine differentiation in adenocarcinoma of the prostate. *Am J Surg Pathol.* 2006; 30: 980–985.

37. Adlakha H, Bostwick DG. Paneth cell-like change in prostatic adenocarcinoma represents neuroendocrine differentiation: report of 30 cases. *Hum Pathol.* 1994;25:135–139.

38. Freschi M, Colombo R, Naspro R, et al. Primary and pure neuroendocrine tumor of the prostate. *Eur Urol.* 2004;45:166–169.

39. Giordano S, Tolonen T, Tolonen T, et al. A pure primary low-grade neuroendocrine carcinoma (carcinoid tumor) of the prostate. *Int Urol Nephrol.* 2010;42:683–687.

40. Goulet-Salmon B, Berthe E, Franc S, et al. Prostatic neuroendocrine tumor in multiple endocrine neoplasia type 2B. *J Endocrinol Invest.* 2004;27:570–573.

41. Whelan T, Gatfield CT, Robertson S, et al. Primary carcinoid of the prostate in conjunction with multiple endocrine neoplasia IIb in a child. *J Urol.* 1995;153:1080–1082.

42. Zarkovic A, Masters J, Carpenter L. Primary carcinoid tumour of the prostate. *Pathology*. 2005;37:184–186.

43. Slater D. Carcinoid tumour of the prostate associated with inappropriate ACTH secretion. *Br J Urol*. 1985;57:591–592.

44. Tash JA, Reuter V, Russo P. Metastatic carcinoid tumor of the prostate. *J Urol*. 2002; 167:2526–2527.

45. Wasserstein PW, Goldman RL. Primary carcinoid of prostate. *Urology*. 1979;13:318–320.

46. Murali R, Kneale K, Lalak N, et al. Carcinoid tumors of the urinary tract and prostate. *Arch Pathol Lab Med*. 2006;130:1693–1706.

47. Turbat-Herrera EA, Herrera GA, Gore I, et al. Neuroendocrine differentiation in prostatic carcinomas. A retrospective autopsy study. *Arch Pathol Lab Med*. 1988;112: 1100–1115.

48. Egan AJM, Youngskin TP, Bostwick DG. Mixed carcinoid-adenocarcinoma of the prostate with spindle cell carcinoid: the spectrum of neuroendocrine differentiation in prostatic neoplasia. *Pathol Case Rev*. 1996;1:65–69.

49. Lee S, Han JS, Chang A, et al. Small cell-like change in prostatic intraepithelial neoplasia, intraductal carcinoma, and invasive prostatic carcinoma: a study of 7 cases. *Hum Pathol*. 2013;44:427–431.

50. Almagro UA. Argyrophilic prostatic carcinoma. Case report with literature review on prostatic carcinoid and "carcinoid-like" prostatic carcinoma. *Cancer*. 1985;55:608–614.

51. Azumi N, Shibuya H, Ishikura M. Primary prostatic carcinoid tumor with intracytoplasmic prostatic acid phosphatase and prostate-specific antigen. *Am J Surg Pathol*. 1984;8: 545–550.

52. Ghali VS, Garcia RL. Prostatic adenocarcinoma with carcinoidal features producing adrenocorticotropic syndrome. Immunohistochemical study and review of the literature. *Cancer*. 1984;54:1043–1048.

53. Ghannoum JE, DeLellis RA, Shin SJ. Primary carcinoid tumor of the prostate with concurrent adenocarcinoma: a case report. *Int J Surg Pathol*. 2004;12:167–170.

54. Stratton M, Evans DJ, Lampert IA. Prostatic adenocarcinoma evolving into carcinoid: selective effect of hormonal treatment? *J Clin Pathol*. 1986;39:750–756.

55. Rojas-Corona RR, Chen LZ, Mahadevia PS. Prostatic carcinoma with endocrine features. A report of a neoplasm containing multiple immunoreactive hormonal substances. *Am J Clin Pathol*. 1987;88:759–762.

56. Montasser AY, Ong MG, Mehta VT. Carcinoid tumor of the prostate associated with adenocarcinoma. *Cancer*. 1979;44:307–310.

57. Reyes A, Moran CA. Low-grade neuroendocrine carcinoma (carcinoid tumor) of the prostate. *Arch Pathol Lab Med*. 2004;128:e166–e168.

58. Sobin LH, Hjermstad BM, Sesterhenn IA, et al. Prostatic acid phosphatase activity in carcinoid tumors. *Cancer*. 1986;58:136–138.

59. Wang W, Epstein JI. Small cell carcinoma of the prostate. A morphologic and immunohistochemical study of 95 cases. *Am J Surg Pathol*. 2008;32:65–71.

60. Tetu B, Ro JY, Ayala AG, et al. Small cell carcinoma of the prostate. Part I. A clinicopathologic study of 20 cases. *Cancer*. 1987;59:1803–1809.

61. Yao JL, Madeb R, Bourne P, et al. Small cell carcinoma of the prostate: an immunohistochemical study. *Am J Surg Pathol*. 2006;30:705–712.

62. Ro JY, Tetu B, Ayala AG, et al. Small cell carcinoma of the prostate. II. Immunohistochemical and electron microscopic studies of 18 cases. *Cancer*. 1987;59:977–982.

63. Agoff SN, Lamps LW, Philip AT, et al. Thyroid transcription factor-1 is expressed in extrapulmonary small cell carcinomas but not in other extrapulmonary neuroendocrine tumors. *Mod Pathol*. 2000;13:238–242.

64. Ordonez NG. Value of thyroid transcription factor-1 immunostaining in distinguishing small cell lung carcinomas from other small cell carcinomas. *Am J Surg Pathol.* 2000; 24:1217–1223.

65. Tomlins SA, Rhodes DR, Perner S, et al. Recurrent fusion of TMPRSS2 and ETS transcription factor genes in prostate cancer. *Science.* 2005;310:644–648.

66. Lotan TL, Gupta NS, Wang W, et al. ERG gene rearrangements are common in prostatic small cell carcinomas. *Mod Pathol.* 2011;24:820–828.

67. Han B, Mehra R, Lonigro RJ, et al. Fluorescence in situ hybridization study shows association of PTEN deletion with ERG rearrangement during prostate cancer progression. *Mod Pathol.* 2009;22:1083–1093.

68. Guo CC, Dancer JY, Wang Y, et al. TMPRSS2-ERG gene fusion in small cell carcinoma of the prostate. *Hum Pathol.* 2011;42:11–17.

69. Williamson SR, Zhang S, Yao JL, et al. ERG-TMPRSS2 rearrangement is shared by concurrent prostatic adenocarcinoma and prostatic small cell carcinoma and absent in small cell carcinoma of the urinary bladder: evidence supporting monoclonal origin. *Mod Pathol.* 2011; 24:1120–1127.

70. Scheble VJ, Braun M, Wilbertz T, et al. ERG rearrangement in small cell prostatic and lung cancer. *Histopathology.* 2010;56:937–943.

71. Schelling LA, Williamson SR, Zhang S, et al. Frequent TMPRSS2-ERG rearrangement in prostatic small cell carcinoma detected by fluorescence in situ hybridization: the superiority of fluorescence in situ hybridization over ERG immunohistochemistry. *Hum Pathol.* 2013;44:2227–2233.

72. Deorah S, Rao MB, Raman R, et al. Survival of patients with small cell carcinoma of the prostate during 1973-2003: a population-based study. *BJU Int.* 2012;109:824–830.

73. Amato RJ, Logothetis CJ, Hallinan R, et al. Chemotherapy for small cell carcinoma of prostatic origin. *J Urol.* 1992;147:935–937.

74. Rubenstein JH, Katin MJ, Mangano MM, et al. Small cell anaplastic carcinoma of the prostate: seven new cases, review of the literature, and discussion of a therapeutic strategy. *Am J Clin Oncol.* 1997;20:376–380.

75. Aparicio AM, Harzstark AL, Corn PG, et al. Platinum-based chemotherapy for variant castrate-resistant prostate cancer. *Clin Cancer Res.* 2013;19:3621–3630.

76. Papandreou CN, Daliani DD, Thall PF, et al. Results of a phase II study with doxorubicin, etoposide, and cisplatin in patients with fully characterized small-cell carcinoma of the prostate. *J Clin Oncol.* 2002;20:3072–3080.

77. Evans AJ, Humphrey PA, Belani J, et al. Large cell neuroendocrine carcinoma of prostate: a clinicopathologic summary of 7 cases of a rare manifestation of advanced prostate cancer. *Am J Surg Pathol.* 2006;30:684–693.

78. Aparicio A, Tzelepi V, Araujo JC, et al. Neuroendocrine prostate cancer xenografts with large-cell and small-cell features derived from a single patient's tumor: morphological, immunohistochemical, and gene expression profiles. *Prostate.* 2011;71:846–856.

79. Yuan TC, Veeramani S, Lin MF. Neuroendocrine-like prostate cancer cells: neuroendocrine transdifferentiation of prostate adenocarcinoma cells. *Endocr Relat Cancer.* 2007;14:531–547.

80. Beltran H, Rickman DS, Park K, et al. Molecular characterization of neuroendocrine prostate cancer and identification of new drug targets. *Cancer Discov.* 2011;1:487–495.

81. Mosquera JM, Beltran H, Park K, et al. Concurrent AURKA and MYCN gene amplifications are harbingers of lethal treatment-related neuroendocrine prostate cancer. *Neoplasia.* 2013;15:1–10.

13

MUCINOUS DIFFERENTIATION IN THE BENIGN AND MALIGNANT PROSTATE

Benign secretory cells of the prostate contain scant neutral mucin.[1] Although initial reports claimed that benign prostatic glands lacked acid mucin, we have demonstrated that adenosis and occasional atrophic glands can also express acid mucin.[2]

Another form of mucin differentiation in benign prostate is mucous gland metaplasia, which is found in approximately 1% of prostates.[3,4] The lesion consists of tall mucin-filled goblet cells with tiny, dark, basal nuclei (Fig. 13.1, eFigs. 13.1 to 13.18). The cells are positive for prostate-specific antigen (PSA) and are diastase resistant as well as positive for mucicarmine and Alcian blue. The cells are negative for PSA and prostate-specific acid phosphatase (PSAP). These may occur as randomly scattered individual cells or in groups of 5 to 10 cells. Most foci are small, very rarely measuring over 1 mm². Mucous gland metaplasia may be found in normal and hyperplastic prostate glands and in areas of urothelial metaplasia, basal cell hyperplasia, or atrophy. Rarely, it may be seen in high-grade prostatic intraepithelial neoplasia (PIN) (eFig. 13.19). Although it may mimic cancer, it does not appear to be related to cancer or inflammation.

Mucinous (colloid) adenocarcinoma of the prostate gland is one of the least common morphologic variants of prostatic carcinoma.[5–7] A lack of precision in the definition of these mucinous neoplasms has resulted in reports that have overstated the incidence of this rare variant. Much of the confusion in the terminology of this entity arises from the lack of recognition that between 60% and 90% of prostatic adenocarcinomas secrete mucosubstances, depending on the histochemical technique used.[1,8–10] Only when extracellular mucin is secreted in sufficient quantity to result in pools of mucin should the term *mucinous* be employed. If the mucinous area occupies only a small portion of the tumor, it should not be called a "mucinous prostatic carcinoma" but rather a "prostatic adenocarcinoma with focal mucinous features." Using criteria developed for mucinous carcinomas of other organs, the diagnosis of mucinous adenocarcinoma of the prostate gland should be made when at least 25% of the tumor resected

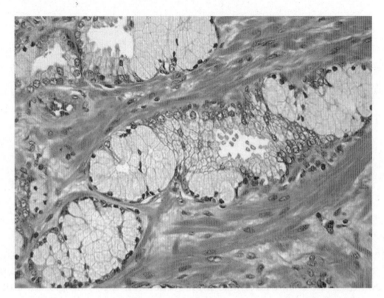

FIGURE 13.1 Extensive mucin cell metaplasia in benign glands.

contains lakes of extracellular mucin.[6] Defined as such, this variant forms less than 1% of all prostate adenocarcinoma.[11] The diagnosis of mucinous adenocarcinoma cannot be established on needle biopsy because the entire tumor is not available for examination. Rather, on needle biopsy, one can diagnose "adenocarcinoma of the prostate with mucinous features."

In a more recent large series from our group, Osunkoya et al.[11] reported the clinicopathologic findings of 47 mucinous adenocarcinomas of the prostate treated by radical prostatectomy. Mean patient age at diagnosis was 56 years. The mean preoperative PSA level was 9.0 ng/mL (range: 1.9 to 34.3 ng/mL). The majority of tumors (72%) were clinical stages T1c and Gleason score 7 (78.7%). Taking into account both the mucinous and nonmucinous tumor components, 43% of cases had extraprostatic extension and 13% had positive margins. Only one case was positive for lymph node metastasis.

The clinical behavior of mucinous prostate adenocarcinomas has been somewhat controversial. Although initial studies, including one from our group, suggested an aggressive biologic behavior,[5–7] our more recent larger series mentioned earlier indicates that mucinous adenocarcinoma of the prostate treated by radical prostatectomy is not more aggressive and possibly is even less aggressive than conventional acinar prostatic adenocarcinoma. With a mean follow-up of 5.6 years, the study by Osunkoya et al.[11] reported progression in only 1 out of 47 patients (2.1%) with a 5-year actuarial progression-free risk of 97% compared to 85% for nonmucinous prostate cancer with matched PSA and postoperative findings. This favorable prognosis is in line with the findings of another recent study by Lane et al.[12]

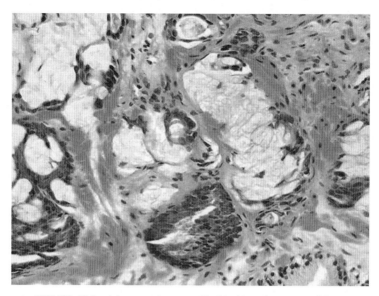

FIGURE 13.2   Adenocarcinoma with focal mucin extravasation.

Mucinous adenocarcinomas of the prostate, similar to usual acinar adenocarcinomas, are associated with elevated serum PSA values, metastasize to bone, and respond to hormonal therapy. Histologically, mucinous adenocarcinomas of the prostate are predominantly Gleason score 7 or 8 as a cribriform pattern tends to predominate in the mucinous areas (see Chapter 9 for grading)[11,13] (Figs. 13.2 to 13.3, eFigs. 13.20 to 13.36).

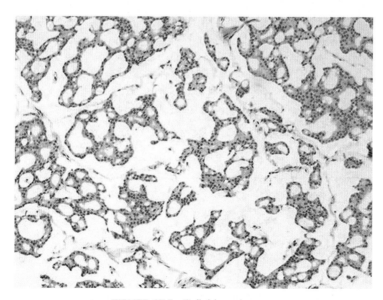

FIGURE 13.3   Colloid carcinoma.

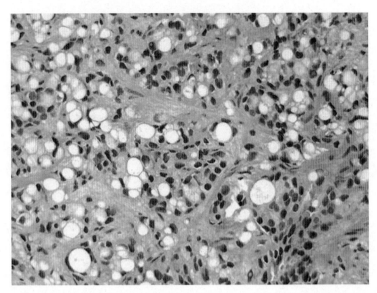

FIGURE 13.4   Adenocarcinoma of the prostate with signet-ring cell features, Gleason pattern 5.

In contrast to bladder adenocarcinomas, mucinous adenocarcinoma of the prostate rarely contains mucin-positive signet cells. Some adenocarcinomas of the prostate will have a signet-ring cell appearance, yet the vacuoles do not contain intracytoplasmic mucin (Fig. 13.4, eFigs. 13.37 to 13.43).[14] Only a few cases of prostate cancer have been reported with mucin-positive

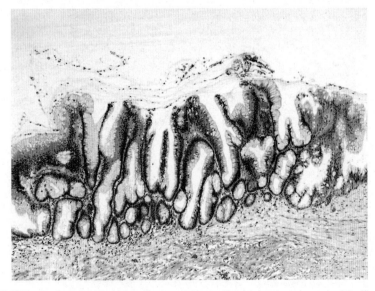

FIGURE 13.5   Surface component of a prostatic urethral adenocarcinoma with villous adenoma arising from prostatic urethra.

signet cells.[15,16] In one of these cases, the signet cell carcinoma appeared to arise from intestinal metaplasia of the overlying urothelium.[17]

At the molecular biologic level, mucinous adenocarcinomas of the prostate demonstrate a higher rate of *TMPRSS2-ERG* gene fusion (83% compared to approximately 50% of usual acinar adenocarcinoma).[18] Mucinous adenocarcinoma of the prostate shows frequent and diffuse expression of MUC2, a "gel-forming" type of mucin that exerts a tumor suppressor role in other exocrine mucinous adenocarcinomas including pancreatic and breast colloid carcinomas. MUC2 is absent in normal prostatic glands and is not expressed in the majority of conventional acinar adenocarcinomas of the prostate. The high rate of MUC2 expression in mucinous adenocarcinoma of the prostate may play a role, not only in its colloid differentiation but also in its relatively indolent behavior that has been recently elucidated as discussed earlier.[19]

Our group and others have described the occurrence of prostatic urethral adenocarcinoma that arises through a process of glandular metaplasia of the prostatic urethral urothelium, sometimes associated with villous adenoma, and subsequent in situ adenocarcinoma with invasion into the prostate (Fig. 13.5, eFigs. 13.44 to 13.54).[20–24] These prostatic adenocarcinomas are analogous to nonurachal adenocarcinomas arising in the bladder in a background of cystitis glandularis. The distinction between usual adenocarcinoma of the prostate, adenocarcinoma from another organ secondarily involving the prostate (typically gastrointestinal [GI] tract), and prostatic urethral adenocarcinoma has significant therapeutic implications, as in the latter two situations, the tumors are not prostatic in origin despite involving the prostate. Our largest recent series included 15 cases of prostatic urethral adenocarcinoma with a mean patient age at diagnosis of 72 years. All men had negative colonoscopies, clinically excluding a colonic primary. Bladder primaries were also ruled out clinically and/or pathologically. On follow-up (mean 50 months), over one-quarter of patients developed metastatic disease and approximately half died of disease. Glandular metaplasia of the prostatic urethra and contiguous transition to adenocarcinoma were identified in approximately half of the cases. Multiple histologic patterns were observed including dissection of the stroma by mucin pools (100%), villous features (47%), necrosis (13.3%), and presence of signet ring cells (20%). On immunohistochemical stains, all cases were negative for PSA, CDX2, and beta-catenin, whereas high molecular weight cytokeratin, CK7, and CK20 were positive in the majority of cases. As prostatic urethral adenocarcinoma is entirely analogous to bladder adenocarcinoma in both morphology and immunophenotype, only clinical studies or, in some cases, pathologic examination of the cystoprostatectomy specimen can exclude infiltration from a primary bladder adenocarcinoma. Ductal adenocarcinomas of the prostate may cytologically resemble these tumors; however, prostatic ductal adenocarcinoma lacks extracellular mucin and is immunohistochemically uniformly positive for PSA.

In a recent immunohistochemistry study evaluating 37 adenocarcinomas of bladder,[25] our group demonstrated that a minority of bladder adenocarcinomas are positive for prostate-specific membrane antigen (PSMA) with diffuse cytoplasmic or membranous staining in 21% of cases including signet ring, urachal, mucinous, and enteric-type variants. This nonspecific staining is one of the reasons why we no longer include PSMA as one of our "prostate-specific" antibodies but rather use PSA, P501S, and NKX3.1, which are negative in bladder adenocarcinomas. Although we have not seen bladder adenocarcinomas labeled with PSA, older studies have reported PSA positivity in primary bladder adenocarcinoma.[26,27] Carcinoembryonic antigen (CEA) staining is of limited use in differentiating between prostate and bladder adenocarcinomas, because 20% to 25% of prostate adenocarcinomas express this substance.

REFERENCES

1. Levine AJ, Foster EA. The relation of mucicarmine-staining properties of carcinomas of the prostate to differentiation, metastases, and prognosis. *Cancer*. 1964;17:21–25.

2. Epstein JI, Fynheer J. Acidic mucin in the prostate: can it differentiate adenosis from adenocarcinoma? *Hum Pathol*. 1992;23:1321–1325.

3. Shiraishi T, Kusano I, Watanabe M, et al. Mucous gland metaplasia of the prostate. *Am J Surg Pathol*. 1993;17:618–622.

4. Grignon DJ, O'Malley FP. Mucinous metaplasia in the prostate gland. *Am J Surg Pathol*. 1993;17:287–290.

5. Epstein JI, Lieberman PH. Mucinous adenocarcinoma of the prostate gland. *Am J Surg Pathol*. 1985;9:299–308.

6. Ro JY, Grignon DJ, Ayala AG, et al. Mucinous adenocarcinoma of the prostate: histochemical and immunohistochemical studies. *Hum Pathol*. 1990;21:593–600.

7. Saito S, Iwaki H. Mucin-producing carcinoma of the prostate: review of 88 cases. *Urology*. 1999;54:141–144.

8. Foster EA, Levine AJ. Mucin production in metastatic carcinomas. *Cancer*. 1963;16:506–509.

9. Franks LM, O'Shea JD, Thomson AE. Mucin in the prostate: a histochemical study in normal glands, latent, clinical, and colloid cancers. *Cancer*. 1964;17:983–991.

10. Hukill PB, Vidone RA. Histochemistry of mucus and other polysaccharides in tumors. II. Carcinoma of the prostate. *Lab Invest*. 1967;16:395–406.

11. Osunkoya AO, Nielsen ME, Epstein JI. Prognosis of mucinous adenocarcinoma of the prostate treated by radical prostatectomy: a study of 47 cases. *Am J Surg Pathol*. 2008;32:468–472.

12. Lane BR, Magi-Galluzzi C, Reuther AM, et al. Mucinous adenocarcinoma of the prostate does not confer poor prognosis. *Urology*. 2006;68:825–830.

13. Grignon DJ. Unusual subtypes of prostate cancer. *Mod Pathol*. 2004;17:316–327.

14. Ro JY, el-Naggar A, Ayala AG, et al. Signet-ring-cell carcinoma of the prostate. Electron-microscopic and immunohistochemical studies of eight cases. *Am J Surg Pathol*. 1988;12:453–460.

15. Hejka AG, England DM. Signet ring cell carcinoma of prostate. Immunohistochemical and ultrastructural study of a case. *Urology*. 1989;34:155–158.

16. Uchijima Y, Ito H, Takahashi M, et al. Prostate mucinous adenocarcinoma with signet ring cell. *Urology*. 1990;36:267–268.

17. Skodras G, Wang J, Kragel PJ. Primary prostatic signet-ring cell carcinoma. *Urology*. 1993;42:338–342.

18. Han B, Mehra R, Suleman K, et al. Characterization of ETS gene aberrations in select histologic variants of prostate carcinoma. *Mod Pathol*. 2009;22:1176–1185.

19. Osunkoya AO, Adsay NV, Cohen C, et al. MUC2 expression in primary mucinous and nonmucinous adenocarcinoma of the prostate: an analysis of 50 cases on radical prostatectomy. *Mod Pathol*. 2008;21:789–794.

20. Tran KP, Epstein JI. Mucinous adenocarcinoma of urinary bladder type arising from the prostatic urethra. Distinction from mucinous adenocarcinoma of the prostate. *Am J Surg Pathol*. 1996;20:1346–1150.

21. Osunkoya AO, Epstein JI. Primary mucin-producing urothelial-type adenocarcinoma of prostate: report of 15 cases. *Am J Surg Pathol*. 2007;31:1323–1329.

22. Ortiz-Rey JA, Dos Santos JE, Rodriguez-Castilla M, et al. Mucinous urothelial-type adenocarcinoma of the prostate. *Scand J Urol Nephrol*. 2004;38:256–257.

23. Curtis MW, Evans AJ, Srigley JR. Mucin-producing urothelial-type adenocarcinoma of prostate: report of two cases of a rare and diagnostically challenging entity. *Mod Pathol*. 2005;18:585–590.

24. Sakamoto N, Ohtsubo S, Iguchi A, et al. Intestinal-type mucinous adenocarcinoma arising from the prostatic duct. *Int J Urol*. 2005;12:509–512.

25. Lane Z, Hansel DE, Epstein JI. Immunohistochemical expression of prostatic antigens in adenocarcinoma and villous adenoma of the urinary bladder. *Am J Surg Pathol*. 2008;32:1322–1326.

26. Heyderman E, Brown BM, Richardson TC. Epithelial markers in prostatic, bladder, and colorectal cancer: an immunoperoxidase study of epithelial membrane antigen, carcinoembryonic antigen, and prostatic acid phosphatase. *J Clin Pathol*. 1984;37:1363–1369.

27. Minkowitz G, Peterson P, Godwin TA. A histochemical and immunohistochemical study of adenocarcinomas involving urinary bladder. *Mod Pathol*. 1990;3:68A.

14

BENIGN AND MALIGNANT PROSTATE FOLLOWING TREATMENT

ANTIANDROGEN THERAPY

There are several different forms of antiandrogen therapy, some are used for treating benign prostatic hyperplasia (BPH) and other more potent ones are used for treating prostate cancer. In the prostate, testosterone is converted to the more potent androgen dihydrotestosterone (DHT) by type 2 5-α-reductase. Finasteride (Proscar) inhibits type 2 5-α-reductase. By blocking the production of DHT, finasteride leads to a shrinkage of the prostate in some men and improves their urinary obstructive symptoms. Because testosterone is still present, this therapy does not result in total androgen withdrawal. We have previously demonstrated that finasteride does not alter the histology of either benign or malignant tissue.[1] It also does not appear that the parameters of tissue composition on needle biopsy (percentage of epithelium, epithelial volume, and stromal/epithelial ratio) can predict a favorable response to hormonal treatment of BPH.[2]

Although 5-α-reductase inhibitors have most commonly been used to reduce prostatic volume in symptomatic BPH, these agents are now used to treat male pattern baldness and there has been considerable interest in examining the ability of these agents to reduce the risk of developing prostate cancer. The Prostate Cancer Prevention Trial reported a 24.8% reduction in the prevalence of prostate cancer in patients receiving finasteride compared to placebo group at 7-year follow-up. The study also reported a higher proportion of Gleason grade 7 and higher cancer in the finasteride group, which raised questions whether 5-α-reductase inhibitors alter prostate cancer morphology and whether Gleason scoring post–5-α-reductase inhibitors therapy might be unreliable. Subsequent studies based on blind histologic review confirmed that 5-α-reductase inhibitors are not associated with morphologic changes that affect Gleason scoring.[3,4] As such, pathologists should provide Gleason scores for such specimens. Most of the available evidence suggests that the increased incidence of higher grade cancers found in the Prostate Cancer Prevention Trial was a result of reductions in biopsy sampling error associated with prostate shrinkage.[5]

The more potent hormonal therapy used to treat prostate cancer consists of a luteinizing hormone-releasing hormone (LHRH) agonist (Lupron) typically in association with the antiandrogen flutamide. This regimen aims at achieving "chemical castration" and is at times referred to as maximal androgen blockade. It is occasionally used prior to radical prostatectomy (neoadjuvant hormone therapy), as it has been demonstrated that it results in less frequent positive margins at radical prostatectomy.[6] This therapy may also be used if a delay of several months between the diagnosis of cancer and radical surgery is anticipated so as to allay any concerns that patients may have not received immediate treatment for their tumor. Despite the less frequently positive margins, this combination neoadjuvant therapy has not been demonstrated to improve the prognosis and has fallen out of favor.[6] Typically, pathologists encounter combination endocrine treated radical prostatectomy specimens, although occasionally, needle biopsies or transurethral resections of the prostate (TURP) may be performed following this therapy.

The histology of both the normal and neoplastic tissue may be significantly altered with this therapy, making the assessment of these specimens difficult[4,7–12] (Table 14.1). Within the nonneoplastic prostate, antiandrogen therapy results in squamous metaplasia in both the overlying urethra as well as diffusely throughout the prostate (Fig. 14.1, eFigs. 14.1 to 14.5). In these areas, the altered glands have the appearance of urothelial metaplasia and basal cell hyperplasia. There is less abundant squamous differentiation than in patients who have been treated in the past with estrogen therapy. Other situations where one may see squamous metaplasia within the urethra is following transurethral resection. The diffuse nature of squamous metaplasia with antiandrogen therapy is characteristic because the only other situation in which squamous metaplasia occurs within the prostate

TABLE 14.1 **Changes in the Prostate Following Hormonal Therapy**
Benign Prostate Tissue
Diffuse squamous metaplasia
Diffuse urothelial metaplasia
Diffuse basal cell hyperplasia
Glandular atrophy
Stromal fibrosis
Malignant Prostate Tissue
Atrophic cancer
Glands with xanthomatous cytoplasm and pyknotic nuclei
Individual tumor cells resembling xanthomatous histiocytes
Individual tumor cells in fibrotic and inflamed stroma

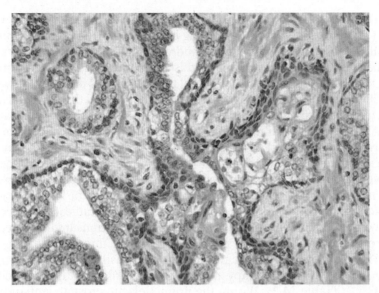

FIGURE 14.1 Squamous metaplasia and basal cell hyperplasia resulting from antiandrogen therapy.

is when it is localized to the immediate vicinity of prostatic infarcts. Other changes with antiandrogen therapy seen in the nonneoplastic tissue include atrophy of the glandular epithelium with some stromal fibrosis.

Therapy with LHRH agonists and flutamide may result in three different histologic patterns in prostate cancer. The neoplastic acini may become atrophic (Fig. 14.2, eFigs. 14.6 to 14.12).[4,7–13] At higher power,

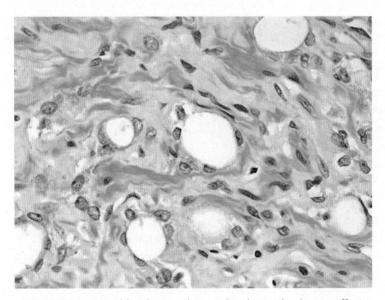

FIGURE 14.2 Atrophic adenocarcinoma showing antiandrogen effect.

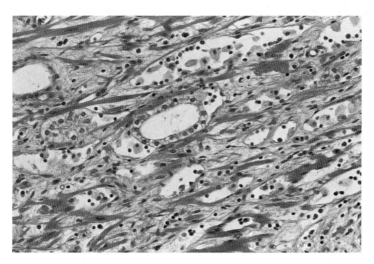

FIGURE 14.3 Adenocarcinoma showing antiandrogen effect.

these neoplastic glands are identical to benign atrophic glands. Only their crowded infiltrative appearance or location outside of the prostate is diagnostic of adenocarcinoma. Furthermore, there may be other areas of the tumor that do not show as prominent response to hormonal therapy and are more recognizable as carcinoma. The second pattern is when the atrophic neoplastic glands develop pyknotic nuclei and abundant xanthomatous cytoplasm (Figs. 14.3 and 14.4). These cells then desquamate into the lumen of the malignant glands where they resemble

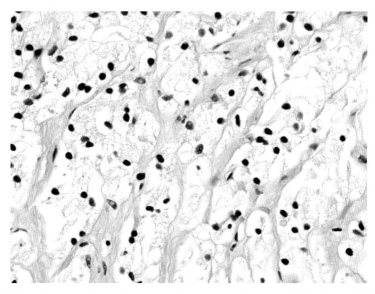

FIGURE 14.4 Adenocarcinoma showing antiandrogen effect resembling foamy histiocytes.

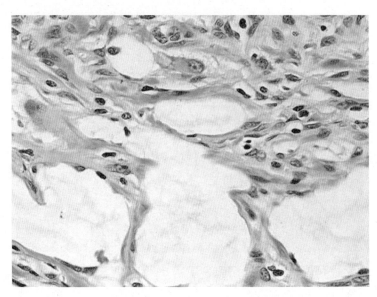

FIGURE 14.5   Acellular clefts resulting from adenocarcinoma showing antiandrogen effect.

histiocytes and lymphocytes (Fig. 14.5, eFigs. 14.13 to 14.17). The fact that they are still identifiable as glandular structures is helpful in establishing the diagnosis. There may be areas where only scattered cells resembling foamy histiocytes with pyknotic nuclei and xanthomatous cytoplasm are visible. These cells, however, are pancytokeratin-positive demonstrating their epithelial nature. The third pattern is when there are individual tumor cells resembling inflammatory cells. At low power, these areas may be difficult to identify, and often, the only clue to areas of hormonally treated carcinoma is a fibrotic background with scattered cells with tumor cells identified at higher magnification. Immunohistochemistry for prostate-specific antigen (PSA) or pancytokeratin can aid in the diagnosis of carcinoma in these cases by identifying the individual cells as epithelial cells of prostatic origin. Cancer cells following hormonal therapy demonstrate a lack of high molecular weight cytokeratin staining, identical to untreated prostate cancer. Following hormonal therapy, there may be a decrease in immunoreactivity with PSA, but most tumors maintain some labeling.[14] Following a response to combination endocrine therapy, the grade of the tumor appears artifactually higher when compared to the grade of the pretreated tumor.[11,15] Consequently, prostatic adenocarcinoma with significant treatment effect should not be assigned a Gleason grade. In a patient with prior hormonal therapy, if there is tumor without treatment affect, it can be graded as usual.

Several studies have demonstrated that the extent and prevalence of high-grade prostatic intraepithelial neoplasia (PIN) is substantially decreased in prostates that have been treated with androgen deprivation for 3 months prior to radical prostatectomy.[16,17] High-grade PIN may still

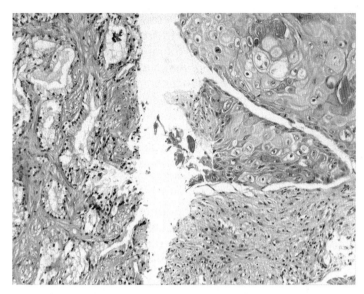

FIGURE 14.6   Adenosquamous carcinoma.

persist following androgen blockade therapy, although tufted PIN may be replaced by flat high-grade PIN.[18]

Treatment with estrogen, such as diethylstilbestrol (DES), is no longer widely used. The typical changes following DES include widespread fully developed squamous metaplasia in the benign prostate and tumor cells with strikingly clear cytoplasm and small pyknotic nuclei.[19] Following estrogen therapy, the prostate may also develop squamous metaplasia in some of the neoplastic glands as well, resulting in adenosquamous carcinomas (Fig. 14.6, eFigs. 14.18 to 14.20).[20] The metastases may be adenosquamous carcinoma or pure squamous carcinoma. There have also been reports of adenosquamous carcinoma of the prostate in which there was no previous estrogen therapy.[21,22] In some cases of adenosquamous carcinoma, the squamous components have been reported to be positive for PSA or prostate-specific acid phosphatase (PSAP).[20]

RADIATION

The use of radiotherapy as a primary treatment for clinically localized prostate cancer has been increasing. Typically, following radiotherapy, the serum PSA level will decrease to a nadir level. In some men, the PSA will then subsequently rise; a rise of ≥ 2 ng/ml above nadir PSA level is the most widely accepted definition of radiotherapy failure. It is controversial whether it is necessary to perform a biopsy to histologically demonstrate carcinoma if the serum PSA is rising after radiotherapy. Some experts argue that one can document that tumor is recurring following radiotherapy solely based on the rising serial PSA measurements and treat the patients, for example, with hormone therapy. Other oncologists feel more comfortable histologically documenting progression of cancer before initiating therapy. For more definitive therapy of postradiotherapy failures (i.e., salvage prostatectomy), where associated morbidity is higher, histologic documentation of recurrent cancer is mandatory. Often, pathologists will not get a history of prior irradiation, such that it is necessary for them to recognize the histologic features of radiation atypia in benign glands so as to avoid a misdiagnosis of cancer.

Within the nonneoplastic prostatic glands, radiation results in glandular atrophy, squamous metaplasia, and cytologic atypia[23] (eFigs. 14.21 to 14.31). Although one may find vascular radiation changes, the stromal atypia characteristic of radiation in other organs is not usually seen. The distinction between irradiated nonneoplastic prostatic glands and carcinoma is best made on the low-magnification architectural pattern of the glands (Table 14.2). Within the radiated normal prostate, glands maintain their normal architectural lobular configuration. In contrast to carcinoma, the nonneoplastic glands are separated by a modest amount of prostatic stroma. On higher magnification, whereas glands of prostatic carcinoma are lined by a single cell layer, there is piling up of the nuclei within irradiated normal prostate as well as an occasional recognizable basal cell layer (Fig. 14.7). This piling up of the cells in radiated benign glands frequently appears slightly spindled resembling urothelial metaplasia. The finding of scattered markedly atypical nuclei within well-formed acini is typical of radiated benign glands and rare in prostate carcinoma. Prostate carcinomas that are sufficiently differentiated to form glands rarely manifest the degree of atypia seen with radiation, and if present, would be more uniformly present in all cells. Radiated nuclei also have a degenerative, hyperchromatic, smudgy appearance as opposed to malignant prostatic nuclei that usually contain prominent nucleoli. Irradiated nonneoplastic glands often are atrophic, in contrast to gland-forming prostatic adenocarcinomas that typically have abundant cytoplasm. It has been demonstrated that high molecular weight cytokeratin, p63, and/or

TABLE 14.2 **Distinction Between Radiated Benign and Malignant Prostate Glands**

Radiated Benign	Radiated Malignant
Lobular	Infiltrative
Glands separated by stroma	Back-to-back
Multilayering	Single cell layer
Atrophic cytoplasm	Abundant cytoplasm
Scattered markedly atypical nuclei in glands	Gland with diffuse atypia

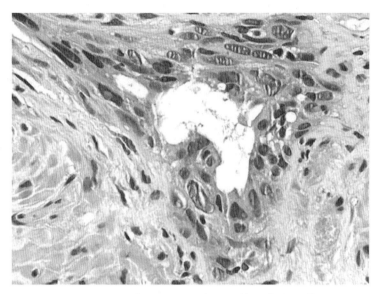

FIGURE 14.7   Benign prostate tissue with radiation effect.

alpha-methylacyl-CoA-racemase (AMACR) immunohistochemistry can aid in the diagnosis of irradiated prostate.[24–27]

Although it may be difficult to diagnose high-grade PIN following radiation therapy, this diagnosis may occasionally be made in this setting.[28] The typical nuclear changes of high-grade PIN characterized by prominent nucleoli are present, which differ from the degenerative smudgy chromatin seen with radiation atypia.

Radiated adenocarcinoma of the prostate may show either no recognizable difference from nonradiated cancer or the effects of radiation damage. In order to diagnose either pattern of cancer, the key feature is that architecturally, the findings are inconsistent with benign glands. The presence of closely packed glands with a haphazard infiltrative growth pattern is typical of adenocarcinoma and cannot be attributed to radiation change (Fig. 14.8). Similarly, the presence of infiltrating individual epithelial cells is diagnostic of carcinoma (Fig. 14.9). Cancers not showing any treatment effect have typical prostate cancer nuclei with prominent nucleoli and glands with a modest amount of cytoplasm (eFig. 14.32). Cancers with radiation effect demonstrate either glands or individual cells with abundant vacuolated cytoplasm or single cells with indistinct cytoplasm (eFigs. 14.33 to 14.56). Nuclei lack apparent nucleoli and are either large with bizarre shapes or pyknotic with smudged chromatin.[4,12,29–32]

There are differences in the effect on the prostate depending on the type of radiation administered. Brachytherapy, also known as interstitial radiotherapy, where radioactive seeds are implanted in the prostate, results in more atypia in benign prostate glands than with external beam radiation

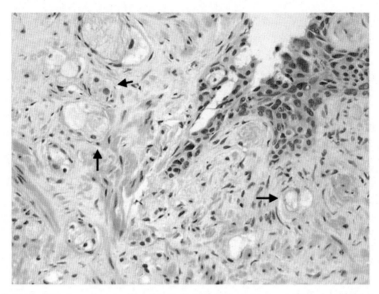

FIGURE 14.8 Adenocarcinoma showing radiation effect *(arrows)*. Note large benign prostate glands showing radiation effect *(upper right)*.

therapy.[32] Similarly, there is less decrease in the atypia in benign glands over time in men with brachytherapy. With external beam radiotherapy, the atypia in benign glands is less apparent after 4 years following therapy. Radiation atypia in benign glands can persist, especially with brachytherapy, for many years with prominent atypia seen as late as 6 years later.

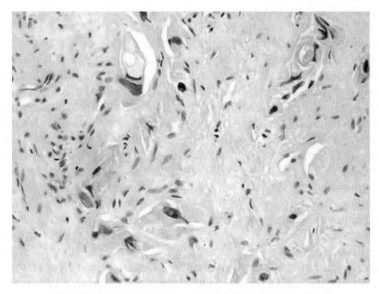

FIGURE 14.9 Adenocarcinoma showing radiation effect.

The best data on the significance of cancer with treatment effect is from Crook et al.[33] They revealed that 2-year posttreatment biopsy status is a strong predictor of 5-year disease-free survival rate: 82% and 83% for negative and indeterminate (cancer with treatment effect) biopsies, respectively, versus 27% for positive biopsies without treatment effect.[33]

When signing out postradiotherapy biopsies, we diagnose them as "benign," "cancer without significant treatment effect" (a Gleason grade is assigned), or "cancer showing significant treatment effect" (no Gleason grade assigned).

The expression of proliferation markers (PCNA/MIB-1) in postradiated cancer can also help predict clinical failure.[34] Relatively few studies have been done on the immunohistochemistry of radiated prostate, with most cases showing retention of their PSAP and PSA positivity in almost all cases.[14,29,35]

POSTRADICAL PROSTATECTOMY BIOPSIES

Following radical prostatectomy, a needle biopsy of the prostatic fossa may be performed to detect recurrence. There are no uniform guidelines as to when postradical prostatectomy biopsies are performed to document postoperative failure. Practices range from routine biopsies in men with rising postoperative serum PSA levels to reliance on clinical findings to establish a diagnosis of recurrent prostate cancer. Several investigators have demonstrated the difficulty in diagnosing recurrent adenocarcinoma on biopsy, sometimes requiring the patient to have several needle biopsies over time.[36–38] We have demonstrated that recurrent cancer on needle biopsy may be focal and difficult to diagnose, in part due to the limited extent of cancer seen on biopsy (Fig. 14.10, eFigs. 14.57 to 14.61).[39]

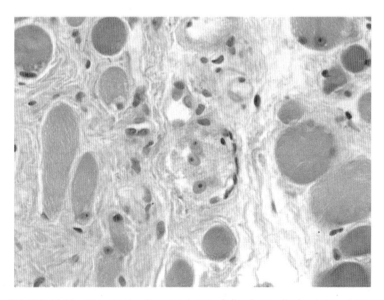

FIGURE 14.10   Recurrent adenocarcinoma following radical prostatectomy.

Another factor that leads to diagnostic difficulties is that the usual clues for the diagnosis of prostate cancer are often not present. We believe that there should be a lower histologic threshold for diagnosing recurrent prostate cancer in men who have had a prior radical prostatectomy. First, these men have a history of prostate cancer, where rare malignant-appearing glands may be consistent with recurrent cancer, yet insufficient to establish a primary diagnosis. Secondly, the prostate has been removed, such that the finding of a few atypical glands in soft tissue without surrounding benign prostate tissue is not expected and indicates recurrent cancer. Although in 14% of our postoperative biopsies we found benign prostate tissue, these glands were histologically bland and typically away from the recurrent cancer. Consequently, the presence of a few atypical glands is often diagnostic of recurrent prostate cancer, although those same glands sampled on a needle biopsy of the intact prostate might be called suspicious but not diagnostic of cancer. One cannot rely on the clinical, radiologic, or prior radical prostatectomy data to establish a diagnosis of locally recurrent prostate cancer. The diagnosis of locally recurrent cancer must be based on a constellation of the histologic findings along with the history of prior surgery.

Several prior studies have noted the presence of benign glands in biopsies following radical prostatectomy. Foster et al.[40] reported on eight patients with benign glands on biopsy following radical prostatectomy. Of six patients who underwent repeat biopsies, four were eventually shown to have, in addition, recurrent adenocarcinoma of the prostate. Fowler et al.[37] describes six patients who had benign prostate glands on biopsy following radical prostatectomy. The only patient who underwent repeat biopsy was also found to have carcinoma. Benign glands on biopsy after radical prostatectomy imply that the prostate was not removed in its entirety. It remains unknown whether and how frequently the presence of only benign prostate glands left after radical prostatectomy can give rise to an elevated postoperative serum PSA level and the false impression of recurrent prostate cancer.

EMERGING FOCAL/ABLATIVE THERAPIES

In addition to currently established therapeutic management options such as radical prostatectomy, radiation therapy, and active surveillance, several forms of "focal" ablative therapies precisely targeting locations where positive biopsy cores are obtained on detailed mapping biopsies are being investigated.[41-43] Focal ablative therapy modalities include cryotherapy, high-intensity focused ultrasound (HIFU),[44,45] vascular-targeted photodynamic therapy (PDT), interstitial laser therapy, and microwave thermotherapy.[42,46] None of these modalities have gained universal acceptance as first-line therapies and are still regarded as investigational treatments. The histologic changes associated with these treatments in benign and malignant prostate tissue are being better defined. Given the energy-based nature of these treatments, in general, the changes are more confined to well-demarcated areas of coagulative necrosis, hemorrhage, granulation tissue, inflammatory or histiocytic infiltrates, calcification, hemosiderin, and fibrosis in areas where the treatment has been effective. Ghosts of malignant glands may be appreciated in areas showing coagulative necrosis. Tissue obtained from untreated or suboptimally treated areas will show normal prostate tissue and/or adenocarcinoma with no apparent morphologic changes (Fig. 14.11, eFig. 14.62).[4,47–49]

HIFU therapy uses ultrasonic waves with frequencies in the range of 0.8 to 3.5 MHz to ablate tissue by raising its temperature to greater than 60°C, causing coagulative necrosis followed by cavitation as a consequence of alternating cycles of compression and rarefaction.[43–45] Outside the United States, it is increasingly used as a salvage therapy following failed radiation therapy or as a primary method of therapy. HIFU is not U.S. Food and Drug Administration (FDA)–approved as a primary therapy for prostate cancer. Biopsies obtained 3 to 6 months post-HIFU are negative in up to 90% of patients. Only few studies have addressed the histologic changes post-HIFU. Van Leenders et al.[50] described central necrosis and hemorrhage in prostatectomy specimens obtained 2 weeks after receiving HIFU therapy. The histologic features in post-HIFU biopsies, taken 6 months after treatment, were described by Biermann et al.[51] They include the presence of chronic inflammation, reactive fibroblastic proliferation, glandular atrophy, hemosiderin deposition, acute inflammation, focal coagulation necrosis, and stromal edema and fibrosis in benign tissue. Residual adenocarcinoma was identified in 44% of patients with cancer involving an average of 5% of the biopsy tissue. The adenocarcinoma showed no apparent treatment-related changes and thus it is recommended to assign Gleason scores to

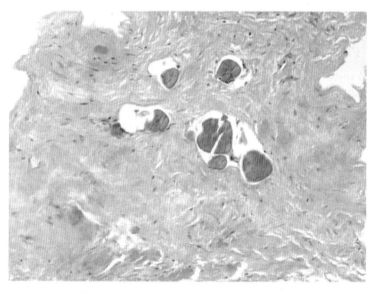

FIGURE 14.11 Dense fibrous tissue with residual corpora amylacea following cryotherapy.

these biopsies. High molecular weight cytokeratin remained useful in confirming the benign nature of atypical/reactive glands in post-HIFU biopsies.

Vascular-targeted PDT involves the intravenous administration of bacteriochlorophyll-derived, pharmacologically inactive photosensitizers. Activating light is delivered to the prostate, triggering the formation of reactive oxygen species. This leads to thrombosis in the vascular bed resulting in localized necrosis.[52] Biopsies obtained 6 months after PDT show sharply demarcated tissue damage. The areas of damage are characterized by well-demarcated areas of dense fibrosis often with an absence of prostatic glands. Less frequently, organizing granulation tissue or coagulative necrosis is present. Areas of viable adenocarcinoma located immediately adjacent to the foci of damage show no obvious morphologic changes that would preclude the use of Gleason scoring.

HYPERTHERMIA

Hyperthermia is used primarily to treat BPH. This therapy results in areas of hemorrhagic coagulative necrosis and occasionally reactive changes (eFig. 14.63).[53]

PHYTOTHERAPY

The use of alternative medicines, such as various plant extracts, to treat prostatic diseases has gained widespread popularity in recent years. One of the most frequently used is that of saw palmetto. We have demonstrated that this therapy does not significantly alter the histology of benign prostate tissue.[54] Sabal, another plant extract that is in widespread use for treating BPH in Germany, similarly does not alter the histology of benign or neoplastic epithelium.[55]

POST-TEFLON INJECTION GRANULOMAS

Teflon is injected into the periurethral tissues and submucosa of the bladder for the treatment of incontinence. On occasion, the foreign material may migrate into the prostate. Teflon has a very basophilic appearance, is birefringent, and induces a marked granulomatous reaction.[56]

POSTNEEDLE BIOPSY CHANGES

Needle biopsy tracts of the prostate in radical prostatectomy specimens manifest differently depending on the plane of section and location in the prostate. At the edge of the prostate, hemosiderin, recent hemorrhage, and fibrosis are noted in the periprostatic tissue. Within the prostate, one can visualize an irregular stellate defect surrounded by fibrosis or a linear fibrous tract (eFigs. 14.64 and 14.65). Although there is literature on the tracking of cancer into the periprostatic tissue with larger core needle biopsies, there is no evidence that contemporary thin-gauge needle biopsy instruments result in local cancer seeding.[57,58]

REFERENCES

1. Yang XJ, Lecksell K, Short K, et al. Does long-term finasteride therapy affect the histologic features of benign prostatic tissue and prostate cancer on needle biopsy? PLESS Study Group. Proscar Long-Term Efficacy and Safety Study. *Urology*. 1999;53:696–700.
2. Eri LM, Svindland A. Can prostate epithelial content predict response to hormonal treatment of patients with benign prostatic hyperplasia? *Urology*. 2000;56:261–265.
3. Lucia MS, Epstein JI, Goodman PJ, et al. Finasteride and high-grade prostate cancer in the Prostate Cancer Prevention Trial. *J Natl Cancer Inst*. 2007;99:1375–1383.
4. Evans AJ, Ryan P, Van der Kwast T. Treatment effects in the prostate including those associated with traditional and emerging therapies. *Adv Anat Pathol*. 2011;18:281–293.
5. Wilt TJ, Macdonald R, Hagerty K, et al. 5-alpha-Reductase inhibitors for prostate cancer chemoprevention: an updated Cochrane systematic review. *BJU Int*. 2010;106: 1444–1451.
6. Van Poppel H, De Ridder D, Elgamal AA, et al. Neoadjuvant hormonal therapy before radical prostatectomy decreases the number of positive surgical margins in stage T2 prostate cancer: interim results of a prospective randomized trial. The Belgian Uro-Oncological Study Group. *J Urol*. 1995;154:429–434.
7. Tetu B, Srigley JR, Boivin JC, et al. Effect of combination endocrine therapy (LHRH agonist and flutamide) on normal prostate and prostatic adenocarcinoma. A histopathologic and immunohistochemical study. *Am J Surg Pathol*. 1991;15:111–120.
8. Balaji KC, Rabbani F, Tsai H, et al. Effect of neoadjuvant hormonal therapy on prostatic intraepithelial neoplasia and its prognostic significance. *J Urol*. 1999;162:753–757.
9. Murphy WM, Soloway MS, Barrows GH. Pathologic changes associated with androgen deprivation therapy for prostate cancer. *Cancer*. 1991;68:821–828.
10. Armas OA, Aprikian AG, Melamed J, et al. Clinical and pathobiological effects of neoadjuvant total androgen ablation therapy on clinically localized prostatic adenocarcinoma. *Am J Surg Pathol*. 1994;18:979–991.
11. Smith DM, Murphy WM. Histologic changes in prostate carcinomas treated with leuprolide (luteinizing hormone-releasing hormone effect). Distinction from poor tumor differentiation. *Cancer*. 1994;73:1472–1477.
12. Petraki CD, Sfikas CP. Histopathological changes induced by therapies in the benign prostate and prostate adenocarcinoma. *Histol Histopathol*. 2007;22:107–118.
13. Roznovanu SL, Radulescu D, Novac C, et al. The morphologic changes induced by hormone and radiation therapy on prostate carcinoma. *Rev Med Chir Soc Med Nat Iasi*. 2005;109:337–342.
14. Vernon SE, Williams WD. Pre-treatment and post-treatment evaluation of prostatic adenocarcinoma for prostatic specific acid phosphatase and prostatic specific antigen by immunohistochemistry. *J Urol*. 1983;130:95–98.
15. Grignon D, Troster M. Changes in immunohistochemical staining in prostatic adenocarcinoma following diethylstilbestrol therapy. *Prostate*. 1985;7:195–202.
16. Vailancourt L, Ttu B, Fradet Y, et al. Effect of neoadjuvant endocrine therapy (combined androgen blockade) on normal prostate and prostatic carcinoma. A randomized study. *Am J Surg Pathol*. 1996;20:86–93.
17. Ferguson J, Zincke H, Ellison E, et al. Decrease of prostatic intraepithelial neoplasia following androgen deprivation therapy in patients with stage T3 carcinoma treated by radical prostatectomy. *Urology*. 1994;44:91–95.
18. van der Kwast TH, Labrie F, Tetu B. Persistence of high-grade prostatic intra-epithelial neoplasia under combined androgen blockade therapy. *Hum Pathol*. 1999;30: 1503–1507.
19. Franks LM. Estrogen-treated prostatic cancer: the variation in responsiveness of tumor ells. *Cancer*. 1960;13:490–501.

20. Accetta PA, Gardner WA. Squamous metastases from prostatic adenocarcinoma. *Prostate*. 1982;3:515–521.

21. Accetta PA, Gardner WA Jr. Adenosquamous carcinoma of prostate. *Urology*. 1983;22: 73–75.

22. Bassler TJ Jr, Orozco R, Bassler IC, et al. Adenosquamous carcinoma of the prostate: case report with DNA analysis, immunohistochemistry, and literature review. *Urology*. 1999;53:832–834.

23. Bostwick DG, Egbert BM, Fajardo LF. Radiation injury of the normal and neoplastic prostate. *Am J Surg Pathol*. 1982;6:541–551.

24. Brawer MK, Nagle RB, Pitts W, et al. Keratin immunoreactivity as an aid to the diagnosis of persistent adenocarcinoma in irradiated human prostates. *Cancer*. 1989;63:454–460.

25. Martens MB, Keller JH. Routine immunohistochemical staining for high-molecular weight cytokeratin 34-beta and alpha-methylacyl CoA racemase (P504S) in postirradiation prostate biopsies. *Mod Pathol*. 2006;19:287–290.

26. Yang XJ, Laven B, Tretiakova M, et al. Detection of alpha-methylacyl-coenzyme A racemase in postradiation prostatic adenocarcinoma. *Urology*. 2003;62:282–286.

27. Beach R, Gown AM, De Peralta-Venturina MN, et al. P504S immunohistochemical detection in 405 prostatic specimens including 376 18-gauge needle biopsies. *Am J Surg Pathol*. 2002;26:1588–1596.

28. Arakawa A, Song S, Scardino PT, et al. High grade prostatic intraepithelial neoplasia in prostates removed following irradiation failure in the treatment of prostatic adenocarcinoma. *Pathol Res Pract*. 1995;191:868–872.

29. Crook JM, Bahadur YA, Robertson SJ, et al. Evaluation of radiation effect, tumor differentiation, and prostate specific antigen staining in sequential prostate biopsies after external beam radiotherapy for patients with prostate carcinoma. *Cancer*. 1997;79:81–89.

30. Gaudin PB, Zelefsky MJ, Leibel SA, et al. Histopathologic effects of three-dimensional conformal external beam radiation therapy on benign and malignant prostate tissues. *Am J Surg Pathol*. 1999;23:1021–1031.

31. Pisansky TM. External-beam radiotherapy for localized prostate cancer. *N Engl J Med*. 2006;355:1583–1591.

32. Magi-Galluzzi C, Sanderson H, Epstein JI. Atypia in nonneoplastic prostate glands after radiotherapy for prostate cancer: duration of atypia and relation to type of radiotherapy. *Am J Surg Pathol*. 2003;27:206–212.

33. Crook JM, Malone S, Perry G, et al. Twenty-four-month postradiation prostate biopsies are strongly predictive of 7-year disease-free survival: results from a Canadian randomized trial. *Cancer*. 2009;115:673–679.

34. Crook J, Malone S, Perry G, et al. Postradiotherapy prostate biopsies: what do they really mean? Results for 498 patients. *Int J Rad Onc Biol Phys*. 2000;48:355–367.

35. Mahan DE, Bruce AW, Manley PN, et al. Immunohistochemical evaluation of prostatic carcinoma before and after radiotherapy. *J Urol*. 1980;124:488–491.

36. Connolly JA, Shinohara K, Presti JC Jr, et al. Local recurrence after radical prostatectomy: characteristics in size, location, and relationship to prostate-specific antigen and surgical margins. *Urology*. 1996;47:225–231.

37. Fowler JE Jr, Brooks J, Pandey P, et al. Variable histology of anastomotic biopsies with detectable prostate specific antigen after radical prostatectomy. *J Urol*. 1995;153: 1011–1014.

38. Saleem MD, Sanders H, Abu El Naser M, et al. Factors predicting cancer detection in biopsy of the prostatic fossa after radical prostatectomy. *Urology*. 1998;51:283–286.

39. Ripple MG, Potter SR, Partin AW, et al. Needle biopsy of recurrent adenocarcinoma of the prostate after radical prostatectomy. *Mod Pathol*. 2000;13:521–527.

40. Foster LS, Jajodia P, Fournier G Jr, et al. The value of prostate specific antigen and transrectal ultrasound guided biopsy in detecting prostatic fossa recurrences following radical prostatectomy. *J Urol*. 1993;149:1024–1028.

41. Mouraviev V, Polascik TJ. New frontiers in imaging and focal therapy: highlights from the Third International Symposium on Focal Therapy and Imaging of Prostate and Kidney Cancer, February 24–27, 2010, Washington, DC. *Rev Urol*. 2011;13:104–111.

42. Lindner U, Lawrentschuk N, Weersink RA, et al. Focal laser ablation for prostate cancer followed by radical prostatectomy: validation of focal therapy and imaging accuracy. *Eur Urol*. 2010;57:1111–1114.

43. Lindner U, Trachtenberg J, Lawrentschuk N. Focal therapy in prostate cancer: modalities, findings and future considerations. *Nat Rev Urol*. 2010;7:562–571.

44. Ahmed HU, Zacharakis E, Dudderidge T, et al. High-intensity-focused ultrasound in the treatment of primary prostate cancer: the first UK series. *Br J Cancer*. 2009;101:19–26.

45. Blana A, Murat FJ, Walter B, et al. First analysis of the long-term results with transrectal HIFU in patients with localised prostate cancer. *Eur Urol*. 2008;53:1194–1201.

46. Raz O, Haider MA, Davidson SR, et al. Real-time magnetic resonance imaging-guided focal laser therapy in patients with low-risk prostate cancer. *Eur Urol*. 2010;58:173–177.

47. Borkowski P, Robinson MJ, Poppiti RJ Jr, et al. Histologic findings in postcryosurgical prostatic biopsies. *Mod Pathol*. 1996;9:807–811.

48. Ellis DS, Manny TB Jr, Rewcastle JC. Focal cryosurgery followed by penile rehabilitation as primary treatment for localized prostate cancer: initial results. *Urology*. 2007;70:9–15.

49. Pisters LL. Cryotherapy for prostate cancer: ready for prime time? *Curr Opin Urol*. 2010;20:218–222.

50. Van Leenders GJ, Beerlage HP, Ruijter ET, et al. Histopathological changes associated with high intensity focused ultrasound (HIFU) treatment for localised adenocarcinoma of the prostate. *J Clin Pathol*. 2000;53:391–394.

51. Biermann K, Montironi R, Lopez-Beltran A, et al. Histopathological findings after treatment of prostate cancer using high-intensity focused ultrasound (HIFU). *Prostate*. 2010;70:1196–1200.

52. Trachtenberg J, Bogaards A, Weersink RA, et al. Vascular targeted photodynamic therapy with palladium-bacteriopheophorbide photosensitizer for recurrent prostate cancer following definitive radiation therapy: assessment of safety and treatment response. *J Urol*. 2007;178:1974–1979.

53. Orihuela E, Motamedi M, Pow-Sang M, et al. Histopathological evaluation of laser thermocoagulation in the human prostate: optimization of laser irradiation for benign prostatic hyperplasia. *J Urol*. 1995;153:1531–1536.

54. Marks LS, Partin AW, Epstein JI, et al. Effects of a saw palmetto herbal blend in men with symptomatic benign prostatic hyperplasia. *J Urol*. 2000;163:1451–1456.

55. Helpap B, Oehler U, Weisser H. Morphology of benign prostatic hyperplasia after treatment with Sabal Extract IDS89 or placebo: results of a prospective, randomized, double-blind trial. *J Urol Path*. 1995;3:175–182.

56. Orozco RE, Peters RL. Teflon granuloma of the prostate mimicking adenocarcinoma: report of two cases. *J Urol Path*. 1995;3:365–368.

57. Bostwick DG, Vonk J, Picado A. Pathologic changes in the prostate following contemporary 18-gauge needle biopsy: no apparent risk of local cancer seeding. *J Urol Path*. 1994;2:203–212.

58. Bastacky SS, Walsh PC, Epstein JI. Needle biopsy associated tumor tracking of adenocarcinoma of the prostate. *J Urol*. 1991;145:1003–1007.

15

UROTHELIAL CARCINOMA

Prostatic urothelial carcinoma seen in association with bladder urothelial neoplasia may be invasive via direct stromal extension from the bladder, purely intraductal, or intraductal and invasive.

DISTINCTION OF HIGH-GRADE PROSTATIC ADENOCARCINOMA FROM UROTHELIAL CARCINOMA

Prostatic involvement by urothelial carcinoma in a patient with bladder urothelial neoplasia may result from direct invasion of an infiltrating bladder cancer into the stroma of the prostate.[1,2] In this situation, the prognosis of the urothelial carcinoma of the bladder worsens dramatically and is equivalent in survival to cases of bladder carcinoma with regional lymph node metastases.

In these cases, a common diagnostic problem is in differentiating on transurethral resection of the prostate (TURP) between a poorly differentiated urothelial carcinoma of the bladder and a poorly differentiated prostatic adenocarcinoma. The differences in therapy between these two diseases differ significantly, making the distinction between these two entities crucial. Even in poorly differentiated prostatic carcinomas, there is relatively little pleomorphism or mitotic activity compared to poorly differentiated urothelial carcinoma (Figs. 15.1 and 15.2). Poorly differentiated prostate cancers may have enlarged nuclei and prominent nucleoli, yet there is little variability in nuclear shape or size from one nucleus to another (Fig. 15.1). High-grade urothelial carcinomas often reveal marked pleomorphism with tumor giant cells (Fig. 15.2, eFig. 15.1). A subtler finding is that the cytoplasm of prostatic adenocarcinoma is often very foamy and pale, imparting a "soft" appearance. In contrast, urothelial carcinomas may demonstrate hard, glassy eosinophilic cytoplasm or more prominent squamous differentiation (Fig. 15.3). The findings of infiltrating cords of cells (Fig. 15.4) or focal cribriform glandular differentiation are other features more typical of prostatic adenocarcinoma than urothelial carcinoma, which tends to form nests (Fig. 15.5, eFig. 15.2). However, very poorly differentiated urothelial carcinomas can grow in sheets of cells resembling poorly differentiated prostatic adenocarcinoma (Fig. 15.6). Another useful differentiating feature in high-grade prostatic adenocarcinoma is a subtle

(text continues on p. 318)

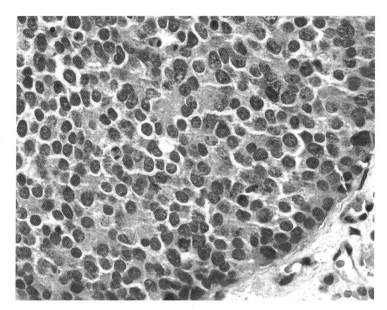

FIGURE 15.1   Poorly differentiated (high-grade) prostatic adenocarcinoma with relatively little anaplasia, as opposed to poorly differentiated transitional cell carcinoma. Note paucity of mitotic figures despite the tumor's poor differentiation. Tumor shows primitive attempts at glandular differentiation resembling rosettes.

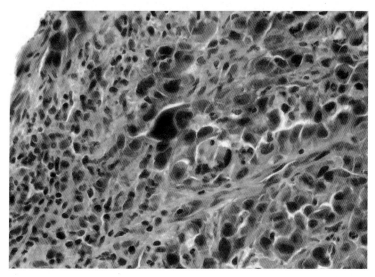

FIGURE 15.2   Infiltrating, poorly differentiated transitional cell carcinoma within the prostate showing marked nuclear atypia and associated inflammation.

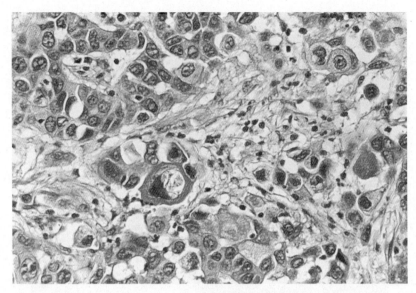

FIGURE 15.3 Infiltrating urothelial carcinoma showing a cell with densely eosinophilic, hard cytoplasm.

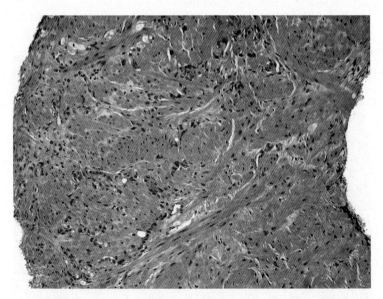

FIGURE 15.4 Infiltrating cords of cells more typical of prostatic adenocarcinoma versus urothelial carcinoma.

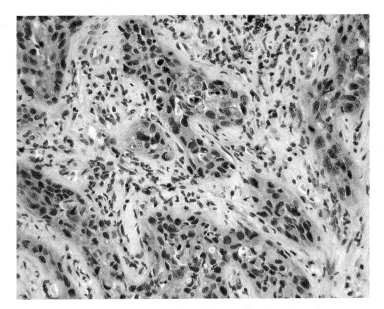

FIGURE 15.5   Nests of infiltrating urothelial carcinoma.

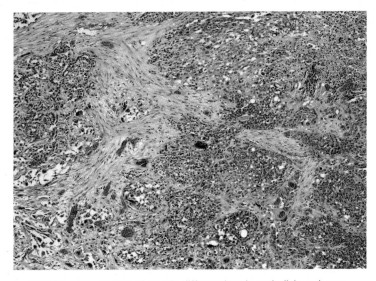

FIGURE 15.6   Sheets of poorly differentiated urothelial carcinoma.

attempt at cribriform gland formation. The tumor is so poorly differentiated that it cannot form true lumina but there are rosette-like areas of cytoplasm in an attempt at glandular differentiation. Urothelial carcinoma lacks this morphology (Fig. 15.1, eFig. 15.3). Another pitfall is that poorly differentiated prostatic adenocarcinoma can fall apart away from its blood supply, giving rise to pseudopapillary structures closely mimicking papillary urothelial carcinoma (Fig. 15.7).

Although for most cases, the distinction between urothelial carcinoma and poorly differentiated prostatic adenocarcinoma can be made on morphologic grounds, there is overlap in a minority of cases. Whereas usual prostate adenocarcinoma has relatively bland cytology as opposed to the greater pleomorphism in urothelial carcinoma, there is a small subset of prostate adenocarcinomas with giant cell pleomorphic features indistinguishable from urothelial carcinoma[3] (Fig. 15.8). Given the crucial difference in management and prognosis, resorting to immunostains is a must if the distinction between urothelial carcinoma and prostatic adenocarcinoma cannot be made with absolute certainty on morphologic features alone.

With only a few exceptions, immunoperoxidase staining for prostate-specific antigen (PSA) and prostate-specific acid phosphatase (PSAP) is very specific for prostatic tissue. Situations that can cause diagnostic difficulty include PSA and PSAP within periurethral glands as well as cystitis cystica and cystitis glandularis in both men and women.[4,5] Other examples of cross-reactive staining include anal glands in men (PSA, PSAP) and urachal remnants (PSA).[6,7] Some intestinal carcinoids and pancreatic islet cell tumors are strongly reactive with antibodies to PSAP, yet are negative

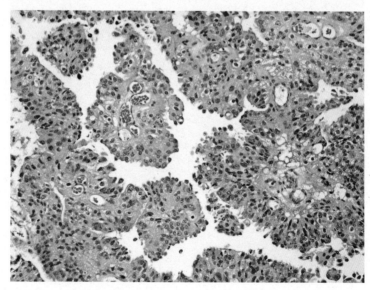

FIGURE 15.7 Prostatic adenocarcinoma with dyscohesive areas away from blood vessels mimicking papillary urothelial carcinoma.

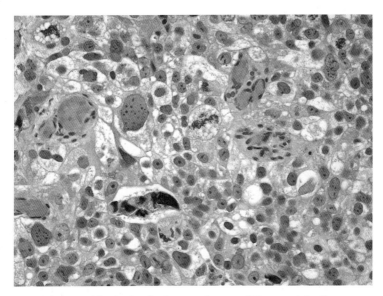

FIGURE 15.8 Pleomorphic giant cell adenocarcinoma of the prostate. Tumor was positive for all prostatic markers and negative for urothelial markers.

with antibodies to PSA.[8] Periurethral gland carcinomas in women and various salivary gland tumors may also be PSA and PSAP positive.[9,10] Weak false-positive staining for PSAP has been reported in several breast and renal cell carcinomas, and we have seen some cases where PSA was focally and weakly positive though the patient was subsequently shown to have a nonprostatic tumor. This suggests that weak focal positive staining for either antigen should be interpreted with caution.

Although PSA and PSAP have proven to be useful in identifying prostate lineage, their sensitivity decreases in poorly differentiated prostate adenocarcinoma. In three studies addressing PSA and the latter issue, 35% to 70% and 25% to 50% of the cases showed less than 25% of the tumor cells staining with PSAP and PSA, respectively.[11–13] The same studies found 5% to 13% of cases to be completely negative to PSAP or PSA. The significance of these figures is that given the, at times, limited amount of tissue sampled, up to 50% of the prostate adenocarcinoma may be interpreted as negative for PSA or PSAP, owing to only focal positivity that may not be sampled. Even when both PSA and PSAP are employed, the lack of immunoreactivity in a poorly differentiated tumor within the prostate, especially on limited amount of sample, does not exclude the diagnosis of a poorly differentiated prostatic adenocarcinoma. In such scenario, newer prostate lineage markers such as prostein (P501S), prostate-specific membrane antigen (PSMA), NKX3.1,[14] HOXB13,[15] and androgen receptor[16] could be of added use. Of these markers, PSMA has lower specificity and androgen receptor can also be positive in urothelial carcinoma.[17] HOXB13 has not been used in routine surgical pathology practice. P501S has the benefit of distinctive clumpy granular immunoreactivity and NKX3.1 is a very sensitive and specific nuclear antibody (Fig. 15.9). Combining some of the aforementioned markers with urothelial lineage markers will further facilitate resolving a urothelial versus prostatic carcinoma differential diagnosis (Table 15.1). Recent studies have documented high molecular weight cytokeratin (HMWCK) positivity in over 90% of urothelial carcinoma.[14,18] HMWCK is only rarely and focally expressed in prostate carcinoma (8%).[14] A cautionary note is warranted given that HMWCK labels squamous epithelia including areas of squamous differentiation in post-therapy recurrent prostate carcinoma lesions. HMWCK positivity that is restricted to areas of squamous differentiation does not exclude the diagnosis of adenocarcinoma of the prostate.[19] P63 has a greater specificity albeit lower sensitivity for urothelial carcinoma compared to HMWCK (100% specificity and 83% sensitivity).[14]

Uroplakins are urothelium-specific transmembrane proteins expressed by the majority of noninvasive and up to two-thirds of advanced invasive and metastatic urothelial carcinomas as assessed by uroplakin III (UP III).[20–24] Although highly specific for urothelial differentiation, UP III is only of moderate degree of sensitivity (as low as 40%) in high-grade urothelial carcinoma.[25] Thrombomodulin is an endothelial cell–associated cofactor for thrombin-mediated activator of protein C. Its expression, predominantly as membranous staining, has been found in 69% to 100% of urothelial carcinoma.[14,22,26,27] Thrombomodulin is only rarely positive in prostate adenocarcinoma.[14,27] It is also expressed by nonurothelial tumors such as vascular tumors, mesotheliomas, and squamous cell carcinomas.[27] Compared to UP III, thrombomodulin has a higher degree of sensitivity

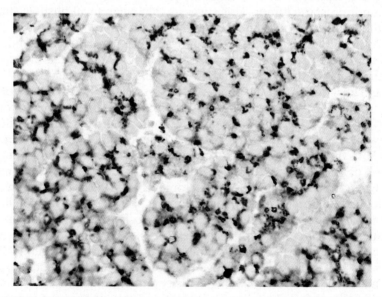

FIGURE 15.9 Poorly differentiated adenocarcinoma of the prostate with distinctive P501S (prostein) cytoplasmic granular immunoreactivity.

TABLE 15.1 Urothelial and Prostatic Markers in the Differential of Prostate Carcinoma versus Urothelial Carcinoma

	HMWCK	p63	Thrombomodulin	GATA3		
Prostate carcinoma	7.9%	0%	5.3%	0%		
Urothelial carcinoma	91.4%	82.9%	68.6%	86%		

	PSA	P501S	PSMA	NKX3.1	pPSA
Prostate carcinoma	97.4%	100%	92.1%	94.7%	94.7%
Urothelial carcinoma	0%	5.7%	0%	0%	0%

HMWCK, high molecular weight cytokeratin; PSA, prostate-specific antigen; PSMA, prostate-specific membrane antigen; pPSA, pro–prostate-specific antigen.

Modified from Chuang AY, De Marzo AM, Veltri RW, et al. Immunohistochemical differentiation of high-grade prostate carcinoma from urothelial carcinoma. *Am J Surg Pathol.* 2007;31:1246–1255; Liu H, Shi J, Wilkerson ML, et al. Immuhistochemical evaluation of GATA3 expression in tumors and normal tissues: a useful immunomarker for breast and urothelial carcinomas. *Am J Clin Pathol.* 2012;138:57–64.

but lower specificity as a marker for urothelial carcinoma. In a recent study, we also found p63 to be superior to thrombomodulin as a urothelial marker in high-grade tumors.[14]

GATA3 (GATA binding protein 3 to DNA sequence [A/T]GATA[A/G]) is a member of a zinc finger transcription factor family. Several recent studies have confirmed its use as a marker of urothelial carcinoma.[28–31] In the two largest studies, by Liu et al.[30] and Miettinen et al.,[31] 86% and more than 90% of urothelial carcinomas were positive for GATA3, respectively. The nuclear staining is usually diffuse in more than 50% of cells. Less than 10% of prostatic adenocarcinomas were positive for GATA3.[31] In our experience, GATA3 is specific in the differential diagnosis of urothelial carcinoma versus prostatic adenocarcinoma and is the marker of choice for identifying a poorly differentiated tumor in this region as being of urothelial origin[14,32] (Table 15.1). Finally, in our experience, CK7 and CK20 are of limited use in this differential, given that they may be both positive in a subset of adenocarcinoma of the prostate.[33,34]

Distinguishing primary urothelial carcinoma with focal glandular differentiation (Fig. 15.10) and bladder adenocarcinoma extending to prostate is also of important clinical and management implications. In general, adenocarcinomas of the bladder resemble adenocarcinomas of the intestine, although signet ring and nonintestinal types also exist. Immunohistochemical markers of prostate lineage are again of great use in this regard.

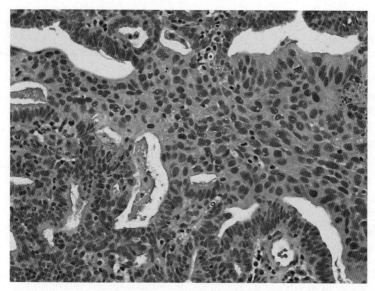

FIGURE 15.10   Urothelial carcinoma with areas of glandular differentiation.

Adenocarcinomas of the bladder, whether as a pure tumor or with mixed urothelial carcinoma, have been reported to be occasionally positive for PSA or PSAP; however, there has yet to be a case reported positive for both.[35,36]

Although the specificity of newer prostate lineage markers has been tested against bladder urothelial carcinoma, the same could not be said about their pattern of reactivity in bladder adenocarcinoma. In a recent immunohistochemistry study evaluating 37 adenocarcinomas of bladder, our group demonstrated that a minority of bladder adenocarcinomas are positive for prostate antigens P501S and PSMA.[37] P501S showed moderate diffuse cytoplasmic staining in 11% of cases including enteric-type and rare mucinous adenocarcinomas. The granular perinuclear staining pattern of P501S typically seen in prostatic adenocarcinoma was absent in all cases of bladder adenocarcinoma. In addition, PSMA showed diffuse cytoplasmic or membranous staining in 21% of bladder adenocarcinomas including signet ring, urachal, mucinous, and enteric-type variants. All cases were negative for PSA and PSAP. Therefore, immunoreactivity for P501S and PSMA should be interpreted with caution in such settings. The lack of granular perinuclear staining for P501S and the absence of membranous PSMA staining both favor a bladder adenocarcinoma. Membranous PSMA staining indistinguishable from that seen in prostate cancer can be seen in less than 10% of bladder adenocarcinoma. Our group has recently evaluated the expression of GATA-3 in primary bladder adenocarcinoma.[38] Diffuse nuclear GATA-3 labeling was seen in 41% of signet ring adenocarcinoma of bladder but only in 7% of conventional adenocarcinomas, making the marker only helpful in the differential of tumors with signet ring features.

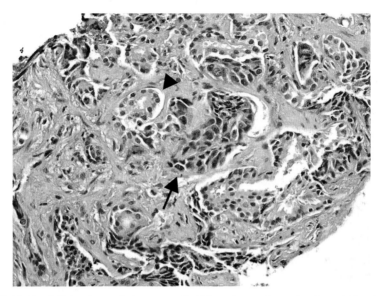

FIGURE 15.11 Collision tumor between urothelial carcinoma *(arrow)* and prostatic adenocarcinoma *(arrowhead)*. Each tumor expressed lineage-specific immunohistochemical staining.

Almost 50% of cystoprostatectomy specimens performed for urothelial carcinoma also contain adenocarcinoma of the prostate.[1,39–41] Therefore, the finding in a TURP of a small focus of well-differentiated adenocarcinoma of the prostate should not necessarily influence whether a separate focus of poorly differentiated tumor is urothelial carcinoma or adenocarcinoma of the prostate. We have even seen rare cases of collision tumors between prostatic adenocarcinoma and urothelial carcinoma (Fig. 15.11).

INTRADUCTAL UROTHELIAL CARCINOMA INVOLVING THE PROSTATE

Most commonly, urothelial carcinoma involves the prostate in a setting of a patient with bladder urothelial carcinoma. Although topical chemotherapy and immunotherapy for superficial bladder carcinomas appear to act by direct contact with neoplastic epithelium, it has become critical to identify those cases of bladder urothelial carcinomas with prostatic involvement, because conservative management will not treat these cases effectively. Currently, biopsies of the prostatic urethra and suburethral prostate tissue are often recommended as a staging procedure in patients undergoing conservative treatment for superficial bladder tumors. It is also important to evaluate the urothelium in routine TURP specimens, because we have seen several cases of carcinoma in situ (CIS) where no history of bladder cancer was present. Several studies have shown that by examining random sections of the prostate at the time of cystectomy for urothelial carcinoma of the bladder, between 12% and 20% of the cases will be shown to have prostatic involvement by urothelial carcinoma. If serial sections of the prostate in cystoprostatectomy specimens with bladder urothelial carcinoma are performed, involvement of the prostate by urothelial carcinoma may be found in 37% to 45% of the cases.[1,42,43] If intraductal urothelial carcinoma is identified on TURP or transurethral biopsy, patients usually will be recommended for radical cystoprostatectomy. The finding of intraductal urothelial carcinoma also has been demonstrated to increase the risk of urethral recurrence following cystoprostatectomy, such that its identification may also result in prophylactic total urethrectomy.

Intraductal urothelial carcinoma of the prostate is usually accompanied by CIS of the prostatic urethra. Involvement of the prostate appears to be by direct extension from the overlying urethra, because in the majority of cases, the more centrally located prostatic ducts are involved by urothelial neoplasia to a greater extent than the peripheral ducts and acini. Intraductal urothelial carcinoma of the prostatic ducts initially consists of malignant urothelial cells insinuating themselves between the basal cell layer and the columnar to cuboidal luminal epithelium of the prostatic ducts. More peripherally, urothelial carcinoma spreads in a pagetoid fashion within the ducts. Similar to that seen in the breast, large tumor cells with clear cytoplasm are seen in the midst of otherwise normal urothelium. With more extensive involvement, urothelial carcinoma fills and expands ducts and often develops central comedonecrosis (Fig. 15.12, eFigs. 15.4 to 15.17). Intraductal urothelial carcinoma of the prostatic ducts without prostatic stromal invasion tends to be seen in lower stage bladder urothelial carcinomas. Once resected by cystoprostatectomy, the noninvasive involvement of the prostate by urothelial carcinoma does not adversely affect survival; the prognosis is determined by the stage of the bladder tumor.[1,2,44] In prostates with intraductal urothelial carcinoma and stromal invasion, the associated bladder tumors tend to be high-stage, in which case the already poor prognosis is not affected by the prostatic involvement.[1] However, intraductal and infiltrating prostatic urothelial carcinoma may also be associated with low-stage bladder tumors.

The differentiation between extensive intraductal urothelial carcinoma from intraductal and invasive urothelial carcinoma may be difficult. With intraductal urothelial carcinoma of the prostate, nests of urothelial carcinoma have the contours and distribution of prostatic ducts and acini. The nests are circumscribed with a smooth discrete edge between the epithelium and the adjacent stroma, and the stroma lacks a desmoplastic response (Figs. 15.12 and 15.13). Infiltrating urothelial carcinoma is characterized by small cords, nests, or individual cells eliciting a desmoplastic stromal response (Fig. 15.14, eFigs. 15.18 to 15.23). In some instances, numerous closely packed irregular large nests and small nests are diagnosable as infiltrating urothelial carcinoma, because this architectural pattern is not consistent with intraductal growth of urothelial carcinoma. In approximately one-third of cases, urothelial carcinoma is negative for

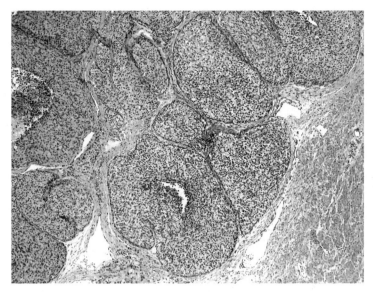

FIGURE 15.12 Intraductal urothelial carcinoma filling up and expanding several prostatic ducts and acini with areas of central necrosis.

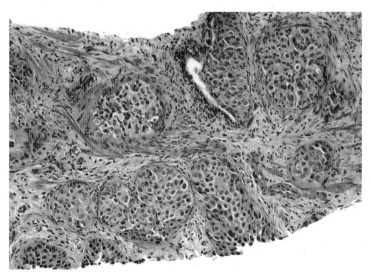

FIGURE 15.13 Intraductal urothelial carcinoma on needle biopsy. Note lack of desmoplastic response surrounding these nests.

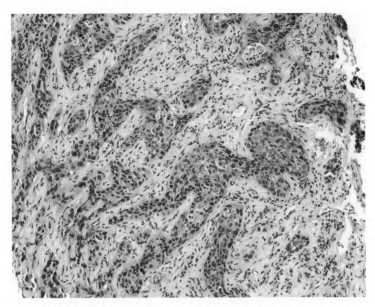

FIGURE 15.14 Infiltrating nests of urothelial carcinoma with a desmoplastic stromal response and irregular borders in the infiltrating tumor nests.

HMWCK and p63, such that the outlining of residual prostatic basal cells can help establish the diagnosis of intraductal urothelial carcinoma (Fig. 15.15). However, in the majority of cases, urothelial carcinoma expresses HMWCK and p63 such that the antibodies are not helpful in clarifying the intraductal nature of the process (Fig. 15.16).

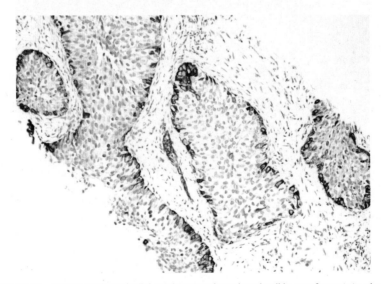

FIGURE 15.15 Intraductal urothelial carcinoma where basal cell layer of prostate glands are positive and urothelial carcinoma is negative.

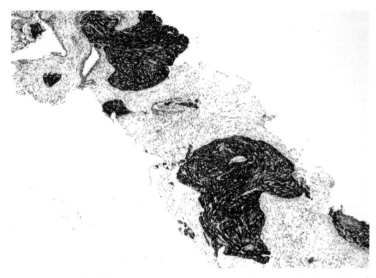

FIGURE 15.16   Urothelial carcinoma on prostate needle biopsy labeled with HMWCK.

UROTHELIAL CARCINOMA SEEN ON NEEDLE BIOPSY

The diagnosis of urothelial carcinoma on prostate needle biopsy is especially difficult for several reasons. First, urothelial carcinoma on prostate biopsy is rare, especially relative to the frequency with which adenocarcinoma of the prostate is diagnosed on needle biopsy. Second, we have shown that urothelial carcinoma involving the prostate clinically can mimic prostatic adenocarcinoma in terms of findings on digital rectal exam and ultrasound, along with the potential for an elevated serum PSA level.[45] Third, there may be no prior or concurrent history of urothelial carcinoma in the bladder (47% of our cases).

Histologic features and immunohistochemical studies (see earlier discussion) are therefore essential to establish the correct diagnosis. Urothelial carcinoma involving the prostate differs from adenocarcinoma of the prostate both architecturally and cytologically. Urothelial carcinoma in the prostate typically forms nests of tumor, whereas poorly differentiated prostate cancer tends to form sheets, individual cells, or cords. Urothelial carcinoma involving the prostate in our study contained areas of necrosis in 43% of cases. Necrosis is an unusual finding in even high-grade adenocarcinoma of the prostate. The presence of an intraductal growth where preexisting benign prostate glands are filled with solid nests of tumor also differs from high-grade prostatic intraepithelial neoplasia, although can be seen in intraductal carcinoma of the prostate. The presence of squamous differentiation seen in 14% of our cases would also be unusual for adenocarcinoma of the prostate. Cytologically, urothelial carcinomas involving the prostate tend to show greater nuclear pleomorphism, variably prominent nucleoli, and increased mitotic activity compared to even poorly differentiated prostate adenocarcinoma, although as noted earlier, there is overlap in some cases. In high-grade adenocarcinomas of the prostate, nuclei tend to be more uniform from one to another with centrally located prominent eosinophilic nucleoli. Mitotic figures in high-grade prostate cancer are typically not as frequent compared to what is seen in urothelial carcinoma on biopsy. Finally, the presence of stromal inflammation, seen in 76% of our cases of urothelial carcinoma on biopsy, differs from the typical lack of associated inflammation seen with ordinary adenocarcinoma of the prostate. The overall prognosis of urothelial cell carcinoma diagnosed on prostatic needle biopsy is poor, even in cases without histologic evidence of stromal invasion on biopsy.[45] In these cases with intraductal cancer on biopsy, most likely invasive cancer is present elsewhere in the prostate that was not sampled. Although the prognosis is poor, even with only apparent intraductal involvement, histologic recognition is essential because the only opportunity for improved outcome is early and aggressive therapy.

PRIMARY UROTHELIAL CARCINOMA

Primary urothelial carcinoma of the prostate without bladder involvement is a rare lesion.[46-50] Primary urothelial carcinoma of the prostate should not be called periurethral prostatic duct carcinoma, as sometimes reported in the literature, because this term may be confused with prostatic duct adenocarcinomas. Histologically, primary urothelial carcinoma of the prostate is characterized by intraductal urothelial carcinoma, almost always accompanied by infiltration. A continuum from urothelial hyperplasia without atypia to atypical urothelial hyperplasia to CIS can also be identified.[51] Rarely, urothelial CIS may be papillary within enlarged dilated prostatic ducts.[46] Although Greene et al.[46] claims that one-third of the cases of primary urothelial carcinoma of the prostate have areas of adenocarcinoma, this number is probably overstated. This study predated the use of immunohistochemistry for PSA and PSAP, and these cases may have been adenocarcinomas of the prostate with areas of poor differentiation, resembling urothelial carcinoma.

Primary urothelial carcinomas of the prostate tend to infiltrate the bladder neck and surrounding soft tissue such that over 50% of the patients present with tumors extending out of the prostate. Twenty percent of the patients present with distant metastases; bone and liver being the most common sites. In contrast to adenocarcinoma of the prostate, bone metastases are usually osteolytic. Rubenstein and Rubnitz[49] described 10 cases of urothelial cell carcinoma arising within the large periurethral prostatic ducts. These patients all died within 2 years of diagnosis, with 8 (80%) dying within 1 year.[49] Greene et al.[46] reported a series of 39 patients with primary urothelial cell carcinoma of the prostate. Again, the prognosis was poor with 34 (87%) patients dying within 5 years.[46] Average survival was only 17 months.[47] In their review of three additional cases, Nicolaisen and

Williams[48] emphasized clinical presentation (obstructive symptoms in younger patients) and an aggressive course with a propensity for local invasion and stressed radical surgery as the only hope for survival. In 2010, the American Joint Committee on Cancer revised the classification of prostatic urothelial carcinoma according to the depth and mode of invasion.[52] Specifically, the revised staging classification assigns patients with extravesical (transmural) invasion of the prostate from a bladder tumor as pT4a. Involvement of the prostate by subepithelial urethral invasion is no longer classified as pT4 but rather given a separate pathologic tumor stage according to depth invasion as pTis for noninvasive disease and pT2 for prostatic stromal invasion. Two recent studies by Patel et al.[53] and Knoedler et al.[54] validated the new classification. The latter study reported the Mayo clinic experience with urothelial carcinoma involving the prostate in light of the revised staging and addressed the prognostic significance of coexistent bladder cancer following radical cystectomy. Median follow-up was 10.5 years. Five-year cancer-specific survival for patients with pTis, pT2, and pT4a prostate urothelial carcinoma was 73%, 57%, and 20%, respectively. On multivariable analysis, higher prostate tumor stage, positive lymph node status, and concurrent ≥pT3 bladder cancer were significantly associated with an increased risk of death from urothelial carcinoma. The findings validated the recently suggested staging reclassification. The negative impact on survival of the coexisting bladder tumor stage suggested a potential role for assigning a secondary tumor stage in such cases.

REFERENCES

1. Schellhammer PF, Bean MA, Whitmore WF Jr. Prostatic involvement by transitional cell carcinoma: pathogenesis, patterns and prognosis. *J Urol.* 1977;118:399–403.
2. Chibber PJ, McIntyre MA, Hindmarsh JR, et al. Transitional cell carcinoma involving the prostate. *Br J Urol.* 1981;53:605–609.
3. Parwani AV, Herawi M, Epstein JI. Pleomorphic giant cell adenocarcinoma of the prostate: report of 6 cases. *Am J Surg Pathol.* 2006;30:1254–1259.
4. Nowels K, Kent E, Rinsho K, et al. Prostate specific antigen and acid phosphatase-reactive cells in cystitis cystica and glandularis. *Arch Pathol Lab Med.* 1988;112:734–737.
5. Pollen JJ, Dreilinger A. Immunohistochemical identification of prostatic acid phosphatase and prostate specific antigen in female periurethral glands. *Urology.* 1984;23:303–304.
6. Kamoshida S, Tsutsumi Y. Extraprostatic localization of prostatic acid phosphatase and prostate-specific antigen: distribution in cloacogenic glandular epithelium and sex-dependent expression in human anal gland. *Hum Pathol.* 1990;21:1108–1111.
7. Golz R, Schubert GE. Prostatic specific antigen: immunoreactivity in urachal remnants. *J Urol.* 1989;141:1480–1482.
8. Sobin LH, Hjermstad BM, Sesterhenn IA, et al. Prostatic acid phosphatase activity in carcinoid tumors. *Cancer.* 1986;58:136–138.
9. Spencer JR, Brodin AG, Ignatoff JM. Clear cell adenocarcinoma of the urethra: evidence for origin within paraurethral ducts. *J Urol.* 1990;143:122–125.
10. van Krieken JH. Prostate marker immunoreactivity in salivary gland neoplasms. A rare pitfall in immunohistochemistry. *Am J Surg Pathol.* 1993;17:410–414.

11. Svanholm H. Evaluation of commercial immunoperoxidase kits for prostatic specific antigen and prostatic specific acid phosphatase. *Acta Pathol Microbiol Immunol Scand [A]*. 1986;94:7–12.

12. Ellis DW, Leffers S, Davies JS, et al. Multiple immunoperoxidase markers in benign hyperplasia and adenocarcinoma of the prostate. *Am J Clin Pathol*. 1984;81:279–284.

13. Ford TF, Butcher DN, Masters JR, et al. Immunocytochemical localisation of prostate-specific antigen: specificity and application to clinical practice. *Br J Urol*. 1985;57: 50–55.

14. Chuang AY, DeMarzo AM, Veltri RW, et al. Immunohistochemical differentiation of high-grade prostate carcinoma from urothelial carcinoma. *Am J Surg Pathol*. 2007;31: 1246–1255.

15. Varinot J, Cussenot O, Roupret M, et al. HOXB13 is a sensitive and specific marker of prostate cells, useful in distinguishing between carcinomas of prostatic and urothelial origin. *Virchows Arch*. 2013;463:803–809.

16. Downes MR, Torlakovic EE, Aldaoud N, et al. Diagnostic utility of androgen receptor expression in discriminating poorly differentiated urothelial and prostate carcinoma. *J Clin Pathol*. 2013;66:779–786.

17. Miyamoto H, Yao JL, Chaux A, et al. Expression of androgen and oestrogen receptors and its prognostic significance in urothelial neoplasm of the urinary bladder. *BJU Int*. 2012;109:1716–1726.

18. Varma M, Morgan M, Amin MB, et al. High molecular weight cytokeratin antibody (clone 34betaE12): a sensitive marker for differentiation of high-grade invasive urothelial carcinoma from prostate cancer. *Histopathology*. 2003;42:167–172.

19. Parwani AV, Kronz JD, Genega EM, et al. Prostate carcinoma with squamous differentiation: an analysis of 33 cases. *Am J Surg Pathol*. 2004;28:651–657.

20. Kaufmann O, Volmerig J, Dietel M. Uroplakin III is a highly specific and moderately sensitive immunohistochemical marker for primary and metastatic urothelial carcinomas. *Am J Clin Pathol*. 2000;113:683–687.

21. Ohtsuka Y, Kawakami S, Fujii Y, et al. Loss of uroplakin III expression is associated with a poor prognosis in patients with urothelial carcinoma of the upper urinary tract. *BJU Int*. 2006;97:1322–1326.

22. Parker DC, Folpe AL, Bell J, et al. Potential utility of uroplakin III, thrombomodulin, high molecular weight cytokeratin, and cytokeratin 20 in noninvasive, invasive, and metastatic urothelial (transitional cell) carcinomas. *Am J Surg Pathol*. 2003;27:1–10.

23. Huang HY, Shariat SF, Sun TT, et al. Persistent uroplakin expression in advanced urothelial carcinomas: implications in urothelial tumor progression and clinical outcome. *Hum Pathol*. 2007;38:1703–1713.

24. Moll R, Wu XR, Lin JH, et al. Uroplakins, specific membrane proteins of urothelial umbrella cells, as histological markers of metastatic transitional cell carcinomas. *Am J Pathol*. 1995;147:1383–1397.

25. Logani S, Oliva E, Amin MB, et al. Immunoprofile of ovarian tumors with putative transitional cell (urothelial) differentiation using novel urothelial markers: histogenetic and diagnostic implications. *Am J Surg Pathol*. 2003;27:1434–1441.

26. Wang HL, Lu DW, Yerian LM, et al. Immunohistochemical distinction between primary adenocarcinoma of the bladder and secondary colorectal adenocarcinoma. *Am J Surg Pathol*. 2001;25:1380–1387.

27. Ordonez NG. Thrombomodulin expression in transitional cell carcinoma. *Am J Clin Pathol*. 1998;110:385–390.

28. Higgins JP, Kaygusuz G, Wang L, et al. Placental S100 (S100P) and GATA3: markers for transitional epithelium and urothelial carcinoma discovered by complementary DNA microarray. *Am J Surg Pathol*. 2007;31:673–680.

29. Esheba GE, Longacre TA, Atkins KA, et al. Expression of the urothelial differentiation markers GATA3 and placental S100 (S100P) in female genital tract transitional cell proliferations. *Am J Surg Pathol.* 2009;33:347–353.

30. Liu H, Shi J, Wilkerson ML, et al. Immunohistochemical evaluation of GATA3 expression in tumors and normal tissues: a useful immunomarker for breast and urothelial carcinomas. *Am J Clin Pathol.* 2012;138:57–64.

31. Miettinen M, McCue PA, Sarlomo-Rikala M, et al. GATA3: a multispecific but potentially useful marker in surgical pathology: a systematic analysis of 2500 epithelial and nonepithelial tumors. *Am J Surg Pathol.* 2014;38:13–22.

32. Chang A, Amin A, Gabrielson E, et al. Utility of GATA3 immunohistochemistry in differentiating urothelial carcinoma from prostate adenocarcinoma and squamous cell carcinomas of the uterine cervix, anus, and lung. *Am J Surg Pathol.* 2012;36:1472–1476.

33. Genega EM, Hutchinson B, Reuter VE, et al. Immunophenotype of high-grade prostatic adenocarcinoma and urothelial carcinoma. *Mod Pathol.* 2000;13:1186–1191.

34. Mhawech P, Uchida T, Pelte MF. Immunohistochemical profile of high-grade urothelial bladder carcinoma and prostate adenocarcinoma. *Hum Pathol.* 2002;33:1136–1140.

35. Epstein JI, Kuhajda FP, Lieberman PH. Prostate-specific acid phosphatase immunoreactivity in adenocarcinomas of the urinary bladder. *Hum Pathol.* 1986;17:939–942.

36. Grignon DJ, Ro JY, Ayala AG, et al. Primary adenocarcinoma of the urinary bladder. A clinicopathologic analysis of 72 cases. *Cancer.* 1991;67:2165–2172.

37. Lane Z, Hansel DE, Epstein JI. Immunohistochemical expression of prostatic antigens in adenocarcinoma and villous adenoma of the urinary bladder. *Am J Surg Pathol.* 2008;32:1322–1326.

38. Ellis CL, Chang AG, Cimino-Mathews A, et al. GATA-3 immunohistochemistry in the differential diagnosis of adenocarcinoma of the urinary bladder. *Am J Surg Pathol.* 2013;37:1756–1760.

39. Wood DP Jr, Montie JE, Pontes JE, et al. Transitional cell carcinoma of the prostate in cystoprostatectomy specimens removed for bladder cancer. *J Urol.* 1989;141:346–349.

40. Mahadevia PS, Koss LG, Tar IJ. Prostatic involvement in bladder cancer. Prostate mapping in 20 cystoprostatectomy specimens. *Cancer.* 1986;58:2096–2102.

41. Bruins HM, Djaladat H, Ahmadi H, et al. Incidental prostate cancer in patients with bladder urothelial carcinoma: comprehensive analysis of 1,476 radical cystoprostatectomy specimens. *J Urol.* 2013;190:1704–1709.

42. Nadji M, Tabei SZ, Castro A, et al. Prostatic-specific antigen: an immunohistologic marker for prostatic neoplasms. *Cancer.* 1981;48:1229–1232.

43. Esrig D, Freeman JA, Elmajian DA, et al. Transitional cell carcinoma involving the prostate with a proposed staging classification for stromal invasion. *J Urol.* 1996;156: 1071–1076.

44. Wishnow KI, Ro JY. Importance of early treatment of transitional cell carcinoma of prostatic ducts. *Urology.* 1988;32:11–12.

45. Oliai BR, Kahane H, Epstein JI. A clinicopathologic analysis of urothelial carcinomas diagnosed on prostate needle biopsy. *Am J Surg Pathol.* 2001;25:794–801.

46. Greene LF, O'Dea MJ, Dockerty MB. Primary transitional cell carcinoma of the prostate. *J Urol.* 1976;116:761–763.

47. Goebbels R, Amberger L, Wernert N, et al. Urothelial carcinoma of the prostate. *Appl Pathol.* 1985;3:242–254.

48. Nicolaisen GS, Williams RD. Primary transitional cell carcinoma of prostate. Urology. 1984;24:544–549.

49. Rubenstein AB, Rubnitz ME. Transitional cell carcinoma of the prostate. *Cancer.* 1969; 24:543–546.

50. Sawczuk I, Tannenbaum M, Olsson CA, et al. Primary transitional cell carcinoma of prostatic periurethral ducts. *Urology.* 1985;25:339–343.

51. Ullmann AS, Ross OA. Hyperplasia, atypism, and carcinoma in situ in prostatic periurethral glands. *Am J Clin Pathol.* 1967;47:497–504.

52. Edge S, Byrd D, Compton C, et al. *AJCC Cancer Staging Manual.* 7th ed. New York, NY: Springer; 2010.

53. Patel AR, Cohn JA, Abd El Latif A, et al. Validation of new AJCC exclusion criteria for subepithelial prostatic stromal invasion from pT4a bladder urothelial carcinoma. *J Urol.* 2013;189:53–58.

54. Knoedler JJ, Boorjian SA, Tollefson MK, et al. Urothelial carcinoma involving the prostate: the Association of Revised Tumor Stage and Coexistent Bladder Cancer with Survival Following Radical Cystectomy [published online ahead of print October 7, 2013]. *BJU Int.* 2013. doi:10.1111/bju.12486.

16

MESENCHYMAL TUMORS AND TUMOR-LIKE CONDITIONS

STROMAL TUMORS OF UNCERTAIN MALIGNANT POTENTIAL AND STROMAL SARCOMAS

Prostatic stromal tumors arising from the specialized prostatic stroma are rare and distinct tumors with diverse histologic patterns (eFigs. 16.1 to 16.28). In the past, these tumors have been reported under a variety of terms including atypical stromal (smooth muscle) hyperplasia, phyllodes type of atypical stromal hyperplasia, phyllodes tumor, and cystic epithelial-stromal tumors. Because the phyllodes "leaflike" pattern is only seen in a subset of both benign and malignant stromal tumors, we prefer to designate stromal tumors of the prostates in more general descriptive terms such as *stromal tumors of uncertain malignant potential* (STUMPs) and *stromal sarcomas*, as has also been recommended by the 2004 World Health Organization Classification of Tumours of the Urinary System and Male Genital Organs.[1] To date, there have been three large studies on these lesions.[2-4] STUMPs have been reported to occur between the ages of 27 and 83 years, with a median age of 58 years and a peak incidence in the sixth and seventh decades. Patients present most commonly with lower urinary tract obstruction, followed by an abnormal digital rectal examination, hematuria, hematospermia, rectal fullness, a palpable rectal mass, or elevated serum prostate-specific antigen (PSA) levels. On gross examination, STUMPs appear white-tan and may demonstrate a solid or solid-cystic pattern with smooth-walled cysts filled with bloody, mucinous, or clear fluid. These tumors may involve either the transition zone or the peripheral zone and may range in size from microscopic lesions (which are typically incidentally found) to large, cystic lesions up to 15 cm in size.

Microscopically, four patterns of STUMP have been described and include (a) hypercellular stroma with scattered atypical but degenerative-appearing cells admixed with benign prostatic glands (Fig. 16.1), (b) hypercellular stroma consisting of bland fusiform stromal cells with eosinophilic cytoplasm admixed with benign glands (Fig. 16.2), (c) leaflike hypocellular fibrous stroma covered by benign-appearing prostatic epithelium similar in morphology to a benign phyllodes tumor of the

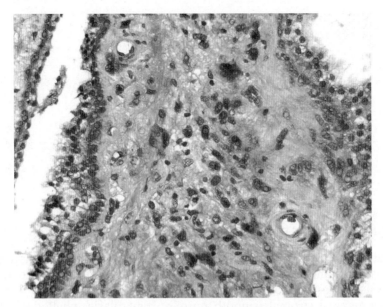

FIGURE 16.1   STUMP with scattered stromal cells with enlarged but degenerative-appearing nuclei.

breast (Fig. 16.3), and (d) myxoid stroma containing bland stromal cells and often lacking admixed glands (Fig. 16.4). Cases can exhibit a mixture of the aforementioned patterns. Areas of benign prostatic hyperplasia (BPH) can have microscopic fibroadenoma-like foci, which should not be designated as STUMP (Fig 16.5, eFig. 16.29).

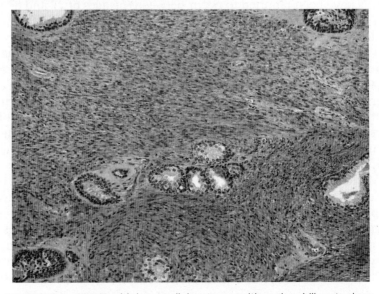

FIGURE 16.2   STUMP with hypercellular stroma with eosinophilic cytoplasm.

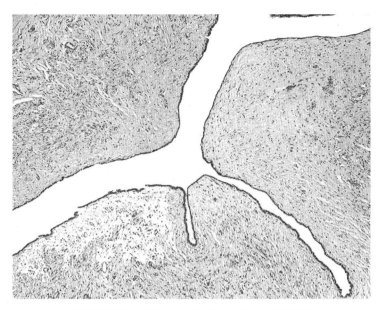

FIGURE 16.3 Benign phyllodes pattern of STUMP.

Approximately half of all reported cases of STUMP demonstrate the first pattern of hypercellular stroma containing atypical cells intermixed with, but not compressing, benign glands. The atypical stromal cells in these cases are pleomorphic and hyperchromatic, with a marked degenerative appearance. Mitotic figures are typically absent and

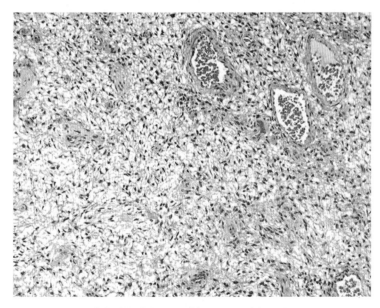

FIGURE 16.4 Myxoid pattern of STUMP.

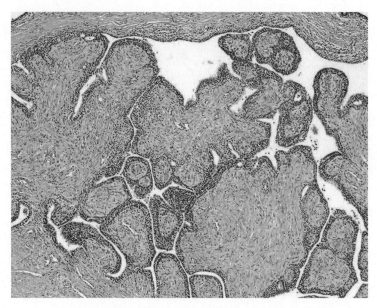

FIGURE 16.5 Incidental finding of small focus of fibroadenomatoid change in BPH.

atypical mitoses should not be seen. Cases of STUMP demonstrating hypercellular, elongated, bland stromal cells with admixed glands may be occasionally misdiagnosed as a cellular stromal proliferation associated with BPH, although the extent of hypercellularity and often more eosinophilic nature of the cytoplasm are unique. The benign phyllodes pattern of STUMP may also contain atypical, degenerative-appearing stromal cells and may be associated with a variety of benign epithelial proliferations, including basal cell hyperplasia, adenosis, and sclerosing adenosis. Finally, the myxoid pattern of STUMP may be confused with stromal nodules of BPH, although the myxoid pattern of STUMP consists of extensive sheets of myxoid stroma without the nodularity identified in BPH. Occasionally, the extensive myxoid stroma is admixed with benign prostate glands.[4] In contrast to myxoid STUMPs, stromal BPH is nodular and contains thick-walled arterioles cut in cross section (Figs. 16.6 and 16.7).

STUMPS and stromal sarcomas, although the neoplastic cells are mesenchymal, often have associated epithelial proliferations. These include adenosis, glandular crowding and complexity, prostatic intraepithelial neoplasia (PIN), squamous metaplasia, urothelial metaplasia, basal cell hyperplasia, adenosis, and clear cell cribriform hyperplasia (Fig. 16.8). Within these tumors, there is epithelial-mesenchymal crosstalk, as has been described in benign prostate and in prostatic carcinogenesis. In unusual cases of STUMP, the epithelial proliferation may predominate to the extent that it can mask the diagnosis of STUMP.[5]

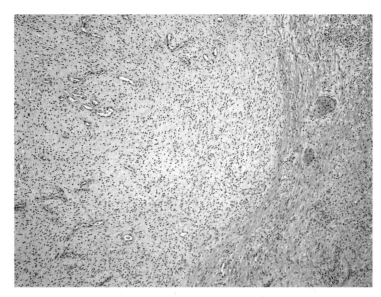

FIGURE 16.6   Myxoid stromal nodular of BPH with multiple thick-walled capillaries cut in cross section.

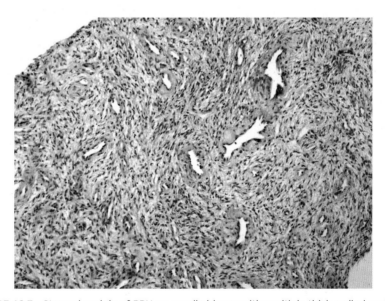

FIGURE 16.7   Stromal nodule of BPH on needle biopsy with multiple thick-walled capillaries cut in cross section.

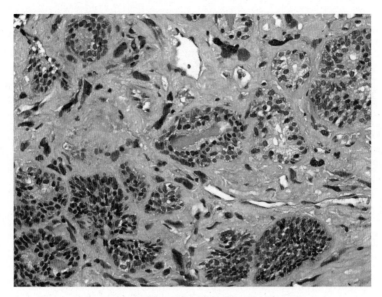

FIGURE 16.8   STUMP with basal cell hyperplasia.

Most cases of STUMP are positive for CD34 and vimentin and variably positive for smooth muscle actin and desmin (Table 16.1).[6] Due to the derivation of these tumors from the prostatic stroma, progesterone receptor is frequently present on immunostaining, although estrogen receptor is less commonly positive. C-kit and S100 have been negative in all cases

TABLE 16.1							
Immunohistochemical Characteristics of Nonepithelial Prostatic Spindle Cell Lesions							
	STUMP	**SS**	**Leiomyo-sarcoma**	**Rhabdomyo-sarcoma**	**IMT**	**SFT**	**GIST**
CD34	+	+	−	−	−	+	+
SMA	+/−	−	+	+	+	−	+/−
Desmin	+/−	−	+	+	+	−	+/−
Myogenin	−	−	−	+	−	−	−
c-kit	−	−	−	−	+/−	−	+
ALK-1	−	−	−	−	+	−	−
PR	+	+	+/−	−	−	+/−	−

STUMP, stromal tumor of uncertain malignant potential; SS, stromal sarcoma; IMT, inflammatory myofibroblastic tumor; SFT, solitary fibrous tumor; GIST, gastrointestinal stromal tumor; SMA, smooth muscle actin; PR, progesterone receptor; +/−, variably positive.

examined. Most STUMPs carry chromosomal alterations consistent with a neoplastic process, disproving earlier proposals that STUMPs were BPH with degenerative atypia.[7]

Although STUMPs are generally considered to represent a benign neoplastic stromal process, a subset of STUMPs has been associated with stromal sarcoma on concurrent biopsy material or has demonstrated stromal sarcoma on repeat biopsy, suggesting a malignant progression in at least some cases[2] (Fig. 16.9). There appears to be no correlation between the pattern of STUMP and association with stromal sarcoma. As most STUMPs are confined to the prostate and rarely progress to sarcoma, STUMPs are in general associated with a good prognosis.

In contrast to STUMPs, stromal sarcomas tend to affect a slightly younger population, with a reported age range of 25 to 86 years (eFigs. 16.30 to 16.37). Approximately half of all reported cases of stromal sarcoma occur before the age of 50 years. Stromal sarcomas may arise de novo or may exist in association with either a preexistent or concurrent STUMP.

Gross examination of stromal sarcomas demonstrates predominantly tan-white, solid, fleshy lesions ranging in size from 2 to 18 cm. Occasionally, areas of edema, hemorrhage, or small cysts may be identified. Microscopically, stromal sarcomas demonstrate either a solid growth of neoplastic stromal cells, which may have storiform, epithelioid, fibrosarcomatous, or patternless patterns, or may infiltrate between benign prostatic glands (Figs. 16.10 and 16.11). Less commonly, stromal sarcomas may demonstrate leaflike glands with underlying hypercellular

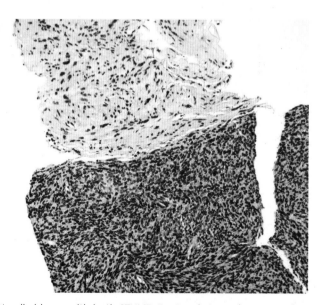

FIGURE 16.9 Needle biopsy with both STUMP *(top)* and stromal sarcoma *(bottom)*.

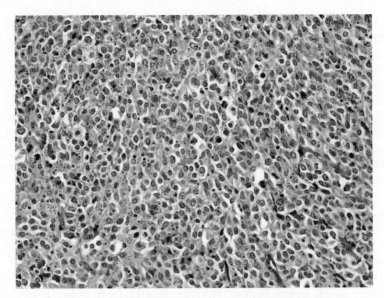

FIGURE 16.10   Stromal sarcoma with epithelioid pattern.

stroma, which are also termed *malignant phyllodes tumors* (Fig. 16.12). Stromal sarcomas have one or more of the following features within the spindle cell component: hypercellularity, cytologic atypia, mitotic figures, and necrosis. The finding of even a single atypical mitotic figure rules out a STUMP and leads to the diagnosis of stromal sarcoma (Fig. 16.13).

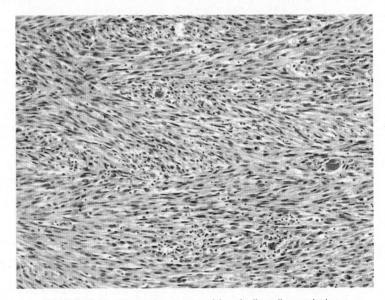

FIGURE 16.11   Stromal sarcoma with spindle cell morphology.

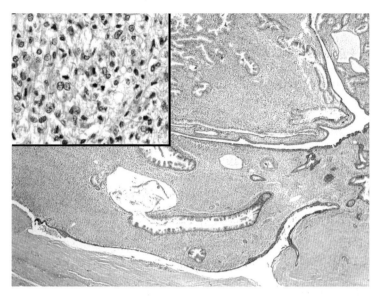

FIGURE 16.12 Malignant phyllodes pattern of STUMP with hypercellular stroma containing increased mitotic figures *(inset)*.

Stromal sarcomas may additionally be subclassified into low and high grades, with high-grade tumors defined by moderate-marked pleomorphism and hypercellularity, often with increased mitotic activity and occasional necrosis. Rarely, adenocarcinomas of the prostate can involve a stromal sarcoma.

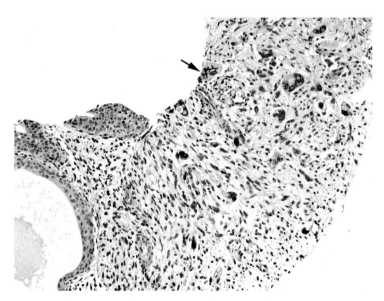

FIGURE 16.13 Stromal sarcoma with atypical mitotic figure *(arrow)*.

Immunohistochemical findings are similar to those of STUMPs, with strong vimentin reactivity and positivity for CD34 and progesterone receptor. In a subset of cases studied, pancytokeratin and CAM5.2 stains were negative. One case of stromal sarcoma was reported to demonstrate nuclear reactivity for beta-catenin, although the significance of this finding is unclear. Stromal sarcomas can extend out of the prostate and metastasize to distant sites such as bone, lung, abdomen, and retroperitoneum.

The variability in behavior of STUMPs and stromal sarcomas and their occasional coexistence lead to challenges in patient management. Although many STUMPs may behave in an indolent fashion, their unpredictability in a minority of cases and the lack of correlation between different histologic patterns of STUMPs and sarcomatous dedifferentiation warrant close follow-up and consideration of definitive resection in younger individuals. Factors to consider in deciding whether to proceed with definitive resection for STUMPs diagnosed on biopsy include patient age and treatment preference, presence and size of the lesion on rectal exam or imaging studies, and extent of the lesion on tissue sampling. Expectant management with close clinical follow-up could be considered in an older individual with a limited lesion on biopsy where there is no lesion identified on digital rectal exam or on imaging studies.

LEIOMYOMA/LEIOMYOSARCOMA (eFIGS. 16.38 TO 16.45)

It is difficult to diagnose a leiomyoma of the prostate, mainly because it is difficult to distinguish from a stromal nodule of benign hyperplasia.[8] Both entities may contain abundant smooth muscle, although leiomyomas typically demonstrate well-organized fascicles and may have other degenerative features such as hyalinization and calcification that are not commonly seen in stromal nodules. Large single leiomyomas that are symptomatic are rare, with the largest measuring 12 cm.[9,10] Leiomyomas demonstrate virtually no mitotic activity and minimal to no nuclear atypia, with the exception of occasional scattered degenerative nuclei in a normocellular background (eFig. 16.38).

Sarcomas of the prostate account for 0.1% to 0.2% of all malignant prostatic tumors.[11] Leiomyosarcoma is the most common sarcoma involving the prostate in adults, yet is still rare, affecting men between the ages of 40 and 78 years. It most frequently presents with urinary obstruction, as well as perineal/pelvic pain, urinary frequency, hematuria, constipation, rectal pain, and pain or burning on ejaculation.[11–14] Tumors vary from 1 to 25 cm, with the majority of reports of lesions between 5 and 10 cm. Microscopically, these hypercellular lesions are composed of intersecting bundles of spindled cells with moderate to severe atypia (Fig 16.14, eFigs. 16.36 to 16.44). The vast majority of leiomyosarcomas in the literature have been high grade with frequent mitoses and necrosis, although we have also seen rare cases of low-grade prostatic leiomyosarcoma.[15] Epithelioid leiomyosarcomas have been reported in the prostate.[12] Low-grade

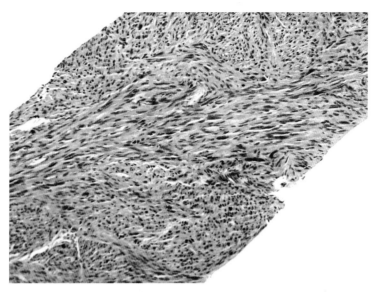

FIGURE 16.14   Prostatic leiomyosarcoma.

leiomyosarcomas are distinguished from leiomyomas by moderate amount of atypia, focal areas of increased cellularity, scattered mitotic figures, and/ or a focally infiltrative growth pattern around benign prostate glands at the perimeter. Symplastic leiomyomas have, in contrast, scattered atypia of a degenerative nature with an overall low cellularity (eFig 16.45). As opposed to some stromal sarcomas, leiomyosarcomas lack admixed normal glands, except entrapped glands at the periphery.

Leiomyosarcomas commonly express vimentin, actin, and desmin. Cytokeratin expression is observed in about one-quarter of cases.[12] In addition, some leiomyosarcomas have been reported to express the progesterone receptor, similar to STUMPs and stromal sarcomas[16] (Table 16.1).

Patients with leiomyosarcoma commonly have a poor outcome, with the clinical course characterized by multiple recurrences. The majority (50% to 75%) of patients die from disease within 2 to 5 years with metastatic spread most commonly to the lungs, often several years following initial diagnosis. In the study by Sexton et al.,[11] the prognosis for leiomyosarcoma of the prostate, as for sarcomas of the prostate in general, was not dependent on stage, with the exception of a better prognosis for those men who presented without distant metastases. The only other variable that these authors found to be predictive of a favorable prognosis was complete surgical resection with microscopically negative margins. Optimal treatment requires a multimodal approach rather than surgery alone. They also noted that survival of patients with isolated local recurrences could be prolonged with salvage surgery. In a report of dedifferentiated leiomyosarcomas from all sites, there was one prostate leiomyosarcoma metastatic to the lungs with 36 months' survival with disease.[17]

INFLAMMATORY MYOFIBROBLASTIC TUMOR (eFIGS. 16.46 TO 16.61)

A controversial spindle cell lesion arising most commonly in the bladder but rarely also seen in the prostate has been described by a variety of terms in the literature, including *pseudosarcomatous fibromyxoid tumor, myofibroblastoma, nodular fasciitis of bladder, pseudosarcomatous myofibroblastic proliferation, inflammatory pseudotumor*, and most recently *inflammatory myofibroblastic tumor* (IMT).[18–23] A smaller subset of these lesions occurs following recent transurethral resection for BPH and has been designated postoperative spindle cell nodule.[20,22] Although lesions occurring in the setting of prior injury and those arising as de novo prostatic lesions have in the past been considered as separate entities, it is now considered that both are the same lesion. Regardless of whether there is or there is not a prior history of instrumentation, lesions have overlapping morphologic, immunohistochemical, and molecular features and demonstrate the same clinical behavior. Of the two largest series of these lesions, one has designated them as pseudosarcomatous fibromyxoid tumor and the other as IMT. As a result of their morphology and genetic changes, we prefer the designation of IMT.

IMTs of the prostate have been reported in men ranging in age from 42 to 67 years, although IMTs within the bladder have been reported in patients between 3 and 86 years of age.[19,21] In contrast to many other spindle cell lesions of the prostate, IMTs may be fairly small, with many cases less than 1 cm in size. Other cases may be very large IMTs of the prostate, which are, for the most part, morphologically identical to those found at other sites. Spindle cells may be composed into intersecting fascicles resembling a smooth muscle tumor or appear more haphazard in their distribution (Table 16.2). The spindle cells have abundant eosinophilic to amphophilic long tapering cytoplasm resembling reactive fibroblasts (Fig. 16.15). Nuclei are elongated and uniform, containing delicate chromatin patterns and one or two distinct nucleoli. Occasionally, there may be prominent nucleoli with occasional moderately pleomorphic cells, yet an important distinguishing feature from sarcomas is that nuclei are not hyperchromatic. Prominent myxoid change in sarcomas arising within the prostate is also unusual. There is a scattering of chronic inflammatory cells, which along with the presence of prominent dilated capillaries throughout the lesion, bear some similarities to granulation tissue. Mitotic figures may be variable, ranging from 1 to 25 per 10 high power fields (HPF), yet atypical mitotic figures are not seen.

IMTs commonly express ALK, pancytokeratin (81%), Cam5.2 (56%), actin (100%), desmin (80%), and p53 (93%) by immunohistochemistry.[24] ALK gene fusion at chromosome 2p23 is identified by fluorescence in situ hybridization (FISH) in approximately 75% of IMTs of the genitourinary tract and often correlates with protein expression by immunohistochemistry.[21,24] The genetic changes support their designation as IMT as opposed to

TABLE 16.2 Inflammatory Myofibroblastic Tumor versus Sarcoma and Sarcomatoid Carcinoma

Features Favoring IMT over Sarcoma and Sarcomatoid Carcinoma

- In some cases onset following prior benign resection
- Some cases small (<1 cm)
- Typically uniform cytology with appearance of tissue–culture fibroblasts
- Lacks nuclear hyperchromasia
- Myxoid stromal change
- In some cases haphazard growth pattern—less fascicular
- Prominent vascularity
- Scattered inflammatory cells and extravasated red blood cells
- No atypical mitotic figures
- Majority express ALK immunohistochemically

Features of IMT Resembling Sarcoma and Sarcomatoid Carcinoma

- Can be large (>9 cm)
- Occasional fascicular growth pattern resembling leiomyosarcoma
- Occasional moderate nuclear pleomorphism
- Numerous mitotic figures
- Can invade detrusor muscle
- Expresses muscle markers and variably keratin by immunohistochemistry
- ALK negative by immunohistochemistry in one-third of cases

IMT, inflammatory myofibroblastic tumor.

the other more descriptive names that have been proposed for this lesion. IMTs are generally negative for S100, CD34, CD117, CD21, and CD23. Most IMTs follow a benign course, although incomplete surgical resection may lead to recurrence in approximately one-quarter of cases. Lesions may extend outside of the prostate. With the exception of the following unique case, IMTs have not been reported to metastasize. We have seen a case involving the prostatic urethra with the overall morphology of IMT and having an ALK gene rearrangement, yet had malignant features with atypical mitotic figures and hypercellularity. The tumor recurred following cystoprostatectomy and the patient subsequently developed intra-abdominal metastases and died 9 months following surgery. The differential diagnosis of IMT is sarcomatoid carcinoma and leiomyosarcoma. The cells in IMT are uniform without pleomorphism or hyperchromasia in contrast to sarcomatoid carcinoma and leiomyosarcoma. Although mitotic figures may be frequent in all three entities, abnormal mitotic figures are not seen in IMT.

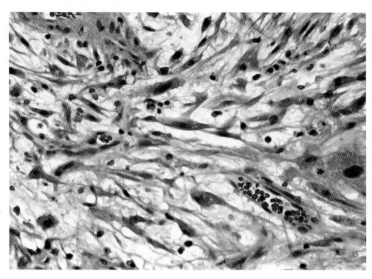

FIGURE 16.15 IMT with tissue culture–like fibroblasts in a myxoid stroma with scattered inflammatory cells.

A pitfall is that sarcomatoid carcinoma, prostatic leiomyosarcoma, and IMT can all express keratin and desmin. Although ALK immunoreactivity is positive in only two-thirds of cases of IMT, it is diagnostic of this entity.

SOLITARY FIBROUS TUMOR (eFIGS. 16.62 TO 16.66)

There are fewer than 20 cases of solitary fibrous tumor (SFT) involving the prostate reported as single cases and one series of 12 cases.[25] Some older reported cases of hemangiopericytoma of the prostate may also be today classified as SFT. Prostatic SFTs have been reported in patients ranging in age from 21 to 75 years and the most common clinical findings include lower urinary retention, urinary frequency, dysuria, constipation, incontinence, and groin pain.

These tumors demonstrate a broad size distribution, ranging from 2 to 14 cm, with many reported to be greater than 5 cm. Microscopically, prostatic SFTs appear similar to those identified in extraprostatic sites. Uniform spindled cells with bland nuclei are arranged in a "patternless" pattern in a background of variable ropy collagen (Fig. 16.16). Many cases demonstrate a hemangiopericytomatous appearance. Admixed prostatic tissue is not commonly associated with these lesions. None of the prostatic SFTs has behaved in an aggressive fashion. However, based on the behavior of SFTs in other sites and the finding in some prostatic SFTs of hypercellularity, pleomorphism, necrosis, and infiltrative margins, careful long-term clinical follow-up is warranted regardless of their histology. We do not designate them as "benign" or "malignant,"

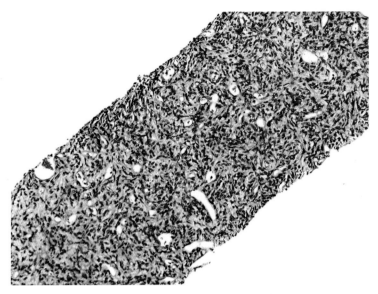

FIGURE 16.16   SFT on prostate needle biopsy.

but rather note whether there are any features particularly worrisome for aggressive behavior.

Immunohistochemistry generally reveals diffuse reactivity for CD34, vimentin, and bcl-2, although rare SFTs may lack some of these markers (Table 16.1). Staining for CD99, beta-catenin, p53, smooth muscle actin, and muscle-specific actin has also been reported. These tumors are typically negative for pancytokeratin, S100, and CD117 (c-kit).

GASTROINTESTINAL STROMAL TUMOR (eFIGS. 16.67 TO 16.69)

Although gastrointestinal stromal tumors (GISTs) lesions may clinically present as primary prostatic processes on imaging studies and clinical exam, such cases are typically large masses arising from the rectum or perirectal space that compress but do not invade the prostate. Exceptionally, they may also invade the prostate.[25-28] Most cases of "prostatic" GISTs are sampled on prostatic needle biopsy, although we have seen one case sampled on a transurethral resection. There is only one prior case reported in the English literature of a GIST that appeared to be localized to the prostate based on computed tomography (CT) and magnetic resonance imaging (MRI).[28] This patient presented simultaneously with multiple liver metastases and the prostatic mass was not resected. It is doubtful whether this neoplasm was truly a prostatic primary, because studies have demonstrated that imaging studies cannot reliably determine the origin of large GISTs. Consequently, to date, there is no fully documented example of a GIST arising within the prostate.

Typically, GIST is not considered in the differential diagnosis of spindle cell lesions of the prostate, although the unique management of these tumors underscores the importance of recognizing these tumors. Misdiagnosis of GISTs involving the prostate is not uncommon, and several patients have undergone pelvic exenteration, irradiation, and chemotherapy for a misdiagnosis of pelvic sarcoma.[27] Patients range in age from 42 to 65 years and present with urinary obstructive symptoms, rectal fullness, and abnormal digital rectal examination. Tumor size ranges from 1 to 14 cm. Microscopically, "prostatic" GISTs are morphologically identical to those found within the gastrointestinal tract. GIST is composed of spindled cells with a fascicular growth pattern (Fig. 16.17). Additional histologic findings include focal epithelioid features, focal dense collagenous stroma, areas with a patternless pattern, and perinuclear halos. When present, a fascicular or palisading growth pattern and perinuclear vacuoles along with a lack of collagen deposition aids in the discrimination of GIST from SFT and STUMP. Tumors with malignant potential show elevated mitotic rates of more than 5 per 50 HPF, cytologically malignant features (high cellularity and overlapping nuclei), or necrosis.

CD117/c-kit is uniformly expressed in all cases and CD34 is positive in almost all cases studied (Table 16.1). S100, desmin, and smooth muscle actin are negative. On prostate biopsy, it may be difficult to distinguish a GIST from other spindle cell tumors due to limited material. Consequently, prior to rendering a diagnosis of SFT, schwannoma, leiomyosarcoma, or stromal sarcoma, GIST should be considered in the differential diagnosis.

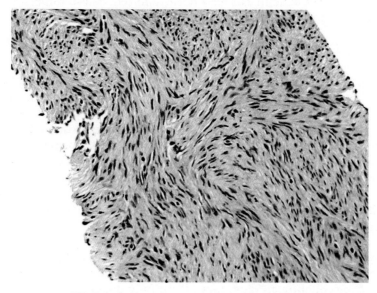

FIGURE 16.17   GIST on "prostate" needle biopsy.

Furthermore, immunostains for CD117 should be performed to verify the diagnosis. If one does not consider GIST in the differential diagnosis on prostate needle biopsy and does not include CD117 (c-kit) in the immunohistochemical panel, there exists the possibility of misdiagnosis as other antigens are often coexpressed among mimickers of GIST. CD34 is not discriminatory as it is positive in GISTs, SFTs, and specialized prostatic stromal tumors and variably positive in schwannomas. It is, however, typically negative in smooth muscle tumors. Strong positive staining for desmin can help discriminate smooth muscle tumors from the other lesions. Similarly, positive immunoreactivity to S100 may aid in diagnosing neural tumors. Smooth muscle actin is typically expressed in smooth muscle tumors and is variably positive in STUMPs and GISTs and typically negative in SFT and schwannoma.

A subset of patients treated with the c-kit tyrosine kinase inhibitor imatinib (Gleevec) following the diagnosis of "prostatic" GIST has demonstrated a subsequent reduction in tumor size.[26] No long-term follow-up is currently available on these patients to determine if the biologic behavior of GISTs secondarily involving the prostate is different than that described in other sites.

RHABDOMYOSARCOMA

The vast majority of rhabdomyosarcomas of the prostate occur in the pediatric population with an average age at diagnosis of 5 years.[29,30] There are rare prostatic rhabdomyosarcomas that have been reported in adults ranging in age from 17 to 68 years old.[31,32] Because of their large size at the time of diagnosis, distinction between rhabdomyosarcoma originating in the bladder and that originating in the prostate may be difficult.

Histologically, about three-quarters of prostate rhabdomyosarcomas are of the embryonal subtype with the remaining alveolar (Fig. 16.18, eFigs. 16.70 to 16.74). A single case of botryoid subtype of embryonal rhabdomyosarcoma has also been reported.[33] Embryonal rhabdomyosarcomas of the prostate are similar to those seen in other organs and may assume a wide variety of histologic patterns. Embryonal rhabdomyosarcoma cells may vary from primitive cells with scant cytoplasm to more well-differentiated tumors with abundant eosinophilic cytoplasm in which cross striations may be seen by light microscopy. Embryonal rhabdomyosarcomas may also assume a cellular spindle cell appearance with a tendency to encircle preserved prostatic glands or a myxoid growth pattern. The use of immunohistochemical, ultrastructural, and molecular techniques may be useful in the diagnosis of embryonal rhabdomyosarcoma involving the prostate. Prostate/bladder rhabdomyosarcomas can be subdivided into low, intermediate, and unfavorable risk prognostic groups.[34] Low risk is the embryonal subtype, either completely resected or with microscopic residual disease. Intermediate risk is embryonal with

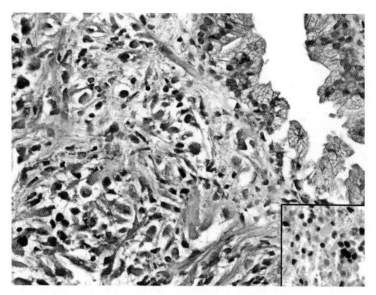

FIGURE 16.18   Prostatic rhabdomyosarcoma with cells labeling with myogenin *(inset)*.

either (a) embryonal with gross residual disease, (b) embryonal in patients younger than 10 years old with metastases, or (c) alveolar subtype with no metastases. Unfavorable risk is alveolar with metastases or embryonal in patients older than 10 years of age with metastases. The 5-year survival is 90%, 65% to 75%, and 40% to 55% for low, intermediate, and unfavorable risk groups, respectively. Metastases typically go to lung and bone. Treatment is initially chemotherapy with or without radiation and, if tumors are made resectable, then surgery. One may see only mature rhabdomyoblasts following chemotherapy, which in general is associated with a favorable response. However, due to sampling, there could be more active disease elsewhere such that patients are closely followed with additional tissue sampling.

MISCELLANEOUS

Other rare mesenchymal lesions of the prostate are hemangioma,[35] chondroma,[36] cartilaginous metaplasia,[37] malignant peripheral nerve sheath tumor,[38] schwannoma,[39] chondrosarcoma,[40] synovial sarcoma (Fig. 16.19, eFig. 16.75),[41–43] granular cell tumor,[44] angiosarcoma (Fig. 16.20, eFig. 16.76),[45–47] neurofibroma (Fig. 16.20),[48] malignant fibrous histiocytoma,[11,49–51] and hemangiopericytoma.[52] The one case reported of an osteosarcoma was in a patient with a prior history of adenocarcinoma of the prostate treated with radiotherapy and most likely represents a sarcomatoid carcinoma with an osteogenic sarcoma component.[53]

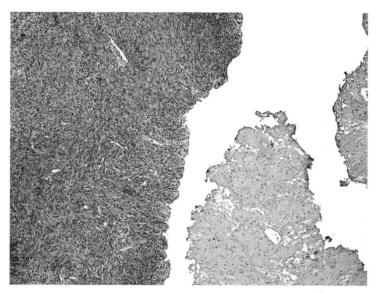

FIGURE 16.19   Prostatic synovial sarcoma on transurethral resection of the prostate (TURP).

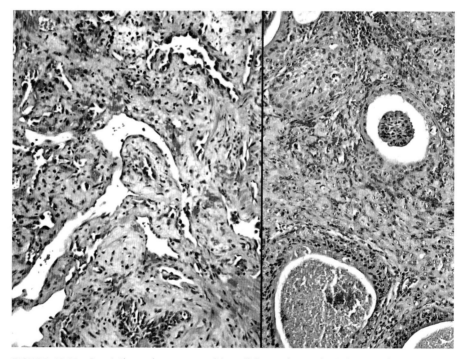

FIGURE 16.20   Prostatic angiosarcoma with well-formed vessels **(left)**. Another case with more poorly differentiated morphology **(right)**, verified as vascular by immunohistochemistry.

REFERENCES

1. Eble JN, Sauter G, Epstein JI, et al. *The World Health Organization Classification of Tumours of the Urinary System and Male Genital System.* Lyon, France: IARC Press; 2004.

2. Gaudin PB, Rosai J, Epstein JI. Sarcomas and related proliferative lesions of specialized prostatic stroma: a clinicopathologic study of 22 cases. *Am J Surg Pathol.* 1998;22: 148–162.

3. Bostwick DG, Hossain D, Qian J, et al. Phyllodes tumor of the prostate: long-term followup study of 23 cases. *J Urol.* 2004;172:894–899.

4. Herawi M, Epstein JI. Specialized stromal tumors of the prostate: a clinicopathologic study of 50 cases. *Am J Surg Pathol.* 2006;30:694–704.

5. Nagar M, Epstein JI. Epithelial proliferations in prostatic stromal tumors of uncertain malignant potential (STUMP). *Am J Surg Pathol.* 2011;35:898–903.

6. Hansel DE, Herawi M, Montgomery E, et al. Spindle cell lesions of the adult prostate. *Mod Pathol.* 2007;20:148–158.

7. Pan CC, Epstein JI. Common chromosomal aberrations detected by array comparative genomic hybridization in specialized stromal tumors of the prostate. *Mod Pathol.* 2013;26:1536–1543.

8. Moore R. Benign hypertrophy of the prostate: a morphologic study. *J Urol.* 1943;50: 680–710.

9. Michaels MM, Brown HE, Favino CJ. Leiomyoma of prostate. *Urology.* 1974;3:617–620.

10. Regan JB, Barrett DM, Wold LE. Giant leiomyoma of the prostate. *Arch Pathol Lab Med.* 1987;111:381–382.

11. Sexton WJ, Lance RE, Reyes AO, et al. Adult prostate sarcoma: the M. D. Anderson Cancer Center Experience. *J Urol.* 2001;166:521–525.

12. Cheville JC, Dundore PA, Nascimento AG, et al. Leiomyosarcoma of the prostate. Report of 23 cases. *Cancer.* 1995;76:1422–1427.

13. Mansouri H, Kanouni L, Kebdani T, et al. Primary prostatic leiomyosarcoma. *J Urol.* 2001;165:1676.

14. Tavora F, Kryvenko ON, Epstein JI. Mesenchymal tumours of the bladder and prostate: an update. *Pathology.* 2013;45:104–115.

15. Stenram U, Holby LE. A case of circumscribed myosarcoma of the prostate. *Cancer.* 1969;24:803–806.

16. Kelley TW, Borden EC, Goldblum JR. Estrogen and progesterone receptor expression in uterine and extrauterine leiomyosarcomas: an immunohistochemical study. *Appl Immunohistochem Mol Morphol.* 2004;12:338–341.

17. Chen E, O'Connell F, Fletcher CD. Dedifferentiated leiomyosarcoma: clinicopathological analysis of 18 cases. *Histopathology.* 2011;59:1135–1143.

18. Cespedes RD, Lynch SC, Grider DJ. Pseudosarcomatous fibromyxoid tumor of the prostate. A case report with review of the literature. *Urol Int.* 1996;57:249–251.

19. Harik LR, Merino C, Coindre JM, et al. Pseudosarcomatous myofibroblastic proliferations of the bladder: a clinicopathologic study of 42 cases. *Am J Surg Pathol.* 2006;30: 787–794.

20. Huang WL, Ro JY, Grignon DJ, et al. Postoperative spindle cell nodule of the prostate and bladder. *J Urol.* 1990;143:824–826.

21. Montgomery EA, Shuster DD, Burkart AL, et al. Inflammatory myofibroblastic tumors of the urinary tract: a clinicopathologic study of 46 cases, including a malignant example inflammatory fibrosarcoma and a subset associated with high-grade urothelial carcinoma. *Am J Surg Pathol.* 2006;30:1502–1512.

22. Proppe KH, Scully RE, Rosai J. Postoperative spindle cell nodules of genitourinary tract resembling sarcomas. A report of eight cases. *Am J Surg Pathol.* 1984;8:101–118.

23. Ro JY, el-Naggar AK, Amin MB, et al. Pseudosarcomatous fibromyxoid tumor of the urinary bladder and prostate: immunohistochemical, ultrastructural, and DNA flow cytometric analyses of nine cases. *Hum Pathol.* 1993;24:1203–1210.

24. Tsuzuki T, Magi-Galluzzi C, Epstein JI. ALK-1 expression in inflammatory myofibroblastic tumor of the urinary bladder. *Am J Surg Pathol.* 2004;28:1609–1614.

25. Herawi M, Epstein JI. Solitary fibrous tumor on needle biopsy and transurethral resection of the prostate: a clinicopathologic study of 13 cases. *Am J Surg Pathol.* 2007;31:870–876.

26. Herawi M, Montgomery EA, Epstein JI. Gastrointestinal stromal tumors (GISTs) on prostate needle biopsy: a clinicopathologic study of 8 cases. *Am J Surg Pathol.* 2006;30: 1389–1395.

27. Madden JF, Burchette JL, Raj GV, et al. Anterior rectal wall gastrointestinal stromal tumor presenting clinically as prostatic mass. *Urol Oncol.* 2005;23:268–272.

28. Van der Aa F, Sciot R, Blyweert W, et al. Gastrointestinal stromal tumor of the prostate. *Urology.* 2005;65:388.

29. Lobe TE, Wiener E, Andrassy RJ, et al. The argument for conservative, delayed surgery in the management of prostatic rhabdomyosarcoma. *J Pediatr Surg.* 1996;31:1084–1087.

30. Raney RB, Anderson JR, Barr FG, et al. Rhabdomyosarcoma and undifferentiated sarcoma in the first two decades of life: a selective review of intergroup rhabdomyosarcoma study group experience and rationale for Intergroup Rhabdomyosarcoma Study V. *J Pediatr Hematol Oncol.* 2001;23:215–220.

31. Waring PM, Newland RC. Prostatic embryonal rhabdomyosarcoma in adults. A clinicopathologic review. *Cancer.* 1992;69:755–762.

32. Nabi G, Dinda AK, Dogra PN. Primary embryonal rhabdomyosarcoma of prostate in adults: diagnosis and management. *Int Urol Nephrol.* 2002;34:531–534.

33. Nuwal P, Solanki RL, Jain S, et al. Botryoid rhabdomyosarcoma of prostate—a case report. *Indian J Pathol Microbiol.* 2001;44:65–66.

34. Ferrer FA, Isakoff M, Koyle MA. Bladder/prostate rhabdomyosarcoma: past, present and future. *J Urol.* 2006;176:1283–691.

35. Sundarasivarao D, Banerjea S, Nageswararao A, et al. Hemangioma of the prostate: a case report. *J Urol.* 1973;110:708–709.

36. Sloan SE, Rapoport JM. Prostatic chondroma. *Urology.* 1985;25:319–321.

37. Bedrosian SA, Goldman RL, Sung MA. Heterotopic cartilage in prostate. *Urology.* 1983;21:536–537.

38. Rames RA, Smith MT. Malignant peripheral nerve sheath tumor of the prostate: a rare manifestion of neurofibromatosis type 1. *J Urol.* 1999;162:165–166.

39. Jiang R, Chen JH, Chen M, et al. Male genital schwannoma, review of 5 cases. *Asian J Androl.* 2003;5:251–254.

40. Dogra PN, Aron M, Rajeev TP, et al. Primary chondrosarcoma of the prostate. *BJU Int.* 1999;83:150–151.

41. Iwasaki H, Ishiguro M, Ohjimi Y, et al. Synovial sarcoma of the prostate with t(X;18) (p11.2;q11.2). *Am J Surg Pathol.* 1999;23:220–226.

42. Pan CC, Chang YH. Primary synovial sarcoma of the prostate. *Histopathology.* 2006;48: 321–323.

43. Williams DH, Hua VN, Chowdhry AA, et al. Synovial sarcoma of the prostate. *J Urol.* 2004;171:2376.

44. Furihata M, Sonobe H, Iwata J, et al. Granular cell tumor expressing myogenic markers in the prostate. *Pathol Int.* 1996;46:298–300.

45. Chandan VS, Wolsh L. Postirradiation angiosarcoma of the prostate. *Arch Pathol Lab Med*. 2003;127:876–878.

46. Humphrey PA. Angiosarcoma of the prostate. *J Urol*. 2012;187:684–685.

47. Khaliq W, Meyer CF, Uzoaru I, et al. Prostate angiosarcoma: is there any association with previous radiation therapy? *BJU Int*. 2012;110:E819–E825.

48. Chung AK, Michels V, Poland GA, et al. Neurofibromatosis with involvement of the prostate gland. *Urology*. 1996;47:448–451.

49. Bain GO, Danyluk JM, Shnitka TK, et al. Malignant fibrous histiocytoma of prostate gland. *Urology*. 1985;26:89–91.

50. Chin W, Fay R, Ortega P. Malignant fibrous histiocytoma of prostate. *Urology*. 1986; 27:363–365.

51. Kulmala RV, Seppanen JH, Vaajalahti PJ, et al. Malignant fibrous histiocytoma of the prostate. Case report. *Scand J Urol Nephrol*. 1994;28:429–431.

52. Reyes JW, Shinozuka H, Garry P, et al. A light and electron microscopic study of a hemangiopericytoma of the prostate with local extension. *Cancer*. 1977;40:1122–1126.

53. Nishiyama T, Ikarashi T, Terunuma M, et al. Osteogenic sarcoma of the prostate. *Int J Urol*. 2001;8:199–201.

17

MISCELLANEOUS BENIGN AND MALIGNANT LESIONS

BENIGN LESIONS

Prostatic Cysts

Prostatic cysts may be subdivided in utricle cysts and retention cysts.[1,2] Utricle cysts usually lie outside the prostate between the bladder and rectum, with the orifice located at the prostatic utricle. The average age of patients with utricle cysts is 26 years. In approximately 25% of cases, there may be abnormalities of the external genitalia, and in 10% of cases, there is unilateral renal dysgenesis or agenesis. Histologically, the cyst walls may lack an epithelial lining or be composed of columnar, cuboidal, transitional, or less frequently, squamous epithelium. Retention cysts arise when prostatic acini become distended with clear fluid and are lined by flattened prostatic glandular or transitional epithelium. Because small asymptomatic dilated prostatic acini are frequently seen as part of focal atrophic changes in prostate, the term *retention cyst* should only be used for symptomatic cysts. Defined accordingly, retention cysts range in size from 1 to 2 cm, are usually unilocular, and are located adjacent to the urethra. In approximately 10% of cases, the cysts contain calculi. Four cases of cystadenoma and isolated cases of squamous cell carcinoma and adenocarcinoma have been reported arising in prostatic cysts.[1,2]

Multilocular Cysts of the Prostate (Multilocular Prostatic Cystadenoma)

Several reports have described large multilocular cystic lesions between the bladder and the rectum.[3–7] They may either be separate from the prostate or attached to the prostate by a pedicle. These masses have weighed up to 6,500 g, ranging from 7.5 to 20 cm in diameter. On cross section, they are well circumscribed and resemble nodular hyperplasia with multiple cysts, ranging from microscopic to several centimeters in diameter. Atrophic prostatic epithelium, reactive with antibodies to prostate-specific antigen (PSA) and prostate-specific acid phosphatase (PSAP), line the cysts. The lining epithelium may react with alpha-methylacyl-CoA racemase (AMACR). The latter, together with the lack of basal cell demonstration on p63 and/or HMWCK immunostain, may lead to an erroneous diagnosis of carcinoma on a small needle biopsy sample.[8] We have seen one case involved by high-grade prostatic intraepithelial neoplasia.[3] There also have been several reports of similar lesions within the prostate. The distinction of intraprostatic multilocular cysts from cystic nodular hyperplasia may be difficult. The diagnosis of intraprostatic cystadenoma should be restricted to cases where one-half of the prostate resembles normal prostate tissue and the remaining prostate is enlarged by a solitary encapsulated nodule composed of epithelium and/or cysts.[9,10] Prostatic cystadenomas may recur if incompletely excised and may require extensive surgery because of their large size and impingement on surrounding structures.

Melanotic Lesions

Melanotic lesions of the prostate consist of cases with only stromal melanin, only glandular melanin, or both stromal and glandular melanin.[11–16] The term *melanosis*, if not otherwise specified, usually refers to melanin found in any location within the prostate. Blue nevus is used to describe stromal melanin deposition, and glandular melanosis denotes the presence of melanin within epithelial cells. Microscopically, blue nevi are characterized by deeply pigmented melanin-filled spindle cells within the fibromuscular stroma (Fig. 17.1, eFig. 17.1). In two cases, in addition to glandular and stromal melanosis, melanin was also seen in adjacent glands of adenocarcinoma of the prostate. Nonneoplastic and neoplastic prostatic epithelial cells with melanin contain only mature melanosomes,

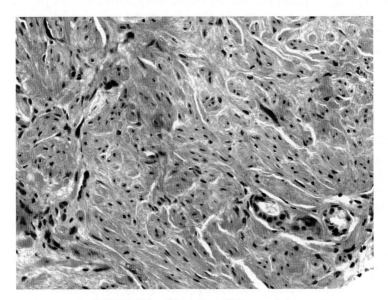

FIGURE 17.1   Blue nevus of the prostate.

suggesting that epithelial melanin results from a transfer of pigment from the stromal melanocytes. The incidence of microscopic focal prostatic blue nevi or glandular melanosis is about 4% each. Cases with more prominent melanosis such as those with grossly visible pigment are much less common and have only been published as isolated case reports. Melanotic lesions of the prostate are incidental findings with no evidence of malignant transformation. There have only been rare case reports of a malignant melanoma with primary prostatic origin.[17,18]

Amyloid

Vascular amyloid can be identified in 2% to 10% of prostates removed for hyperplasia or carcinoma.[19–22] Patients with multiple myeloma, primary amyloidosis of the kidney, or chronic debilitating diseases have a higher incidence of prostatic amyloidosis. In these cases, amyloid is located in subepithelial areas as well as in vessels. Usually, amyloid within the prostate is an incidental finding, although rarely, it may mimic carcinoma on rectal examination. Amyloidosis, which involves the seminal vesicles in about 10% of radical prostatectomy specimens, can also extend into the ejaculatory duct and can be sampled on needle biopsy[19] (Fig. 17.2, eFig. 17.2). Corpora amylacea often stain nonspecifically for amyloid.[23]

Calculi and Calcification

Prostatic calculi are found within the tissues or acini of the gland, in contrast to urinary calculi that are found within the prostatic urethra.[24,25]

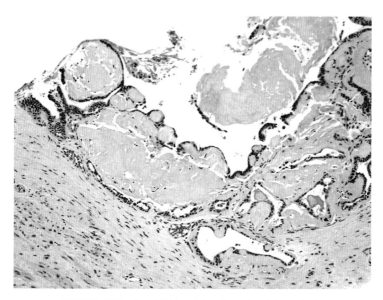

FIGURE 17.2   Amyloid involving the ejaculatory duct.

Prostatic calculi are present in 70% to 100% of the glands studied at autopsy, most commonly in men older than 50 years of age. Generally, prostatic calculi are multiple and small with an average diameter of less than 5 mm. Histologically, calculi are composed of concentric layers resembling calcified corpora amylacea. They form by the consolidation and calcification of corpora amylacea or by calcification of precipitated prostatic secretions. Although prostatic calculi are common, they are usually asymptomatic and are discovered incidentally. Abscesses may occur in patients who have urinary tract infections resistant to antimicrobial therapy in which the prostatic calculi are infected and provide a continual source of infection. Prostatic calculi are also significant in that they may be confused on rectal examination with carcinoma of the prostate.

Basal cell hyperplasia is the most common lesion containing laminated calcifications resembling psammoma bodies. The latter have been encountered in approximately one-fifth of basal cell hyperplasia cases on needle biopsy.[26,27] This finding may be a diagnostic aid, because only rarely do carcinomas contain laminated calcifications. Calcifications within prostate cancers tend to be small stippled granular calcifications in areas of central necrosis, most commonly seen in high-grade carcinomas and ductal adenocarcinomas.

Infarcts

In between 20% and 25% of specimens removed for benign prostatic hyperplasia, prostatic infarcts ranging in size from a few millimeters to 5 cm may be found.[28–30] Patients with acute prostatic infarcts have prostate glands that are twice as large as those without infarcts. Also, patients with infarcts are more prone to acute urinary retention and gross hematuria than those without infarcts. These symptoms, however, may not be due to the infarcts but rather may be due to the larger size of the gland containing them, because the infarcts are often small and not close to the urethra. Acute prostatic infarcts are discrete lesions with a characteristic histologic zonation (Figs. 17.3 and 17.4, eFigs. 17.3 to 17.21). The center of the infarct is characterized by acute coagulative necrosis and some recent hemorrhage. Immediately adjacent to the infarcted tissue, reactive epithelial nests with prominent nucleoli, some pleomorphism, and even atypical mitotic figures can be seen (Fig. 17.4). Progressing away from the center of the infarct, more mature squamous metaplasia is seen. Another finding seen within prostatic infarcts is squamous islands with central cystic formation containing cellular debris. Remote infarcts may also be recognized by finding local areas of densely fibrotic stroma admixed with small glands containing immature squamous metaplasia (eFig. 17.22). Prostatic infarcts may rarely be sampled on needle biopsy, where it may be more difficult to appreciate the zonation.[29] If the infarct is not recognized, the reactive squamous metaplasia cases may be misdiagnosed as urothelial carcinoma.

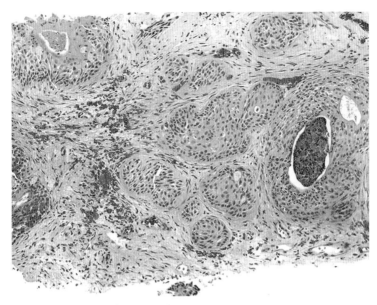

FIGURE 17.3 Prostatic infarct with reactive urothelial metaplasia and recent stromal hemorrhage.

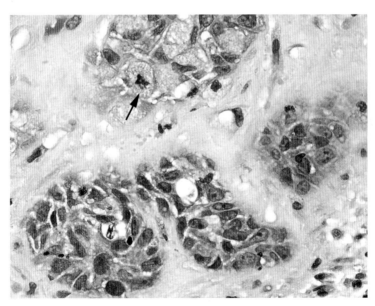

FIGURE 17.4 Same case as Figure 17.3 with reactive nuclear atypia and mitotic figure *(arrow)*. Note densely fibrotic stroma.

Miscellaneous

In a study of prostates from a medical examiner's office, 9% of prostates contained sperm (eFig. 17.23).[31] Spermatozoa have been found in approximately one-quarter of whole mount–examined prostatectomies with the aid of special stains.[32] Rare cases of prostatic endometriosis, hair granuloma, and lymphangiolipomatosis have been diagnosed.[33–35] Vasculitis involving the prostate may occur, including polyarteritis nodosa, Wegener granulomatosis, and giant cell arteritis[36–38] (Fig. 17.5, eFigs. 17.24 to 17.26). Extramedullary hematopoiesis, ganglioneuroma, and ectopic salivary gland tissue have been described in the prostate.[39–41] A form of metaplasia has been designated "Paneth cell-like metaplasia" or "Paneth cell-like change."[42–44] Histologically, it is characterized by bright eosinophilic neuroendocrine granules filling the apical cytoplasm. The cells are immunoreactive with neuroendocrine markers and some have suggested the use of the alternative terminology of *neuroendocrine cells with large eosinophilic granules*.[44,45] We prefer the term *Paneth cell-like neuroendocrine differentiation*, which may also be seen in prostatic adenocarcinoma that was previously discussed in Chapter 12.[46]

Another form of cytoplasmic metaplastic change that occasionally occurs in benign acini is "eosinophilic metaplasia" (Fig. 17.6, eFig. 17.27).[47]

Rarely, the ejaculatory duct may be a site of pathology. Cases of an adenofibroma and an adenomatoid tumor involving this structure have been reported.[48,49]

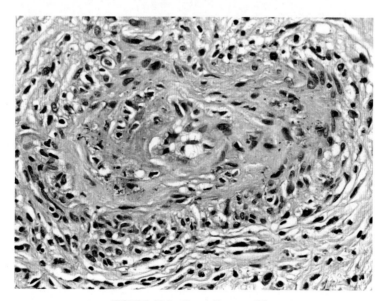

FIGURE 17.5 Prostatic vasculitis.

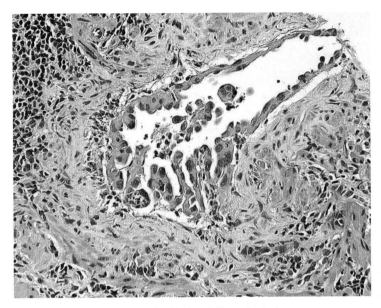

FIGURE 17.6   Eosinophilic metaplasia.

Finally, a rare case of benign prostatic hyperplasia occurring in an adolescent or pediatric patient have been reported and termed *juvenile prostatic hyperplasia.*[50,51]

MALIGNANT LESIONS

Basal Cell Carcinomas

At the other end of the spectrum of basal cell hyperplasia (see Chapter 7) of the prostate is basal cell carcinoma.[52–55] The histologic variability of basal cell carcinomas of the prostate is greater than that of basal cell hyperplasia. They may resemble basal cell carcinomas of the skin with large basaloid nests, peripheral palisading, and necrosis (Fig. 17.7, eFig. 17.28). Other basal cell carcinomas resemble the adenoid basal cell pattern of basal cell hyperplasia[26,56] and have been referred to by some as adenoid cystic carcinoma of the prostate[56,57] (Fig. 17.8, eFigs. 17.29 to 17.34).

In addition to the adenoid cystic pattern and large basaloid nests with necrosis being pathognomonic of basal cell carcinoma, we have noted two other patterns that were only seen with basal cell carcinoma and not basal cell hyperplasia[26,27,52,58] (Table 17.1). One was the finding of anastomosing basaloid nests and tubules centrally lined by eosinophilic cells (Fig. 17.9, eFigs. 17.35 to 17.38). A more subjective assessment of architecture that we identified only in basal cell carcinoma was variably small/medium-sized nests with irregular shapes (Fig. 17.9, eFig. 17.39). Infiltrativeness is another characteristic of basal cell carcinoma that in some cases may be

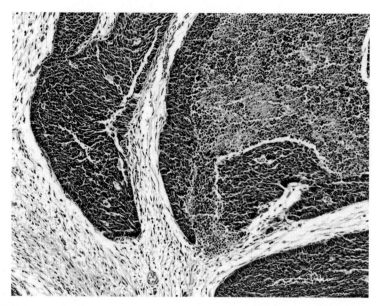

FIGURE 17.7 Basal cell carcinoma with solid sheets of cells and necrosis and associated desmoplastic stroma.

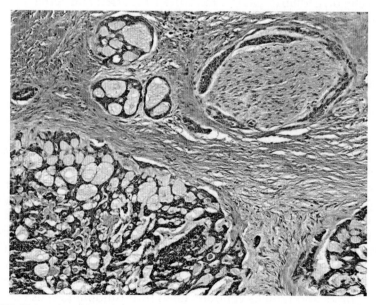

FIGURE 17.8 Adenoid cystic pattern of basal cell hyperplasia with perineural invasion.

TABLE 17.1 Features Seen in Basal Cell Carcinoma as Opposed to Basal Cell Hyperplasia

- Adenoid cystic pattern
- Large basaloid nests with necrosis
- Anastomosing basaloid nests and tubules centrally lined by eosinophilic cells
- Variably small/medium-sized nests with irregular shapes
- Extension into periprostatic adipose tissue or seminal vesicles
- Extension into thick muscle bundles of bladder neck
- Dense stromal response
- Strong, diffuse Bcl-2 staining
- Ki67 labeling index >20%

difficult to assess. Although readily diagnostic of malignancy, extension of basal cell carcinoma into periprostatic adipose tissue or seminal vesicles is typically seen in resection rather than diagnostic specimens. More commonly, infiltration in basal cell carcinoma manifests by extension into the thick muscle bundles of the bladder neck, which is not seen in basal cell hyperplasia (eFig. 17.39). A more problematic diagnostic criterion of basal cell malignancy is widespread infiltration of the malignant basal elements between benign prostatic glands (eFigs. 17.40 to 17.42). Florid basal cell

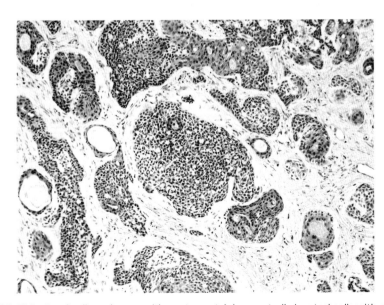

FIGURE 17.9 Basal cell carcinoma with nests containing centrally located cells with eosinophilic cytoplasm. Note associated desmoplastic stroma reaction.

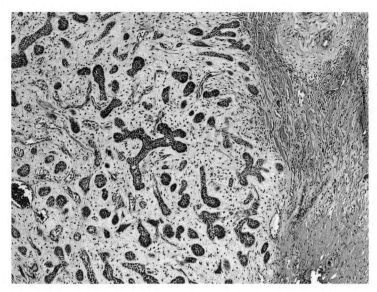

FIGURE 17.10 Basal cell carcinoma composed of small nests of basaloid cells mimicking basal cell hyperplasia, except for the prominent stromal reaction.

hyperplasia may also appear infiltrative between benign glands, although it may represent focal basal cell hyperplasia arising amongst benign prostatic glands, giving the impression of an infiltrative process (eFig 17.43). In contrast to basal cell carcinoma, the nests or tubules of basal cell hyperplasia are more evenly and orderly arranged between benign prostate glands and tend not to infiltrate as isolated units but rather as clusters of nests or tubules. In summary, although basal cell carcinoma can occasionally resemble basal cell hyperplasia, the diagnosis of malignancy is usually based on either (a) extensive infiltration in between normal prostate glands, (b) extension out of the prostate, (c) perineural invasion, (d) necrosis, or (e) the presence of a dense stromal response (Fig. 17.10, eFig. 17.44). Florid basal cell hyperplasia may have a subtle myxoid stromal reaction but lacks the extensive myxoid or desmoplastic reaction that characterizes some basal cell carcinomas.[26] Other findings that may be seen in association with basal cell carcinoma include collagenous globules, squamous differentiation (eFig. 17.45), focal microcalcifications, and vacuoles.

Bcl-2 labels basal cell carcinoma more strongly and diffusely than basal cell hyperplasia[55] (eFig. 17.46). Ki67 staining is greater than 20% in approximately one-half of basal cell carcinomas[52] (eFig. 17.47). Immunohistochemistry for ki67 can be helpful in differentiating basal cell carcinoma from florid basal cell hyperplasia, as basal cell hyperplasia typically shows less than 5% positivity.[55] Basal cell markers (p63, high molecular weight cytokeratin) may highlight multiple cell layers, just the outermost layers or only a few scattered cells with some basal cell carcinomas being negative for high molecular weight cytokeratin (eFigs. 17.48 and 17.49).

Overall, only a small subset of basal cell carcinomas behaves aggressively with local recurrences and distant metastases. In previously reported cases, these have been of the adenoid cystic variant.[57,59,60] In our more recent series, among those with an aggressive behavior, the predominant pattern were cases with large solid nests more often with central necrosis, high Ki67 percentage, and less staining with basal cell markers (eFig. 17.50).[52]

Carcinomas with Squamous Differentiation

Pure squamous cell carcinomas develop osteolytic metastases, do not respond to estrogen therapy, and do not develop elevated serum acid phosphatase levels with metastatic disease (eFig. 17.51).[61,62] Metastases also are seen in the liver, lung, and lymph nodes. Serum PSA levels are not elevated. The diagnosis of primary prostatic squamous cell carcinomas requires (a) lack of glandular differentiation, (b) no prior hormonal therapy, and (c) absence of secondary involvement of the gland by bladder or urethral squamous carcinomas. Squamous cell carcinoma of the prostate must also be differentiated from squamous metaplasia adjacent to a prostatic infarct (see earlier discussion). Primary prostatic squamous cell carcinomas have a poor prognosis with an average survival of about 1 year. Treatment is multimodal with surgery, chemotherapy, and radiation.

Adenosquamous carcinomas may also be seen in the prostate with and without a prior history of endocrine and/or radiation therapy (Fig. 17.11, eFig. 17.52).[63,64] In the largest series reported on adenosquamous carcinomas of the prostate (33 cases from two institutions), the majority of the tumors occurred in patients with a prior established diagnosis of prostatic

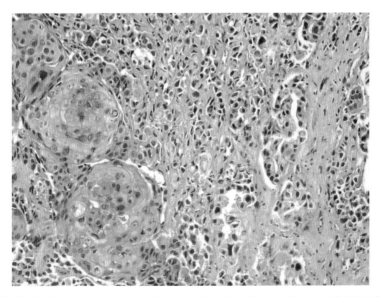

FIGURE 17.11 Adenosquamous carcinoma with both adenocarcinoma *(right)* and squamous *(left)* components.

adenocarcinoma. Approximately one-half of the patients had received prior hormonal therapy and/or radiotherapy.[65] The squamous components only rarely demonstrated focal positivity for PSA or PSAP. Diffuse positivity for high molecular weight cytokeratin was encountered in the squamous components of the tumors. The average survival was 24 months (see also Chapter 14).

Sarcomatoid Carcinoma

Sarcomatoid carcinoma (carcinosarcoma) is a rare type of prostatic cancer with approximately 100 cases reported in the literature, most reported in three large series of 42, 21, and 12 patients, respectively (Figs. 17.12 and 17.13, eFigs. 17.53 to 17.56).[66–68] Tumors are most commonly composed of an admixture of both malignant glandular and spindle cell elements, in which cases with predominantly a sarcomatoid component may be mistaken for a sarcoma. Patients with sarcomatoid carcinoma often have a history of acinar adenocarcinoma of the prostate, although in some cases, the diagnosis may have been as remote as 16 years prior. In our study, the vast majority of patients with known treatment history following the original diagnosis of acinar adenocarcinoma had received external beam radiation, brachytherapy, and/or hormone therapy.[67] The interval between the diagnosis of acinar adenocarcinoma and sarcomatoid carcinoma ranged from 6 months to 16 years (mean 6.8 years). Patients are on average about 70 years old. They typically present with urinary tract obstruction and its symptoms. On digital rectal examination, the palpable prostate is often enlarged, nodular, and hard. PSA elevations are variable.

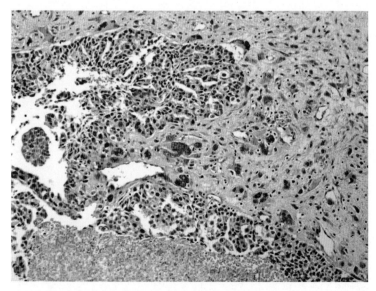

FIGURE 17.12 Sarcomatoid carcinoma with adenocarcinoma and sarcomatous stroma with pleomorphic giant cells.

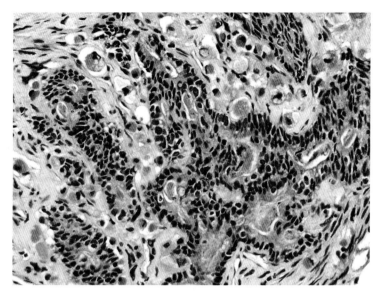

FIGURE 17.13 Sarcomatoid carcinoma with adenocarcinoma and rhabdomyosarcoma stroma.

Morphologically, sarcomatoid carcinoma demonstrates a variety of patterns. Typically, the glandular component is composed of high-grade acinar adenocarcinoma or an unusual subtype of prostatic carcinoma (small cell, foamy gland, basal cell, ductal, or adenosquamous carcinoma). The sarcomatoid component, which may account for as little as 5% of the tumor, usually demonstrates frank malignant features including hypercellularity, nuclear atypia, frequent mitoses, and focal necrosis. Bizarre tumor giant cells may be present. In approximately one-third of cases, a heterologous element such as osteosarcoma, chondrosarcoma, or rhabdomyosarcoma is encountered. We diagnose these lesions as "sarcomatoid carcinoma (carcinosarcoma)." The epithelial component consists of acinar adenocarcinoma, small cell carcinoma, ductal adenocarcinoma, and so forth, and the mesenchymal component consists of nonspecific malignant spindle cells, osteosarcoma, chondrosarcoma, and so forth. Although there is no prognostic significance to the various histologic elements present, we note them in the report so that if there are subsequent metastases with one of the elements other than usual prostatic adenocarcinoma, one would be still be able to recognize that the metastasis came from the prostatic sarcomatoid carcinoma based on its report.

Typically, the spindle component is negative for PSA. It is often at least focally positive for cytokeratin immunostains including cases with heterologous components, with desmosomes seen on electron microscopy.[67,69] The latter features further support a common origin for the sarcomatoid and carcinomatous elements rather than a collision of a sarcoma and a carcinoma. The common origin of the sarcomatoid and carcinomatous component and the fact that the prognosis is the same regardless of whether heterologous elements are present arguments for considering "carcinosarcoma" and sarcomatoid carcinoma as one entity. In support of the use of the term *sarcomatoid carcinoma*, it has been recently demonstrated that both the malignant epithelial and spindle cell components are clonally related.[70] The differential diagnosis of sarcomatoid carcinoma of the prostate is inflammatory myofibroblastic tumor (IMT) and leiomyosarcoma. The cells in IMT are uniform without pleomorphism or hyperchromasia. Although mitotic figures may be frequent, abnormal mitotic figures are not seen in IMT. Sarcomatoid carcinoma lacks the uniform fascicles of spindle cells cut in different planes of section present in leiomyosarcoma. A pitfall is that sarcomatoid carcinoma, prostatic leiomyosarcoma, and IMT can all express keratin and desmin. Although ALK immunoreactivity is positive in only two-thirds of cases of IMT, it is diagnostic of this entity. Sarcomatoid carcinoma has a poor outcome with an actuarial risk of death of 20% within the first year and frequent widespread metastases to bone, liver, and lung.[67] Sarcomatoid carcinoma is also associated with local recurrences and the formation of large pelvic masses. Sites of metastasis include, in order of frequency, the lung, bone, lymph nodes, and brain with either epithelial, mesenchymal, or both elements in metastases.

Finally, in a group of cases, there is a recent history (<2 years) of prostatic carcinoma treated with radiation with the recurrent tumor composed of pure spindle cell population. The tumor may not fit into any of the typical patterns of sarcomas that occur in the prostate (i.e., lacks long intersecting fascicles of fusiform cells of leiomyosarcoma) or may show a heterologous differentiation. Even if such tumors lack evidence of keratin expression, the likelihood is that they represent sarcomatoid carcinomas rather than true sarcomas. Postradiation sarcomas typically occur several years after treatment and it is important to remember that many overt sarcomatoid carcinomas only focally express keratin in the spindle cell component.[71,72]

Hematopoietic Tumors

Lymphomas of the prostate typically present in older men with urinary obstructive symptoms, urinary tract infections, or hematuria. Systemic symptoms are unusual.[73] Primary prostatic lymphoma with or without pelvic lymph node involvement is rare, with less than 200 cases reported in the literature. In the largest most recent series by Chu et al.,[74] only 29 cases were found among over 4,800 cases reviewed (0.6%), including 18 that were primary to the prostate or pelvic lymph nodes. Chronic lymphocytic leukemia (CLL)/small lymphocytic lymphoma (SLL) is incidentally discovered in 0.2% to 1.2% of pelvic lymph node dissections.[73] Most reported primary lymphomas have been B-cell lymphomas of the small lymphocytic, marginal zone, large cell, and small cleaved cell types with a diffuse pattern[74,75] (Figs. 17.14 and 17.15, eFigs. 17.57 to 17.63). Poorly differentiated carcinomas can also mimic large cell lymphomas

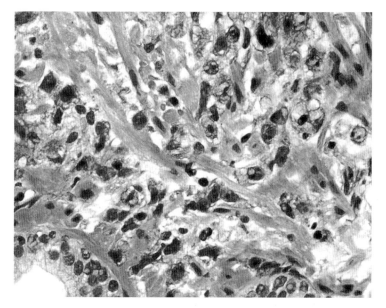

FIGURE 17.14 Large cell lymphoma.

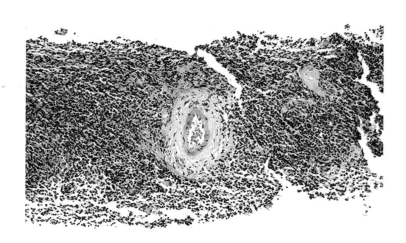

FIGURE 17.15 Small lymphocytic lymphoma.

(eFig. 17.64). The distinction between large cell lymphoma and poorly differentiated prostatic adenocarcinoma can readily be accomplished immunohistochemically with antibodies to PSA, PSAP, and lymphoid markers.

Lymphomas with a nodular pattern involving the prostate are seen infrequently (eFig. 17.65). The entire spectrum of malignant lymphomas seen in other sites may become manifest in the prostate. These include undifferentiated (Burkitt-like) lymphomas, mantle cell lymphoma, intravascular lymphoma, mucosa-associated lymphoid tissue (MALT) lymphomas, Hodgkin disease, and T-cell lymphomas, as well as rare cases of myeloma and pseudolymphoma (eFigs. 17.66 to 17.70).[75–82] Secondary involvement of the prostate and/or pelvic lymph nodes also occur rarely as part of systemic disease dissemination, with SLL/CLL being the most common type found at time of prostatic histologic examination (see the subsequent text). Malignant lymphoma involving the prostate has historically been associated with a poor prognosis, related to the generalized disease that eventually results rather than to the prostatic involvement. It is unclear whether the prognosis of prostatic lymphoma is worse or equal to nodal lymphoma (eFig 17.71). The prognosis probably depends on the histologic type and stage as in other non-Hodgkin lymphomas.[73] The most common form of leukemic involvement of the prostate is that of CLL seen in 0.2% of prostate specimens.[74,83,84] We have seen several cases where the patient was not known to be leukemic. Upon examination of tissue removed for presumed benign prostatic hyperplasia (BPH), there was a dense infiltrate of small mature round lymphocytes extensively infiltrating the prostatic stroma with preservation of prostatic glands. These lesions differed from nonspecific chronic inflammation in the prostate, where the inflammation tends to remain periglandular, is less dense, and often contains an admixture of plasma cells. After raising the possibility of a leukemic infiltrate within the prostate, these patients, upon subsequent workup, were demonstrated to have CLL. Most patients, however, with leukemic involvement of the prostate, are known leukemics or have their diagnosis established at the time of workup for urinary symptoms. It is often unclear whether the prostatic leukemic infiltrate in CLL is an incidental finding in patients with BPH or the cause of their obstructive symptoms. Treatment is not affected by prostatic involvement with CLL/SLL. Other forms of leukemia that have been described in the prostate include monocytic, granulocytic, lymphoblastic leukemias, and myeloid sarcoma.[85]

Miscellaneous Primary Tumors

Other malignant tumors of the prostate include reports of a malignant mixed tumor resembling that seen in the salivary gland,[59] endodermal sinus tumor (yolk sac tumor),[86] seminoma,[87,88] malignant mixed germ cell tumor,[89–91] rhabdoid tumor,[92] papillary cystadenocarcinoma,[93] tubulocystic clear cell adenocarcinoma as seen in the female genital tract,[94] renal-type clear cell carcinoma,[95] ectomesenchymoma with rhab-

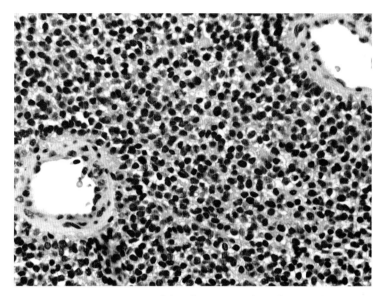

FIGURE 17.16   Peripheral neuroectodermal tumor.

domyosarcoma and ganglioneuroma,[96] peripheral neuroectodermal tumor (PNET) (Fig. 17.16),[97,98] and malignant perivascular epithelioid cell tumor (PECOMA).[99] Prostate adenocarcinomas have also been described with lymphoepithelioma-like,[100,101] pleomorphic giant cell,[102,103] and oncocytic features.[104,105] Finally, postradiation prostatic sarcomas including angiosarcoma have been reported as a rare remote complication following external beam and/or brachytherapy for prostatic adenocarcinoma.[71,72,106]

Involvement of the Prostate by Secondary Tumors

The most common tumor to secondarily infiltrate the prostate is urothelial carcinoma of the bladder (see Chapter 15). Colorectal adenocarcinomas may also directly invade the prostate. Usually, colorectal adenocarcinomas that invade the prostate are not occult, although occasionally they may present in the prostate. Adenocarcinoma of the rectum infiltrating the prostate may resemble one of the patterns of prostatic duct adenocarcinomas (Fig. 17.17, eFigs. 17.72 to 17.77) (see Chapter 11). Histologic features favoring colorectal adenocarcinoma are prominent desmoplasia, "dirty necrosis," chronic inflammatory response, tall columnar epithelium with mucin, or mucin-positive signet ring cells.[107] If there is difficulty in distinguishing colorectal adenocarcinoma from prostatic adenocarcinoma, nuclear beta-catenin and villin positivity are present in the former, with PSA, P501S, and NKX3.1 present in the latter.[108]

Excluding hematopoietic neoplasms, the prostate is rarely involved by metastatic tumor. Metastases from malignant melanoma and carcinoma of the lung predominate (eFig. 17.78).[109]

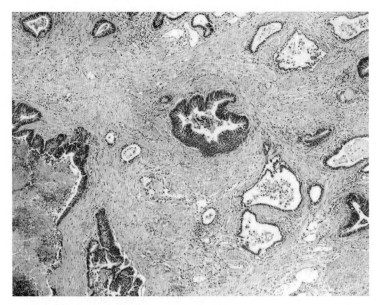

FIGURE 17.17   Adenocarcinoma of the rectum invading the prostate.

REFERENCES

1. Magri J. Cysts of the prostate gland. *Br J Urol.* 1960;32:295–301.
2. Schuhrke TD, Kaplan GW. Prostatic utricle cysts (mullerian duct cysts). *J Urol.* 1978;119:765–767.
3. Allen EA, Brinker DA, Coppola D, et al. Multilocular prostatic cystadenoma with high-grade prostatic intraepithelial neoplasia. *Urology.* 2003;61:644.
4. Hauck EW, Battmann A, Schmelz HU, et al. Giant multilocular cystadenoma of the prostate: a rare differential diagnosis of benign prostatic hyperplasia. *Urol Int.* 2004;73:365–369.
5. Lim DJ, Hayden RT, Murad T, et al. Multilocular prostatic cystadenoma presenting as a large complex pelvic cystic mass. *J Urol.* 1993;149:856–859.
6. Maluf HM, King ME, DeLuca FR, et al. Giant multilocular prostatic cystadenoma: a distinctive lesion of the retroperitoneum in men. A report of two cases. *Am J Surg Pathol.* 1991;15:131–135.
7. Yasukawa S, Aoshi H, Takamatsu M. Ectopic prostatic adenoma in retrovesical space. *J Urol.* 1987;137:998–999.
8. Patriarca C, Zucchini N, Corrada P. Giant multilocular prostate cystoadenoma: an entirely benign prostate neoplasm with some phenotypic features of malignancy. *Am J Surg Pathol.* 2005;29:1252–1254.
9. Kirkland KL, Bale PM. A cystic adenoma of the prostate. *J Urol.* 1967;97:324–327.
10. Melen DR. Multilocular cysts of the prstate. *J Urol.* 1932;27:343–349.
11. Aguilar M, Gaffney EF, Finnerty DP. Prostatic melanosis with involvement of benign and malignant epithelium. *J Urol.* 1982;128:825–827.
12. Botticelli AR, Di Gregorio C, Losi L, et al. Melanosis (pigmented melanocytosis) of the prostate gland. *Eur Urol.* 1989;16:229–232.
13. Jao W, Fretzin DF, Christ ML, et al. Blue nevus of the prostate gland. *Arch Pathol.* 1971;91:187–191.

14. Martínez Martínez CJ, García Gonzalez R, Castañeda Casanova AL. Blue nevus of the prostate: report of two new cases with immunohistochemical and electron-microscopic studies. *Eur Urol.* 1992;22:339–342.

15. Ro JY, Grignon DJ, Ayala AG, et al. Blue nevus and melanosis of the prostate. Electron-microscopic and immunohistochemical studies. *Am J Clin Pathol.* 1988;90:530–535.

16. Ryan J, Crow J. Melanin in the prostate gland. *Br J Urol.* 1988;61:455–456.

17. Wong JA, Bell DG. Primary malignant melanoma of the prostate: case report and review of the literature. *Can J Urol.* 2006;13:3053–3056.

18. Berry NE, Reese L. Malignant melanoma which had its first clinical manifestations in the prostate gland. *J Urol.* 1953;69:286–290.

19. Carris CK, McLaughlin AP III, Gittes RF. Amyloidosis of the lower genitourinary tract. *J Urol.* 1976;115:423–426.

20. Lupovitch A. The prostate and amyloidosis. *J Urol.* 1972;108:301–302.

21. Mattocks S, Molyneux AJ, Doyle P. Localised amyloidosis of the prostate. *Br J Urol.* 1993;72:655–656.

22. Wilson SK, Buchanan RD, Stone WJ, et al. Amyloid deposition in the prostate. *J Urol.* 1973;110:322–323.

23. Cross PA, Bartley CJ, McClure J. Amyloid in prostatic corpora amylacea. *J Clin Pathol.* 1992;45:894–897.

24. Drach GW. Urinary lithiasis: etiology, diagnosis and medical management. In: Walsh PC, Retik AB, Stamey TA, et al, eds. *Campbell's Urology.* 6th ed. Philadelphia, PA: WB Saunders; 1992:2142–2144.

25. Hassler O. Calcifications in the prostate gland and adjacent tissues. A combined biophysical and histological study. *Pathol Microbiol (Basel).* 1968;31:97–107.

26. Hosler GA, Epstein JI. Basal cell hyperplasia: an unusual diagnostic dilemma on prostate needle biopsies. *Hum Pathol.* 2005;36:480–485.

27. Rioux-Leclercq NC, Epstein JI. Unusual morphologic patterns of basal cell hyperplasia of the prostate. *Am J Surg Pathol.* 2002;26:237–243.

28. Baird HH, McKay HW, Kimmelstiel P. Ischemic infarction of the prostate gland. *South Med J.* 1950;43:234–240.

29. Milord RA, Kahane H, Epstein JI. Infarct of the prostate gland: experience on needle biopsy specimens. *Am J Surg Pathol.* 2000;24:1378–1384.

30. Mostofi FK, Morse WH. Epithelial metaplasia in "prostatic infarction." *AMA Arch Pathol.* 1951;51:340–345.

31. Nelson G, Culberson DE, Gardner WA Jr. Intraprostatic spermatozoa. *Hum Pathol.* 1988;19:541–544.

32. Chen X, Zhao J, Salim S, et al. Intraprostatic spermatozoa: zonal distribution and association with atrophy. *Hum Pathol.* 2006;37:345–351.

33. Beckman EN, Pintado SO, Leonard GL, et al. Endometriosis of the prostate. *Am J Surg Pathol.* 1985;9:374–379.

34. Blitz BF, Kramer CE. Lymphangiolipomatosis: a new pathological entity. *J Urol.* 1997;157:1364–1365.

35. Day DS, Carpenter HD Jr, Allsbrook WC Jr. Hair granuloma of the prostate. *Hum Pathol.* 1996;27:196–197.

36. Bretal-Laranga M, Insua-Vilarino S, Blanco-Rodriguez J, et al. Giant cell arteritis limited to the prostate. *J Rheumatol.* 1995;22:566–568.

37. Khattak AQ, Nair M, Haqqani MT, et al. Wegener's granulomatosis: prostatic involvement and recurrent urinary tract infections. *BJU Int.* 1999;84:531–532.

38. Lopez-Beltran A. Vasculitis involving the prostate: report of two cases. *Pathol Case Rev.* 1996;1:70–73.

39. Dikman SH, Toker C. Seromucinous gland ectopia within the prostatic stroma. *J Urol.* 1973;109:852–854.

40. Humphrey PA, Vollmer RT. Extramedullary hematopoiesis in the prostate. *Am J Surg Pathol.* 1991;15:486–490.

41. Nassiri M, Ghazi C, Stivers JR, et al. Ganglioneuroma of the prostate. A novel finding in neurofibromatosis. *Arch Pathol Lab Med.* 1994;118:938–939.

42. Frydman CP, Bleiweiss IJ, Unger PD, et al. Paneth cell-like metaplasia of the prostate gland. *Arch Pathol Lab Med.* 1992;116:274–276.

43. Weaver MG, Abdul-Karim FW, Srigley JR. Paneth cell-like change of the prostate. *Arch Pathol Lab Med.* 1992;116:1101–1102.

44. Weaver MG, Abdul-Karim FW, Srigley JR. Paneth cell-like change and small cell carcinoma of the prostate. Two divergent forms of prostatic neuroendocrine differentiation. *Am J Surg Pathol.* 1992;16:1013–1016.

45. Adlakha H, Bostwick DG. Paneth cell-like change in prostatic adenocarcinoma represents neuroendocrine differentiation: report of 30 cases. *Hum Pathol.* 1994;25:135–139.

46. Tamas EF, Epstein JI. Prognostic significance of paneth cell-like neuroendocrine differentiation in adenocarcinoma of the prostate. *Am J Surg Pathol.* 2006;30:980–985.

47. Cheng L, MacLennan GT, Abdul-Karim FW, et al. Eosinophilic metaplasia of the prostate: a newly described lesion distinct from other eosinophilic changes in prostatic epithelium. *Anal Quant Cytol Histol.* 2008;30:226–230.

48. Fan K, Johnson DE. Adenomatoid tumor of ejaculatory duct. *Urology.* 1985;25:653–654.

49. Mai KT, Walley V. Adenofibroma of the ejaculatory duct. *J Urol Path.* 1994;2:301–305.

50. Choi YD, Cho NH, Kwon DH, et al. Juvenile prostatic hyperplasia. *Urology.* 2005;66:881.

51. Sumiya H, Fuse H, Matsuzaki O, et al. Benign prostatic hypertrophy in a young male. *Eur Urol.* 1987;13:355–357.

52. Ali TZ, Epstein JI. Basal cell carcinoma of the prostate: a clinicopathologic study of 29 cases. *Am J Surg Pathol.* 2007;31:697–705.

53. Denholm SW, Webb JN, Howard GC, et al. Basaloid carcinoma of the prostate gland: histogenesis and review of the literature. *Histopathology.* 1992;20:151–155.

54. Frankel K, Craig JR. Adenoid cystic carcinoma of the prostate. Report of a case. *Am J Clin Pathol.* 1974;62:639–645.

55. Yang XJ, McEntee M, Epstein JI. Distinction of basaloid carcinoma of the prostate from benign basal cell lesions by using immunohistochemistry for bcl-2 and Ki-67. *Hum Pathol.* 1998;29:1447–1450.

56. McKenney JK, Amin MB, Srigley JR, et al. Basal cell proliferations of the prostate other than usual basal cell hyperplasia: a clinicopathologic study of 23 cases, including four carcinomas, with a proposed classification. *Am J Surg Pathol.* 2004;28:1289–1298.

57. Iczkowski KA, Ferguson KL, Grier DD, et al. Adenoid cystic/basal cell carcinoma of the prostate: clinicopathologic findings in 19 cases. *Am J Surg Pathol.* 2003;27:1523–1529.

58. Yang XJ, Tretiakova MS, Sengupta E, et al. Florid basal cell hyperplasia of the prostate: a histological, ultrastructural, and immunohistochemical analysis. *Hum Pathol.* 2003;34:462–470.

59. Manrique JJ, Albores-Saavedra J, Orantes A, et al. Malignant mixed tumor of the salivary-gland type, primary in the prostate. *Am J Clin Pathol.* 1978;70:932–937.

60. Schmid HP, Semjonow A, Eltze E, et al. Late recurrence of adenoid cystic carcinoma of the prostate. *Scand J Urol Nephrol.* 2002;36:158–159.

61. Little NA, Wiener JS, Walther PJ, et al. Squamous cell carcinoma of the prostate: 2 cases of a rare malignancy and review of the literature. *J Urol.* 1993;149:137–139.

62. Arva NC, Das K. Diagnostic dilemmas of squamous differentiation in prostate carcinoma case report and review of the literature. *Diagn Pathol.* 2011;6:46.

63. Bassler TJ Jr, Orozco R, Bassler IC, et al. Adenosquamous carcinoma of the prostate: case report with DNA analysis, immunohistochemistry, and literature review. *Urology.* 1999;53:832–834.

64. Mohan H, Bal A, Punia RP, et al. Squamous cell carcinoma of the prostate. *Int J Urol.* 2003;10:114–116.

65. Parwani AV, Kronz JD, Genega EM, et al. Prostate carcinoma with squamous differentiation: an analysis of 33 cases. *Am J Surg Pathol.* 2004;28:651–657.

66. Lauwers GY, Schevchuk M, Armenakas N, et al. Carcinosarcoma of the prostate. *Am J Surg Pathol.* 1993;17:342–349.

67. Hansel DE, Epstein JI. Sarcomatoid carcinoma of the prostate: a study of 42 cases. *Am J Surg Pathol.* 2006;30:1316–1321.

68. Dundore PA, Cheville JC, Nascimento AG, et al. Carcinosarcoma of the prostate. Report of 21 cases. *Cancer.* 1995;76:1035–1042.

69. Shannon RL, Ro JY, Grignon DJ, et al. Sarcomatoid carcinoma of the prostate. A clinicopathologic study of 12 patients. *Cancer.* 1992;69:2676–2682.

70. Ray ME, Wojno KJ, Goldstein NS, et al. Clonality of sarcomatous and carcinomatous elements in sarcomatoid carcinoma of the prostate. *Urology.* 2006;67:423.e5–423.e8.

71. Chandan VS, Wolsh L. Postirradiation angiosarcoma of the prostate. *Arch Pathol Lab Med.* 2003;127:876–878.

72. Brenner DJ, Curtis RE, Hall EJ, et al. Second malignancies in prostate carcinoma patients after radiotherapy compared with surgery. *Cancer.* 2000;88:398–406.

73. Taleb A, Ismaili N, Belbaraka R, et al. Primary lymphoma of the prostate treated with rituximab-based chemotherapy: a case report and review of the literature. *Cases J.* 2009;2:8875.

74. Chu PG, Huang Q, Weiss LM. Incidental and concurrent malignant lymphomas discovered at the time of prostatectomy and prostate biopsy: a study of 29 cases. *Am J Surg Pathol.* 2005;29:693–699.

75. Bostwick DG, Mann RB. Malignant lymphomas involving the prostate. A study of 13 cases. *Cancer.* 1985;56:2932–2938.

76. Chim CS, Loong F, Yau T, et al. Common malignancies with uncommon sites of presentation: case 2. Mantle-cell lymphoma of the prostate. *J Clin Oncol.* 2003;21:4456–4458.

77. Estrada PC, Scardino PL. Myeloma of the prostate: a case report. *J Urol.* 1971;106:586–587.

78. Hollenberg GM. Extraosseous multiple myeloma simulating primary prostatic neoplasm. *J Urol.* 1978;119:292–294.

79. Klotz LH, Herr HW. Hodgkin's disease of the prostate: a detailed case report. *J Urol.* 1986;135:1261–1262.

80. Peison B, Benisch B, Nicora B, et al. Acute urinary obstruction secondary to pseudolymphoma of prostate. *Urology.* 1977;10:478–479.

81. Quien ET, Wallach B, Sandhaus L, et al. Primary extramedullary leukemia of the prostate: case report and review of the literature. *Am J Hematol.* 1996;53:267–271.

82. Xu M, Yang Q, Li M, et al. Prostate involvement by intravascular large B-cell lymphoma: a case report with literature review. *Int J Surg Pathol.* 2011;19:544–547.

83. Dajani YF, Burke M. Leukemic infiltration of the prostate: a case study and clinicopathological review. *Cancer.* 1976;38:2442–2446.

84. Fehr M, Templeton A, Cogliatti S, et al. Primary manifestation of small lymphocytic lymphoma in the prostate. *Onkologie.* 2009;32:586–588.

85. Spethmann S, Heuer R, Hopfer H, et al. Myeloid sarcoma of the prostate as first clinical manifestation of acute myeloid leukaemia. *Lancet Oncol.* 2004;5:62–63.

86. Tay HP, Bidair M, Shabaik A, et al. Primary yolk sac tumor of the prostate in a patient with Klinefelter's syndrome. *J Urol.* 1995;153:1066–1069.

87. Hayman R, Patel A, Fisher C, et al. Primary seminoma of the prostate. *Br J Urol.* 1995;76:273–274.

88. Hashimoto T, Ohori M, Sakamoto N, et al. Primary seminoma of the prostate. *Int J Urol.* 2009;16:967–970.

89. Han G, Miura K, Takayama T, et al. Primary prostatic endodermal sinus tumor (yolk sac tumor) combined with a small focal seminoma. *Am J Surg Pathol.* 2003;27: 554–559.

90. Michel F, Gattegno B, Roland J, et al. Primary nonseminomatous germ cell tumor of the prostate. *J Urol.* 1986;135:597–599.

91. Namiki K, Tsuchiya A, Noda K, et al. Extragonadal germ cell tumor of the prostate associated with Klinefelter's syndrome. *Int J Urol.* 1999;6:158–161.

92. Ekfors TO, Aho HJ, Kekomaki M. Malignant rhabdoid tumor of the prostatic region. Immunohistological and ultrastructural evidence for epithelial origin. *Virchows Arch A Pathol Anat Histopathol.* 1985;406:381–388.

93. Kojima K, Uehara H, Naruo S, et al. Papillary cystadenocarcinoma of the prostate. *Int J Urol.* 1996;3:511–513.

94. Pan CC, Chiang H, Chang YH, et al. Tubulocystic clear cell adenocarcinoma arising within the prostate. *Am J Surg Pathol.* 2000;24:1433–1436.

95. Singh H, Flores-Sandoval N, Abrams J. Renal-type clear cell carcinoma occurring in the prostate. *Am J Surg Pathol.* 2003;27:407–410.

96. Govender D, Hadley GP. Ectomesenchymoma of the prostate: histological diagnostic criteria. *Pediatr Surg Int.* 1999;15:68–70.

97. Colecchia M, Dagrada G, Poliani PL, et al. Primary primitive peripheral neuro-ectodermal tumor of the prostate. Immunophenotypic and molecular study of a case. *Arch Pathol Lab Med.* 2003;127:e190–e193.

98. Wu T, Jin T, Luo D, et al. Ewing's sarcoma/primitive neuroectodermal tumour of the prostate: a case report and literature review. *Can Urol Assoc J.* 2013;7:E458–E459.

99. Pan CC, Yang AH, Chiang H. Malignant perivascular epithelioid cell tumor involving the prostate. *Arch Pathol Lab Med.* 2003;127:E96–E98.

100. Bostwick DG, Adlakha K. Lymphoepithelioma-like carcinoma of the prostate. *J Urol Path.* 1994;2:319–325.

101. Lopez-Beltran A, Cheng L, Prieto R, et al. Lymphoepithelioma-like carcinoma of the prostate. *Hum Pathol.* 2009;40:982–987.

102. Lopez-Beltran A, Eble JN, Bostwick DG. Pleomorphic giant cell carcinoma of the prostate. *Arch Pathol Lab Med.* 2005;129:683–685.

103. Parwani AV, Herawi M, Epstein JI. Pleomorphic giant cell adenocarcinoma of the prostate: report of 6 cases. *Am J Surg Pathol.* 2006;30:1254–1259.

104. Pinto JA, Gonzalez JE, Granadillo MA. Primary carcinoma of the prostate with diffuse oncocytic changes. *Histopathology.* 1994;25:286–288.

105. Fiandrino G, Lucioni M, Filippin F, et al. Prostatic adenocarcinoma with oncocytic features. *J Clin Pathol.* 2011;64:177–178.

106. Brenner DJ, Hall EJ, Curtis RE, et al. Prostate radiotherapy is associated with second cancers in many organs, not just the colorectum. *Gastroenterology.* 2005;129:773–774.

107. Osunkoya AO, Netto GJ, Epstein JI. Colorectal adenocarcinoma involving the prostate: report of 9 cases. *Hum Pathol.* 2007;38:1836–1841.

108. Bismar TA, Humphrey PA, Grignon DJ, et al. Expression of beta-catenin in prostatic adenocarcinomas: a comparison with colorectal adenocarcinomas. *Am J Clin Pathol.* 2004;121:557–563.

109. Johnson DE, Chalbaud R, Ayala AG. Secondary tumors of the prostate. *J Urol.* 1974; 112:507–508.

18

PROSTATIC URETHRAL LESIONS

PROSTATIC URETHRAL POLYPS

Prostatic urethral polyps are usually single, polypoid lesions growing into the prostatic urethra in and around the verumontanum.[1-3] These lesions typically present with gross and microscopic hematuria and frequently hematospermia, dysuria, and frequency. The lesions may occur over a wide age range, from adolescent to elderly males, with conflicting reports as to the most commonly involved age group. Several of these lesions have also been described within the bladder, usually around the trigone, where they are diagnosed as ectopic prostatic polyps. Histologically, the submucosal component of the urethral polyps is composed of stroma and prostatic glands (Figs. 18.1 and 18.2, eFig. 18.1). The glands may be closely packed, and in some areas, they may be cystically dilated at the periphery. The surface of urethral polyps is often papillary with broad papillae lined by urothelial cells, prostatic epithelial cells, or a combination of both. Rarely, these polyps have broad finger-like villous projections lined by benign prostatic epithelium. Prostatic urethral polyps are totally benign. Cases that have been reported as villous polyps of the urethra represent papillary prostatic duct adenocarcinomas.[4] In lesions reported as villous polyps, the glandular epithelium resembles the cells in colonic villous adenomas. In contrast, the cells lining prostatic urethral polyps are indistinguishable from normal prostatic glandular epithelium. Various proposals for the etiology of urethral polyps include (a) acquired lesions following instrumentation,[3] (b) persistent evagination of glandular epithelium that normally evaginates to form the prostate during embryonic development,[1,5] (c) development from the subcervical glands of Albarran,[6] (d) postpubertal hyperplasia due to hormonal stimulation,[7] (e) extrinsic hyperplasia of the prostate,[8] and (f) prolapse of the prostatic ducts in the posterior urethra.[9]

MISCELLANEOUS URETHRAL POLYPS

A rare type of urethral polyp arising in the prostatic urethra is fibroepithelial polyp (Figs. 18.3 and 18.4, eFigs. 18.2 to 18.7).[10] They are found at all ages, from the newborn to the elderly. Fibroepithelial polyps are typically lined by normal-appearing urothelium, although exceptionally by a columnar epithelial lining. There are three overall architectural patterns

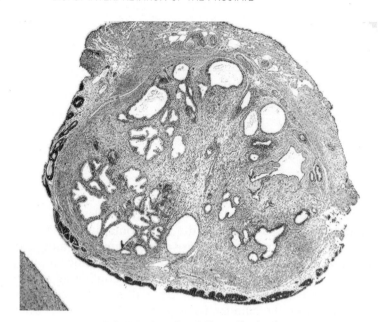

FIGURE 18.1   Prostatic urethral polyp.

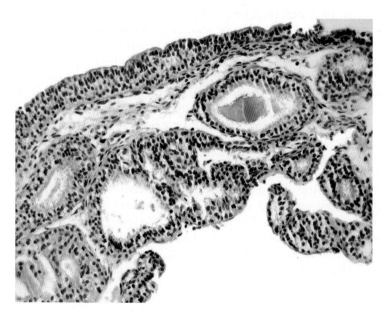

FIGURE 18.2   Prostatic urethral polyp lined both by benign urothelium and prostatic glandular epithelium.

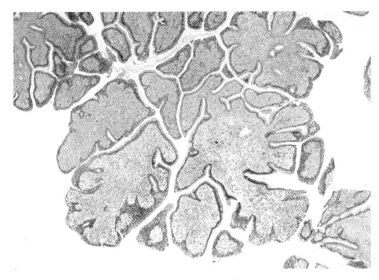

FIGURE 18.3 Fibroepithelial polyp.

seen within fibroepithelial polyps. The most common pattern consists of a polypoid mass with club-like projections resembling a clover leaf with florid cystitis cystica et glandularis of the nonintestinal type in the stalk. The second pattern is that of a papillary tumor composed of numerous small, rounded fibrovascular cores containing dense fibrous tissue. The last morphologic pattern is a polypoid lesion with secondary tall finger-like projections. All lesions lack prominent edema and inflammation seen

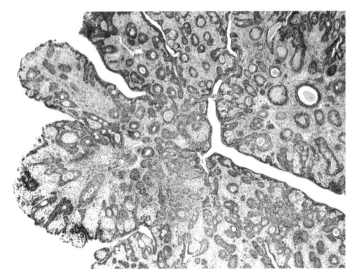

FIGURE 18.4 Fibroepithelial polyp.

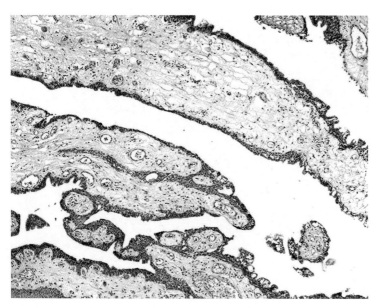

FIGURE 18.5 Polypoid urethritis.

in polypoid cystitis. Fibroepithelial polyps contain broader stalks with dense fibrous tissue, in contrast to the thin delicate loose fibroconnective tissue seen in the stalk of papillomas. Lesions can uncommonly contain atypical degenerative-appearing stromal cells. Although fibroepithelial polyps have been considered to be congenital, we think that some of these polyps could develop after birth because all of our patients first showed clinical symptoms in adulthood. Because fibroepithelial polyps in adults are rare, some of these cases can be misdiagnosed as urothelial neoplasms or reactive conditions.

Posterior urethral polyps are benign polypoid lesions arising from the verumontanum.[11] Most commonly, patients complain of urinary obstruction, hematuria, or complete urinary retention. These lesions almost exclusively occur in boys younger than 10 years of age. Histologically, they are characterized by a polypoid lesion lined by normal urothelium. The lesion has a simple morphology without branching papillae and appears to be a polypoid lesion as a result of edematous stroma.

Reactive polypoid lesions may also result in the prostatic urethra. Identical to polypoid cystitis, these lesions are termed *polypoid urethritis* (Fig. 18.5, eFig. 18.8).

NEPHROGENIC ADENOMAS

Nephrogenic adenomas usually arise in the setting of prior urothelial injury such as past surgery (60%), calculi (14%), or trauma (9%). Eight percent have a history of renal transplantation. In one-third of patients, the lesion is found in patients younger than 30 years of age. Histogenetically, nephrogenic adenomas were thought to have a metaplastic origin in reaction to prior injury and have, therefore, been also designated as nephrogenic metaplasia. Recently, an intriguing and elegant study was able to demonstrate a derivation from renal tubular cells occurring in renal transplant patients.[12] Analyzing sex chromosomes using fluorescence in situ hybridization (FISH) in nephrogenic adenomas occurring in patients who received their renal graft from an opposite sex donor, Mazal et al.[12] were able to show that all nephrogenic adenoma lesions in their study contained the donor kidney sex chromosome makeup. Additional support for nephrogenic adenomas arising from shed renal tubular cells is positivity for PAX2 and PAX8, a transcription factor expressed during renal development.[13]

Nephrogenic adenomas appear as papillary, polypoid, hyperplastic, fungating, friable, or velvety lesions. Typically found in the bladder, 12% are seen in the urethra. Most nephrogenic adenomas measure less than 1 cm, although they may attain dimensions as large as 7 cm. In 18% of cases, multiple lesions are identified. Lesions occurring in the prostatic urethra may be confused with adenocarcinoma of the prostate.[14,15]

Nephrogenic adenomas have a broad histologic spectrum (Table 18.1; eFigs. 18.9 to 18.29). The urothelial surface is often replaced by a flat

TABLE 18.1 Histology of Prostatic Urethral Nephrogenic Adenoma
• Tubules lined by cuboidal cells
• Vascular-like tubules with attenuated or hobnail cells
• Papillary fronds lined by cuboidal epithelium
• Signet-ring–like tubules with mucin
• Tubules with eosinophilic thyroid-like secretions
• Hyaline rim of connective tissue around many tubules
• Degenerative nuclear atypia
• Absent mitotic activity
• Only rare, focal, solid areas
• Only rare, focal cells with clear cytoplasm
• May show muscle involvement
• Associated with acute and chronic inflammation
• Arises in close proximity to overlying urothelium
• Staining for high molecular weight cytokeratin/p63 in over one-half of cases
• Weak immunoreactivity for PSA and PSAP
• Strong cytoplasmic positivity for AMACR
• Nuclear immunoreactivity for PAX2 and PAX8

PSA, prostate-specific antigen; PSAP, prostate-specific acid phosphatase; AMACR, alpha-methylacyl-CoA racemase.

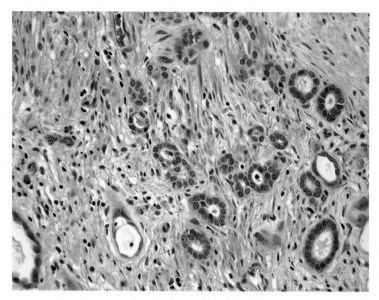

FIGURE 18.6 Nephrogenic adenoma with tubules.

cuboidal line epithelium.[13] Proliferations of small solid to hollow tubules, lined by low columnar to cuboidal epithelial cells with eosinophilic cytoplasm, are identified in the majority of cases (Fig. 18.6). Vascular-like structures with attenuated epithelium, with or without hobnail nuclei, are the second most common pattern (Fig. 18.7). Verification that these

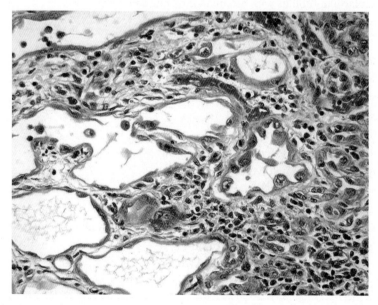

FIGURE 18.7 Nephrogenic adenoma with vascular-like structures lined by atypical hobnail epithelial cells. Note associated prominent inflammation.

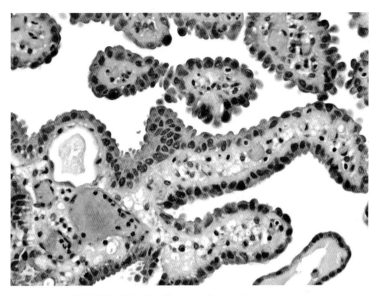

FIGURE 18.8 Papillary nephrogenic adenoma.

vascular-like structures are epithelial can be accomplished with immu-nohistochemistry for cytokeratin, which can help establish the correct diagnosis. Papillary configurations and signet-ring cell–like structures are identified in a decreasing percentage of cases (Figs. 18.8 and 18.9). A dis-tinguishing feature of nephrogenic adenoma is the presence of a thickened

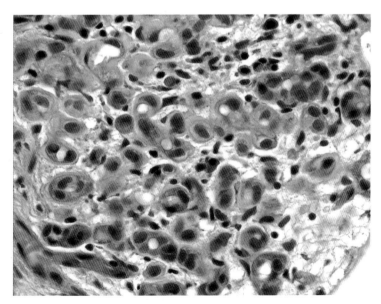

FIGURE 18.9 Nephrogenic adenoma with signet-ring cell features and hyaline sheaths. Cells also contain blue-tinged mucinous secretions.

hyaline sheath around some of the tubules, which may be enhanced with periodic acid-Schiff (PAS) stains (Fig. 18.9). Most cases of nephrogenic adenoma are composed of multiple histologic patterns, with a minority consisting of small tubules alone.

Nuclear atypia, when present, appears degenerative and mitoses are either absent or rare. Nuclei are enlarged and hyperchromatic, yet have a smudged indistinct chromatin pattern. These atypical nuclei often reside in cells with an endothelial or hobnail appearance lining vascular-like dilated tubules (Fig. 18.7). The presence of prominent nucleoli in many cases examined is also a source of possible confusion with prostate cancer. However, prominent nucleoli are usually only focally present within a lesion and often seen in association with degenerative nuclear atypia or with other features not commonly seen in prostate cancer such as hobnail-like cells or peritubular hyaline sheaths. The atypia in nephrogenic adenoma also differs from the atypia seen in clear cell adenocarcinomas of the urethra, which can, in some cases, closely resemble nephrogenic adenoma.[16] In clear cell adenocarcinomas mimicking nephrogenic adenoma, the distinguishing features are diffuse nuclear hyperchromasia, mitotic figures, and more extensive muscle invasion (Fig. 18.10).

Cystic tubules may contain thyroid-like eosinophilic secretions (Fig. 18.11). A possible source of confusion with a malignant lesion of the prostate is the presence of blue-tinged mucinous secretions within tubular lumina. However, this "blue mucin" is seen in structures such as vascular-like tubules or in lesions with other features more typical of nephrogenic

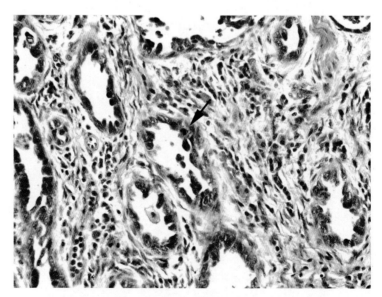

FIGURE 18.10 Clear cell adenocarcinoma mimicking nephrogenic adenoma with hyperchromatic nuclei and mitotic figure (arrow).

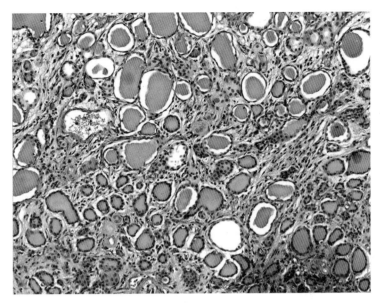

FIGURE 18.11 Nephrogenic adenoma with thyroid-like secretions.

adenoma than of prostate cancer. Nephrogenic adenomas may persist or recur in up to one-third of cases.

We have found that a majority of cases of nephrogenic adenoma arising from the prostatic urethra have some degree of muscle involvement, and in conjunction with a tubule or cord-like architectural pattern, is the most likely source of confusion with prostate cancer[15] (Fig. 18.12). Features helpful to distinguish these cases of nephrogenic adenoma from prostate cancer include the presence of more typical nephrogenic adenoma architectural patterns in other areas of the lesion and that the lesion is located immediately below the urothelial lining, a site unusual for prostate carcinoma.

A more recently described variant is fibromyxoid nephrogenic adenoma.[17] The classic tubular form of nephrogenic adenoma typically composes only a small proportion of the lesion, whereas the remainder consists of compressed spindled cells within a fibromyxoid background with only rare, tubular, and cord-like structures (Fig. 18.13). Immunohistochemistry for pancytokeratin highlights the epithelial component. Most of the patients have a history of prior radiation therapy.

The presence of an acute and/or chronic inflammatory infiltrate within tubular lumina and in association with nephrogenic adenoma structures is seen in almost all nephrogenic adenomas. This intimate association of inflammation is not a feature of most prostate cancers.

As an adjunct to the histologic features of nephrogenic adenoma, immunohistochemical staining patterns that are helpful in identifying nephrogenic adenoma and excluding prostate cancer include cytoplasmic

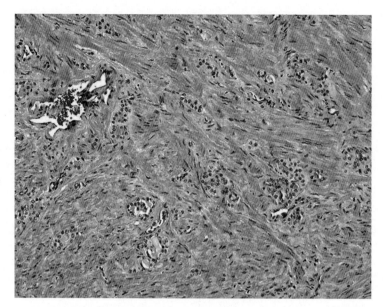

FIGURE 18.12 Nephrogenic adenoma of the prostatic urethra involving prostatic smooth muscle.

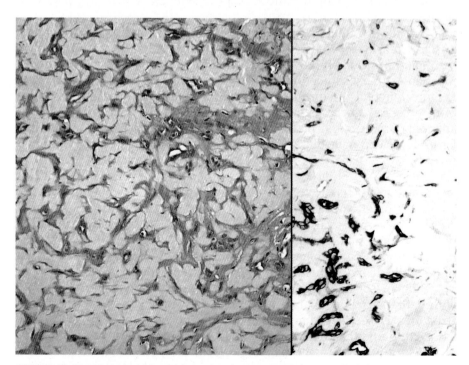

FIGURE 18.13 Fibromyxoid nephrogenic adenoma **(left)**. Pancytokeratin highlights compressed tubules **(right)**.

staining with the antibody clone directed against the high molecular weight cytokeratin (eFigs. 18.30 to 18.34). Cytoplasmic staining for high molecular weight cytokeratin is found in more than one-half of the cases of nephrogenic adenoma. Positive staining for high molecular weight cytokeratin may, therefore, help to establish the correct diagnosis of nephrogenic adenoma, but negative staining should not lead one to a misdiagnosis of prostate cancer.[18] Nephrogenic adenomas show diffuse cytokeratin 7 cytoplasmic localization. Localization of cytokeratin 7 is a sensitive method for identifying nephrogenic adenoma but lacks specificity in that some prostate cancers may show staining with this antibody.[19] Focal cytoplasmic staining and/or positive tubular secretions for prostate-specific antigen (PSA) and prostate-specific acid phosphatase (PSAP) may be seen in almost half of nephrogenic adenomas[15] (Fig. 18.14). The presence of epitopes to PSA and PSAP in nephrogenic adenoma arising from the prostatic urethra may not be surprising. The urothelium that lines this portion of the male urethra and extends into the main prostatic ducts differs histologically, and perhaps embryologically, from that of the bladder and female urethra and can elaborate both PSA and PSAP. In the absence of other diagnostic criteria, the presence of weak positive staining for PSA and/or PSAP in nephrogenic adenoma may lead to confusion with prostate cancer. However, the absence of strong immunoreactivity for PSA and/or PSAP in well-formed tubular structures would be unusual for prostate cancer and should raise the possibility of nephrogenic adenoma. Another pitfall is that alpha-methylacyl-CoA racemase (AMACR) expression can be seen in up to 58% of nephrogenic adenomas.[18,20] AMACR

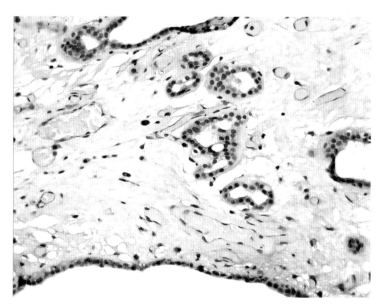

FIGURE 18.14 Nephrogenic adenoma with weak PSA immunoreactivity.

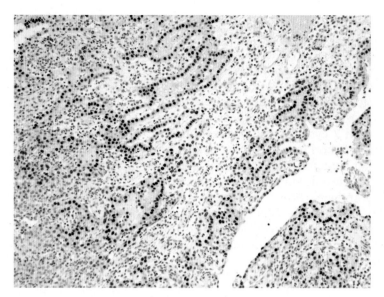

FIGURE 18.15   PAX2 positivity in nephrogenic adenoma.

reactivity coupled with negative basal cell staining (p63, high molecular weight cytokeratin) can further lead to a potential erroneous diagnosis of prostate carcinoma.[20] Fromont et al.,[21] however, report that the AMACR positivity seen in nephrogenic adenoma reflects nonspecific staining relating to a high level of endogenous biotin expression.[21] With the EnVision kit, which is biotin free, AMACR was reportedly negative in nephrogenic adenomas. PAX2 and PAX8 appear to be reliable markers for nephrogenic adenoma that can be used in this differential diagnosis, because prostate cancer lacks PAX2 and PAX8 expression[13,22] (Fig. 18.15).

Ki67 and less so p53 are helpful in differentiating clear cell adenocarcinoma from nephrogenic adenoma[16] (Fig. 18.16). Ki67 nuclear expression averages 33% (range, 10% to 80%) amongst nephrogenic adenoma–like clear cell adenocarcinoma compared to nephrogenic adenoma with an average Ki67 rate of 2% (range, 0% to 5%). p53 nuclear expression averages 4% (range, 0% to 15%) in nephrogenic adenoma–like clear cell adenocarcinoma. In contrast, the p53 nuclear expression rate was 0% in the majority of nephrogenic adenomas or 1% in a minority of cases. PAX2 and PAX8 are expressed in both nephrogenic adenoma and clear cell adenocarcinoma and are not discriminatory.

INVERTED PAPILLOMA OF THE PROSTATIC URETHRA

Although less frequent than their urinary bladder counterparts, inverted papilloma occur in the prostatic urethra (Fig. 18.17). They are usually detected incidentally as part of a workup for prostate carcinoma or benign

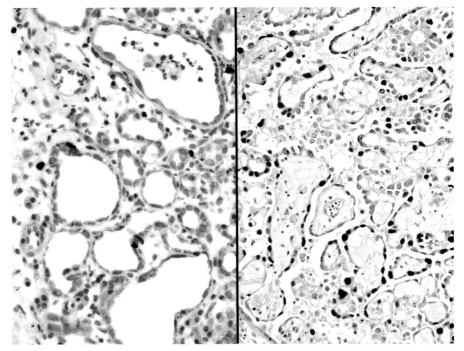

FIGURE 18.16 Nephrogenic adenoma with low Ki67 rate **(left)** compared to clear cell adenocarcinoma mimicking nephrogenic adenoma **(right)**.

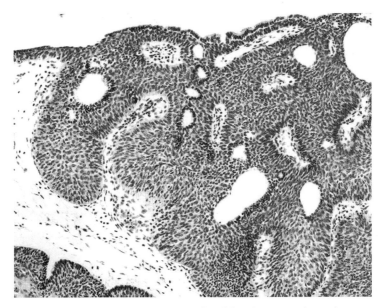

FIGURE 18.17 Inverted papilloma involving the prostatic urethra.

prostatic hyperplasia (BPH). Few cases present with gross hematuria or irritative symptoms.[23] In our series of 21 cases, none of the patients had a prior history of urothelial malignancy, whereas 2 were synchronously diagnosed with a high-grade urothelial carcinoma of the bladder. Histologically, the majority of cases display classic inverted architecture. Rare cases demonstrate focal squamous metaplasia and/or rare true papillary fronds. None of the patients with available follow-up has had a recurrence of their urethral inverted papilloma.

MISCELLANEOUS

Other lesions typically seen in the bladder can also involve the prostatic urethra, including urethral clear cell adenocarcinoma, primary amyloidosis, and paraganglioma.[24–27]

REFERENCES

1. Butterick JD, Schnitzer B, Abell MR. Ectopic prostatic tissue in urethra: a clinocopathological entity and a significant cause of hematuria. *J Urol*. 1971;105:97–104.

2. Mugler KC, Woods JE. Pathologic quiz case: urethral mass in a 62-year-old man. Prostatic-type polyp of verumontanum. *Arch Pathol Lab Med*. 2003;127:e351–e352.

3. Remick DG Jr, Kumar NB. Benign polyps with prostatic-type epithelium of the urethra and the urinary bladder. A suggestion of histogenesis based on histologic and immunohistochemical studies. *Am J Surg Pathol*. 1984;8:833–839.

4. Walker AN, Mills SE, Fechner RE, et al. 'Endometrial' adenocarcinoma of the prostatic urethra arising in a villous polyp. A light microscopic and immunoperoxidase study. *Arch Pathol Lab Med*. 1982;106:624–627.

5. Nesbit RM. The genesis of benign polyps in the prostatic urethra. *J Urol*. 1962;87: 416–418.

6. Gutierrez J, Nesbit RM. Ectopic prostatic tissue in bladder. *J Urol*. 1967;98:474–478.

7. Craig JR, Hart WR. Benign polyps with prostatic-type epithelium of the urethra. *Am J Clin Pathol*. 1975;63:343–347.

8. Goldstein AM, Bragin SD, Terry R, et al. Prostatic urethral polyps in adults: histopathologic variations and clinical manifestations. *J Urol*. 1981;126:129–131.

9. Hara S, Horie A. Prostatic caruncle: a urethral papillary tumor derived from prolapse of the prostatic duct. *J Urol*. 1977;117:303–305.

10. Tsuzuki T, Epstein JI. Fibroepithelial polyp of the lower urinary tract in adults. *Am J Surg Pathol*. 2005;29:460–466.

11. Foster RS, Garrett RA. Congenital posterior urethral polyps. *J Urol*. 1986;136:670–672.

12. Mazal PR, Schaufler R, Altenhuber-Muller R, et al. Derivation of nephrogenic adenomas from renal tubular cells in kidney-transplant recipients. *N Engl J Med*. 2002;347: 653–659.

13. Pina-Oviedo S, Shen SS, Truong LD, et al. Flat pattern of nephrogenic adenoma: previously unrecognized pattern unveiled using PAX2 and PAX8 immunohistochemistry. *Mod Pathol*. 2013;26:792–798.

14. Malpica A, Ro JY, Troncoso P, et al. Nephrogenic adenoma of the prostatic urethra involving the prostate gland: a clinicopathologic and immunohistochemical study of eight cases. *Hum Pathol*. 1994;25:390–395.

15. Allan CH, Epstein JI. Nephrogenic adenoma of the prostatic urethra: a mimicker of prostate adenocarcinoma. *Am J Surg Pathol.* 2001;25:802–808.

16. Herawi M, Drew PA, Pan CC, et al. Clear cell adenocarcinoma of the bladder and urethra: cases diffusely mimicking nephrogenic adenoma. *Hum Pathol.* 2010;41:594–601.

17. Hansel DE, Nadasdy T, Epstein JI. Fibromyxoid nephrogenic adenoma: a newly recognized variant mimicking mucinous adenocarcinoma. *Am J Surg Pathol.* 2007;31:1231–1237.

18. Gupta A, Wang HL, Policarpio-Nicolas ML, et al. Expression of alpha-methylacyl-coenzyme A racemase in nephrogenic adenoma. *Am J Surg Pathol.* 2004;28:1224–1229.

19. Genega EM, Hutchinson B, Reuter VE, et al. Immunophenotype of high-grade prostatic adenocarcinoma and urothelial carcinoma. *Mod Pathol.* 2000;13:1186–1191.

20. Skinnider BF, Oliva E, Young RH, et al. Expression of alpha-methylacyl-CoA racemase (P504S) in nephrogenic adenoma: a significant immunohistochemical pitfall compounding the differential diagnosis with prostatic adenocarcinoma. *Am J Surg Pathol.* 2004;28:701–705.

21. Fromont G, Barcat L, Gaudin J, et al. Revisiting the immunophenotype of nephrogenic adenoma. *Am J Surg Pathol.* 2009;33:1654–1658.

22. Tong GX, Melamed J, Mansukhani M, et al. PAX2: a reliable marker for nephrogenic adenoma. *Mod Pathol.* 2006;19:356–363.

23. Fine SW, Chan TY, Epstein JI. Inverted papillomas of the prostatic urethra. *Am J Surg Pathol.* 2006;30:975–979.

24. Gualco G, Ortega V, Ardao G, et al. Clear cell adenocarcinoma of the prostatic utricle in an adolescent. *Ann Diagn Pathol.* 2005;9:153–156.

25. Badalament RA, Kenworthy P, Pellegrini A, et al. Paraganglioma of urethra. *Urology.* 1991;38:76–78.

26. Vasudevan P, Stein AM, Pinn VW, et al. Primary amyloidosis of urethra. *Urology.* 1981;17:181–183.

27. Young RH, Scully RE. Clear cell adenocarcinoma of the bladder and urethra. A report of three cases and review of the literature. *Am J Surg Pathol.* 1985;9:816–826.

19

EMERGING BIOMARKERS FOR DETECTION AND MANAGEMENT OF PROSTATE CARCINOMA

Numerous molecular biomarkers have been evaluated for their potential role in predicting disease progression, response to therapy, and survival in prostate cancer patients.[1–7] These efforts have been greatly facilitated by the wealth of information garnered from gene expression array studies and by sophisticated bioinformatics tools evaluating the overwhelming datasets generated from genomic, transcriptomic, and proteomic studies. Genomic technologies are yielding new markers that can in turn be evaluated for clinical use in a high-throughput manner using immunohistochemistry (IHC) and fluorescence in situ hybridization (FISH)–labeled tissue micro-arrays and state-of-the-art image analysis systems.[8–11]

Prostate needle biopsy remains the gold standard for establishing the diagnosis of prostate carcinoma in patients with elevated serum prostate-specific antigen (PSA) and/or positive digital rectal exam. As previously pointed out in Chapter 1, the recent debate on whether current serum PSA–based screening strategies are potentially leading to "overtreatment" of at least of a subset of prostate cancer patients[12–15] has further increased the interest in pursuing new molecular markers that may help identify patients with biologically "significant" prostate cancers that calls for active therapy rather than surveillance. A parallel pursuit of clinicopathologic algorithms and criteria that can accurately predict "insignificant" prostate cancers is also gaining momentum. The latter are generally defined as tumors that lack the biologic potential to affect disease-specific mortality and morbidity within a given patient life expectancy. As alternative prostate cancer management approaches such as "active surveillance" are increasingly offered, accurate identification of insignificant prostate cancer becomes more pressing.

EMERGING PROGNOSTIC FACTORS

Firmly established parameters such as clinical stage, pathologic stage, histologic Gleason grade, and serum PSA levels are routinely used for prognostication and guidance of disease management in prostate cancer.[16–18]

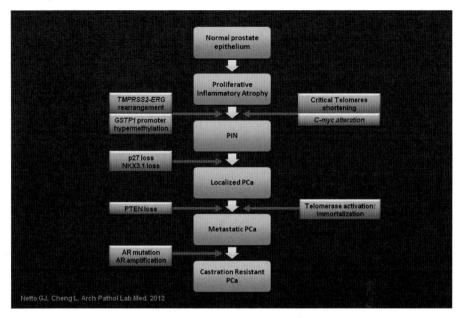

FIGURE 19.1   Somatic genetic alterations involved in the pathogenetic steps of prostate cancer progression. (Reprinted from Netto GJ, Cheng L. Emerging critical role of molecular testing in diagnostic genitourinary pathology. *Arch Path Lab Med.* 2012;136:372–390, with permission.)

As the molecular events underpinning the development of prostate cancer and the pathogenetic steps detailing the epigenetic and genetic alterations involved in the progression of prostate cancer have been brought into focus (Fig. 19.1), an extensive list of molecular biomarkers have been evaluated for their potential role in predicting disease outcome.[1,4–6,8,19–23] The wide array of molecular-based prostate cancer markers include proliferation index (ki67),[24–30] microvessel density,[31–36] nuclear morphometry,[37–40] tumor suppression genes (e.g., p53, p21, p27, NKX3.1, PTEN, retinoblastoma [Rb] gene), oncogenes (e.g., Bcl2, c-myc, EZH2, and HER2/neu), adhesion molecules (CD44, E-cadherin), PI3K/akt/mTOR pathway,[41] apoptosis regulators (e.g., surviving and transforming growth factor β1), androgen receptor status,[42] neuroendocrine differentiation markers,[43–48] and prostate tissue lineage-specific markers expression (PSA, prostate-specific acid phosphatase [PSAP], and prostate-specific membrane antigen [PSMA]). Table 19.1 lists salient genetic and epigenetic alterations in prostate cancer.

Epigenetic Changes in Prostate Cancer

Changes in DNA methylation marks, accompanied by epigenetic gene silencing, appear to be the earliest somatic genome changes in prostate cancer.[21] New generation of assay strategies for detection of specific DNA sequences carrying 5-meC offers promising opportunities for potential clinical tests for prostate cancer screening, detection, diagnosis, staging,

TABLE 19.1 Genetic and Epigenetic Alterations in Prostate Cancer		
Gene and Gene Type	**Location**	**Notes**
Tumor Suppressor Genes		
CDKN1B	12p13.1–p12	Encodes cyclin-dependent kinase inhibitor p27. One allele is frequently deleted in primary prostate cancer.
NKX3.1	8p21.2	Encodes prostate-restricted homeobox protein that can suppress the growth of prostate epithelial cells. One allele is frequently deleted in primary prostate cancer.
PTEN	10q23.31	Encodes phosphatase and tensin homologue, suppresses cell proliferation, and increases apoptosis. One allele is frequently lost in primary prostate cancer tumors. Mutations are found more frequently in metastatic prostate cancer.
TP53	17p13.1	Mutations are uncommon early but occur in about 50% of advanced or castrate-resistant prostate cancer.
Oncogenes		
MYC	8q24	Transcription factor; regulates genes involved in cell proliferation, senescence, apoptosis, and cell metabolism. mRNA levels increased in all stages. Low-level amplification of the MYC locus is common in advanced prostate cancer.
ERG	21q22.3	Fusion transcripts with the 5′ portion of androgen-regulated gene (TMPRSS22) arise from deletion or chromosomal rearrangements commonly found in prostate cancer.
ETV1–4	7p21.3, 19q13.12, 1q21,-q23, 17q21.31	Encodes ETS-like transcription factors 1–4, which are proposed to be new oncogenes for prostate cancer. Fusion transcripts with the 5′ portion of androgen-regulated gene (TMPRSS22) arise from chromosomal rearrangements commonly found in all disease stages.

TABLE 19.1 Genetic and Epigenetic Alterations in Prostate Cancer (Continued)

Gene and Gene Type	Location	Notes
Oncogenes (Continued)		
AR	Xq11–12	Encodes the androgen receptor. Protein is expressed in most prostate cancer. Locus is amplified or mutated in advanced and castrate-resistant prostate cancer.
Activation of the enzyme telomerase		Maintains telomere function and contributes to cell immortalization. Activated in most prostate cancer, mechanism of activation may be through MYC activation.
Caretaker Genes		
GSTP1	11q13	Encodes the enzyme that catalyzes the conjugation of reduced glutathione to electrophilic substrates. Functions to detoxify carcinogens. Inactivated more than 90% of prostate cancer by somatic hypermethylation of the CpG island within the upstream regulatory region.
Telomere dysfunction	Chromosome termini	Contributes to chromosomal instability. Shortened telomeres are found in more than 90% of prostatic intraepithelial neoplasia (PIN) lesions and prostate cancer lesions.
Centrosome abnormalities	N/A	Contributes to chromosomal instability. Centrosomes are structurally and numerically abnormal in most prostate cancers.
Other Somatic Changes		
PTGS2, APC, MDR1, EDNRB, RASSF1α, RARβ2	Various	The hypermethylation of CpG islands within upstream regulatory regions occurs in most primary tumors and metastatic lesions. The functional significance of these changes is not yet known.

Adapted from Netto GJ. Clinical applications of recent molecular advances in urologic malignancies: no longer chasing a "mirage"? *Adv Anat Pathol.* 2013;20:175–203; De Marzo AM, Platz EA, Sutcliffe S, et al. Inflammation in prostate carcinogenesis. *Nat Rev Cancer.* 2007;7:256–269.

and risk stratification. Hypermethylation of glutathione S-transferase-π (GSTP1) transcriptional regulatory sequences has been consistently detected in more than 90% of prostate cancers. GSTP1 encodes an enzyme responsible for detoxifying electrophiles and oxidants, thus shielding cell from genome damage. Loss of GSTP1 expression appears to be an early event in the initiation of prostatic carcinogenesis, as evidenced by the presence of GSTP1 methylation in 5% to 10% of proliferative inflammatory atrophy (PIA) lesions thought by some to be the earliest prostate cancer precursors, and in more than 70% of high-grade prostatic intraepithelial neoplasia (PIN) lesions.[49,50] In addition to GSTP1, more than 40 other genes have been shown to be altered by epigenetic hypermethylation.[51] Yegnasubramanian et al.[52,53] found hypermethylation of GSTP1, APC, RASSF1a, COX2, and MDR1 to be detected both in localized and in metastatic prostate cancer, whereas hypermethylation of other genes such as ERα, hMLH1, and p14/INK4a were more likely to be found in latter stages of prostate cancer progression, suggesting "two waves" of epigenetic alterations in prostate cancer.

ERG-ETS Gene Fusions

In 2005, Tomlins et al.[54,55] identified a recurrent chromosomal rearrangement in over one-half of their analyzed prostate cancer cases. The recurrent chromosomal rearrangements led to a fusion of the androgen-responsive promoter elements of the *TMPRSS2* gene (21q22) to one of three members of the ETS transcription factors family members *ERG*, *ETV1*, and *ETV4* located at chromosomes 21q22, 7p21, and 17q21, respectively. Although the prognostic role of assessing *TMPRSS2-ETS* rearrangements in prostate cancer tissue samples has been called into question by recent well-designed large cohort studies including ours,[56,57] the discovery had great implications in terms of furthering our understanding of the development and pathogenesis of prostate cancer and providing a new marker for molecular diagnosis in prostate cancer.[58–67] The potential diagnostic and prognostic role of detecting *TMPRSS2-ERG* fusion in postprostate massage urine samples requires further investigation.[68–70] Figure 19.2 depicts a commonly used FISH split-apart–based approach for the evaluation of ERG gene fusion.

Recently, commercial anti-ERG monoclonal antibodies became available that makes it possible to use IHC for evaluating ERG protein expression as a surrogate approach to detecting *TMPRSS2-ERG* fusion by FISH. We, and others, have demonstrated a strong correlation between ERG overexpression by IHC and ERG fusion status with over 86% sensitivity and specificity rates. ERG IHC may offer an accurate, simpler, and less costly alternative for evaluation of ERG fusion status in prostate cancer on needle biopsy and radical prostatectomy samples (Fig. 19.3).[71,72]

PI3k/mTOR Pathway

The PI3K/mammalian target of rapamycin (mTOR) pathway plays an important role in cell growth, proliferation, and oncogenesis in prostate

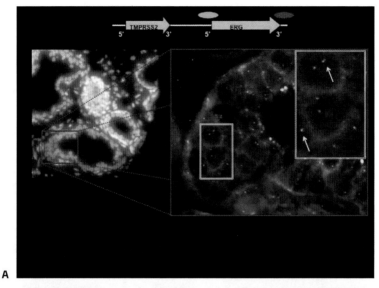

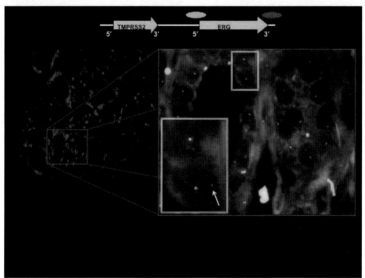

FIGURE 19.2 FISH analysis using ERG split-apart probes. The presence of juxtaposed red and green signals (occasionally forming a yellow signal) indicates lack of *TMPRSS2-ERG* fusion in the benign glands shown in **A**. Loss of green signal in one allele indicates the presence of *TMPRSS2-ERG* fusion by deletion involving 5′ ERG region as shown in the malignant glands in **B**.

cancer.[73–79] *PTEN* is a negative regulator of this pathway. Several recent well-designed retrospective studies have revealed that *loss of PTEN* tumor suppressor gene activity and the ensuing mTOR pathway activation is associated with poor prognosis in prostate cancer. In a recent large nested case–control, tissue microarray–based study from our institution, we were

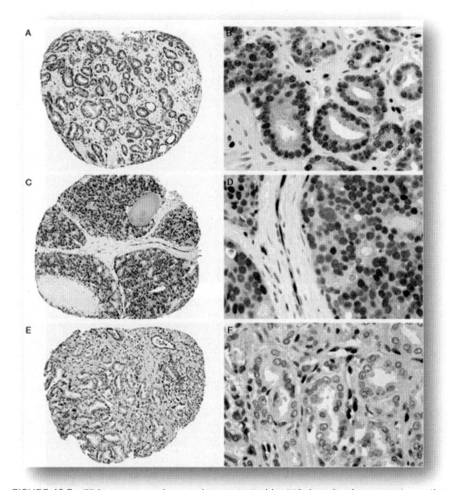

FIGURE 19.3 ERG overexpression, as demonstrated by IHC, is a simple surrogate method for evaluating *TMPRSS2-ERG* fusion in prostate adenocarcinoma. ERG-positive expression in Gleason grades 6 and 8 cases that were also positive for *TMRSS2-ERG* fusion by FISH are shown in **A**, **B**, **C**, and **D**, respectively. **E** and **F** illustrate lack of ERG expression in Gleason grade 6 tumors that lacked *TMRSS2-ERG* fusion by FISH (ERG immunostains; **A**, **C**, **E** 100×; **B**, **D**, **F** 200× magnifications).

able to show loss of immunoexpression of PTEN to be a predictor of biochemical recurrence following radical prostatectomy independent of Gleason grade, cancer stage, and other clinicopathologic parameters.[80] In a second study from our group by Lotan et al.,[81] the prognostic role of PTEN alteration was further linked to adverse pathologic features and decreased time to metastatic disease in a surgical cohort of high-risk prostate cancer patients. The correlation of PTEN immunostains with genomic loss of *PTEN* gene was also established in a later study. The mTOR pathway is also a potential target for prostate cancer treatment and several rapamycin analogs are currently being tested as potential therapeutic agents for prostate cancer.[78,82] We previously reported the results of a pilot study evaluating the pharmacodynamic efficacy of neoadjuvant rapamycin therapy in prostate cancer.[82] Using IHC analysis, we found a significant decrease in Phos-S6 protein, the main downstream effector of mTOR pathway, in patients receiving neoadjuvant mTOR inhibitor agent.[82]

Other Tumor Suppressor Genes and Oncogenes

Among tumor suppressor genes, the role of p53 expression in predicting prognosis in prostate carcinoma has been extensively studied. Brewster et al.[83] found p53 expression and Gleason score in needle biopsy to be independent predictors of biochemical relapse after radical prostatectomy. Another study found p53 status on prostatectomy but not needle biopsies to be predictive raising the issue of sampling.[84] Many studies evaluating prostatectomy specimens found p53 to be of prognostic significance independent of grade, stage, and margin status.[29,36,85-90] As discussed in the following text, more recent genome-wide studies seems to support the prognostic role of p53 alterations.[91] The majority of studies of another tumor suppressor gene p27, a cell cycle inhibitor, have also supported a correlation with progression after prostatectomy. Although less robust evidence exists for the prognostic role of p21,[92] a downstream mediator of p53, and transcription factors such as NKX3.1,[22,93] preponderance of evidence supports a prognostic role for Bcl2[25,83,85,87,89] and myc oncogenes[94,95] as potential adjuncts to histologic prognostic parameters.

It is crucially important to recognize that potential variability in performance characteristics exists even with the new molecular markers. Sources of variability include differences in molecular methodologies, tissue fixation and processing, inter- and intraobserver variability (in IHC-based biomarkers), and differences in cutoff points.[3] Furthermore, illustration of statistical significance for a particular biomarker does not alone assure its utility in a given patient. Therefore, a promising prognostic or therapeutic target biomarker should endure a rigorous "evidence-based" analysis and be validated in large size, prospective clinical trials before transition into standard practice.[96]

Integrated Genomics

In a sentinel gene expression profiling study using cDNA microarrays containing 26,000 genes, Lapointe et al.[9] identified three subclasses of prostate tumors based on distinct patterns of gene expression. High-grade and advanced stage tumors as well as tumors associated with recurrence were disproportionately represented among two of the three subtypes, one of which also included most lymph node metastases. Furthermore, two surrogate genes were differentially expressed among tumor subgroups by IHC. These included (a) *MUC1*, a gene highly expressed in the subgroups with "aggressive" clinicopathologic features and (b) *AZGP1*, a gene highly expressed in the favorable subgroup. The surrogate genes were strong predictors of tumor recurrence independent of tumor grade, stage, and preoperative PSA levels. Such a study suggests that prostate tumors can be usefully classified according to their gene expression patterns, and these tumor subtypes may provide a basis for improved prognostication and treatment stratification. Lapointe et al.[97] complemented their aforementioned gene expression findings by looking for associated copy number alterations using array-based comparative genomic hybridization (array CGH). They were able to identify recurrent copy number genetic aberrations that corresponds to three prognostically distinct groups of prostate cancer: (a) deletions at 5q21 and 6q15 deletion group associated with favorable outcome group, (b) an 8p21 (*NKX3-1*) and 21q22 (resulting in *TMPRSS2-ERG* fusion) deletion group, and (c) 8q24 (*MYC*) and 16p13 gains and loss at 10q23 (*PTEN*) and 16q23 groups correlating with metastatic disease and aggressive outcome.

In a recent genome-wide analysis of prostate cancer, Taylor et al.[98] elegantly illustrated how detailed annotation of prostate cancer genomes can impact our understanding of the disease and its treatment strategy. Assessing DNA copy number, mRNA expression, and focused exon resequencing in 218 prostate cancer tumors, the authors identified the role of nuclear receptor coactivator *NCOA2* as a novel oncogene in 11% of prostate cancer cases. *TMPRSS2-ERG* fusion was associated with novel prostate-specific deletion at chromosome 3p14 that may implicate *FOXP1*, *RYBP*, and *SHQ1* as potential cooperative tumor suppressors. Most intriguing was their ability to define clusters of low-risk and high-risk disease beyond that achieved by Gleason score using DNA copy number data. Six clusters of prostate cancer tumors are identified by unsupervised hierarchical clustering with distinct risk for biochemical recurrence.

Markert et al.[91] also illustrated the potential use of molecular signatures as a prognosticator in prostate cancer. The authors assessed microarray dataset characterizing 281 prostate cancer patients from a Swedish watchful-waiting cohort. mRNA microarray signature profiles for gene signatures reflecting embryonic stem cell (ESC), induced pluripotent stem cell (iPSC), and polycomb repressive complex-2 phenotypes (PRC2), in addition to inactivation of the tumor suppressors *p53* and *PTEN* loss and the *TMPRSS2-ERG* fusion, were assessed. Unsupervised clustering identified prostate cancer subset with "stemlike signatures" combined with *p53* and *PTEN* inactivation to be associated with very poor survival outcome. Prostate cancer tumors characterized by *TMPRSS2-ERG* fusion had intermediate survival outcome, whereas remaining groups demonstrated more favorable outcome (Fig. 19.4). The exciting findings were further validated in an independent clinical cohort at Memorial Sloan-Kettering Cancer Center. This classification was independent of Gleason score and therefore can provide additional added value in prognostication in patients with lower Gleason grade prostate cancer.

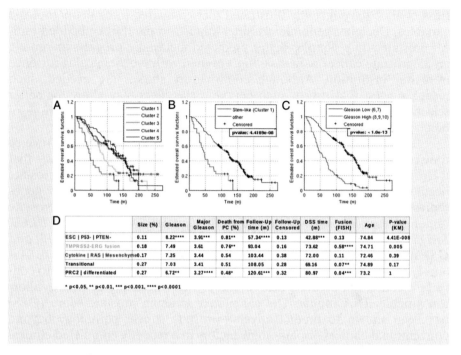

FIGURE 19.4 Clinical outcome data for Swedish watchful-waiting cohort in distinct molecular profile subgroups found by signature profiling. **A–C:** Kaplan–Meier estimates for survival functions for the different subgroups, including side-by-side comparison of survival analysis based on signature profiling **(A,B)** and Gleason score **(C)**. **D:** Clinical variables for the subgroups show a highly significant prognostic value for the stemlike subtype. Significance of assignments is indicated by asterisks adapted from reference. (Reprinted from Markert EK, Mizuno H, Vazquez A, et al. Molecular classification of prostate cancer using curated expression signatures. *Proc Natl Acad Sci U S A.* 2011;108:21276–21281, with permission.)

EMERGING MOLECULAR AND GENOMIC COMMERCIAL PROGNOSTIC ASSAYS

Genomic studies suggest that prostate cancers develop via a limited number of alternative preferred genetic pathways. The resultant molecular genetic subtypes provide a new framework for investigating prostate cancer biology and explain in part the clinical heterogeneity of the disease. Transitioning the aforementioned findings to the clinical arena will no doubt be accelerated by the increasing implementation of genomic and next-generation sequencing (NGS) technologies in clinical molecular diagnostic labs. Only few examples of such burgeoning genomic and molecular tests are discussed in the following text without implying any endorsement for their routine use. Although the role of some of these assays has been supported by initial studies, additional prospective validation studies are ongoing to justify their future implementation as standard of care. GenomeDx Decipher test[99,100] is one example of such genomic classifiers.

Ross et al.[100] have recently illustrated that compared to clinicopathologic variables, Decipher genomic classifier applied to paraffin-embedded radical prostatectomy samples better predicted metastatic progression among an 85 prostate cancer patients cohort of men with biochemical recurrence from our institution. Although confirmatory studies are needed, such results suggest that use of such genomic classifiers may allow for better selection of men requiring earlier initiation of treatment at the time of biochemical recurrence.

The Oncotype DX Prostate Cancer Assay is a multigene reverse transcriptase polymerase chain reaction (RT-PCR) expression assay that was developed for use with fixed paraffin-embedded diagnostic prostate needle biopsies. The assay evaluates the expression of 12 cancer genes representing distinct biologic pathways with a known role in prostate tumorigenesis. These include the androgen pathway (*AZGP1*, *KLK2*, *SRD5A2*, and *FAM13C*), cellular organization (*FLNC*, *GSN*, *TPM2*, *and GSTM2*), proliferation (*TPX2*), and stromal response (*BGN*, *COL1A1*, and *SFRP4*). The expression of five reference genes is also assessed to control for sources of preanalytical and analytical variability as well as allow for variable RNA inputs. The calculated genomic prostate score (GPS) has been shown to predict adverse prostate cancer pathology beyond conventional clinical or pathologic factors in a recently completed clinical validation study.[101,102]

Metamark Genetics Inc, has developed an automated, quantitative, protein-based multiplex imaging platform designated ProMark. Metamark's automated proteomics imaging platform is applied to standard formalin-fixed, paraffin-embedded tissue biopsy sections. The tissue sections are subjected to multiplex immunofluorescent staining with monoclonal antibodies as well as DAPI using a proprietary assay format that enables the quantitative biomarker measurements in the tumor epithelium regions only. Awaiting prospective validation studies, the assay could be of value in predicting indolent disease (organ confined, Gleason grade 3 = 3 or 3 + 4) in patients with positive biopsies that would hence be potential active surveillance candidates. Prospective studies are needed.

EMERGING EARLY DETECTION MARKERS AND TARGETS OF THERAPY

Markers of prostate cancer detection that can be applied to blood, urine, or prostatic secretion fluid (ejaculate or prostate massage fluids) have been the focus of active recent research. Markers that have been investigated in the urine or prostatic secretions include gene promoter hypermethylation profile assays[56,103–105] and differential display code 3 (DD3), also known as PCA3.

DD3 is a noncoding RNA that was initially identified by Bussemakers et al.[106] as one of the most specific markers of prostate cancer. PCA3 gene is

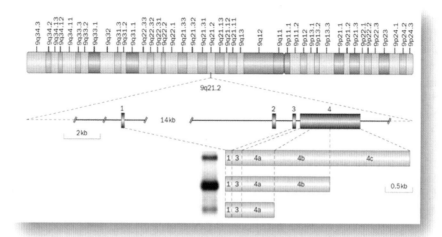

FIGURE 19.5 Structure of the PCA3/DD3 gene. The gene noncoding RNA to chromosome 9q21–22 and consists of four exons. Alternative polyadenylation at three different positions in exon 4 (indicated *4a*, *4b*, and *4c*) gives rise to three different-sized transcripts. The most frequently found transcript contains exons 1, 3, 4a, and 4b.6.

located on chromosome 9q21.2 (Fig. 19.5). Quantitative real-time RT-PCR assay detecting PCA3 can be applied to blood, urine, or prostatic fluid.[107] Evaluation of PCA3 in urine samples, obtained following an "attentive" prostate massage, using transcription-mediated amplification (TMA) technology has shown to be superior to serum PSA in predicting biopsy outcome with sensitivity and specificity approximating 70% and 80%, respectively, and a negative predictive value of 90%[108–111]; it is currently offered by commercial laboratories as a Food and Drug Administration (FDA)–approved assay in the United States. Encouraging data from the Reduction by Dutasteride of Prostate Cancer Events (REDUCE) trial support a role for evaluation of PCA3 in postattentive prostate massage urine sample in predicting positive prostate needle biopsy in immediately subsequent as well as future biopsies following initial negative biopsy. PCA3 may also have a role in predicting the risk for higher Gleason score and larger tumor volume on radical retropubic prostatectomy. If confirmed, the latter could be of great value in treatment options algorithm and delineation of candidates for active surveillance.[112–115] Multiplex urine assays to include *PCA3*, *TMPRSS2-ERG*, SPINK1, and GOLPH2 are also under evaluation with recent data suggesting an improved performance of such assays compared to *PCA3* alone.[116]

In a different approach to early detection, assays that can be applied to negative biopsy tissue samples that may help predict the presence of nonsampled "occult" prostate cancer is gaining some interest. Such approach will help alleviate the morbidity associated with repeat biopsies in patients with a negative initial biopsy triggered by elevated PSA or positive digital rectal exam. ConfirmMDx is an epigenetic assay developed by MDxHealth that assesses the methylation status of three genes: *GSTP1*, *APC*, and *RASSF1* with a multiplexed methylation-specific polymerase chain reaction (MSP) technique. A positive methylation result for any of the tested markers in any of the negative cores signify a positive test that will imply a higher risk of harboring "occult" prostate cancer. Robust prospective studies remain needed.

Finally, several markers are being investigated as potential targets of therapy for prostate cancer. The list includes tyrosine kinase receptors (e.g., epidermal growth factor receptor [EGFR]), angiogenesis targets (e.g., vascular endothelial growth factor [VEGF]),[117] fatty acid synthase (FAS),[118] PI3K/akt/mTOR,[82,119] endothelin receptors,[120,121] and PSMA,[122–125] to name a few.

In summary, a wide array of molecular markers discussed in this chapter may be utilized in the near future as adjuncts to currently established prognostic parameters and early detection markers. *PCA3* and loss of *PTEN* are two such markers that are most likely to soon gain widespread use. Current research efforts in prostate carcinoma are also focused on biologic markers that can serve as targets of therapy.

REFERENCES

1. Srigley JR, Amin M, Boccon-Gibod L, et al. Prognostic and predictive factors in prostate cancer: historical perspectives and recent international consensus initiatives. *Scand J Urol Nephrol Suppl.* 2005;216:8–19.

2. Schalken JA, Bergh A, Bono A, et al. Molecular prostate cancer pathology: current issues and achievements. *Scand J Urol Nephrol Suppl.* 2005;216:82–93.

3. Epstein JI, Amin M, Boccon-Gibod L, et al. Prognostic factors and reporting of prostate carcinoma in radical prostatectomy and pelvic lymphadenectomy specimens. *Scand J Urol Nephrol Suppl.* 2005;216:34–63.

4. DeMarzo AM, Nelson WG, Isaacs WB, et al. Pathological and molecular aspects of prostate cancer. *Lancet.* 2003;361:955–964.

5. Amin M, Boccon-Gibod L, Egevad L, et al. Prognostic and predictive factors and reporting of prostate carcinoma in prostate needle biopsy specimens. *Scand J Urol Nephrol Suppl.* 2005;216:20–33.

6. Nelson WG, De Marzo AM, Isaacs WB. Prostate cancer. *N Engl J Med.* 2003;349:366–381.

7. Netto GJ. Clinical applications of recent molecular advances in urologic malignancies: no longer chasing a "mirage"? *Adv Anat Pathol.* 2013;20:175–203.

8. Prowatke I, Devens F, Benner A, et al. Expression analysis of imbalanced genes in prostate carcinoma using tissue microarrays. *Br J Cancer.* 2007;96:82–88.

9. Lapointe J, Li C, Higgins JP, et al. Gene expression profiling identifies clinically relevant subtypes of prostate cancer. *Proc Natl Acad Sci U S A.* 2004;101:811–816.

10. Khan MA, Sokoll LJ, Chan DW, et al. Clinical utility of proPSA and "benign" PSA when percent free PSA is less than 15%. *Urology.* 2004;64:1160–1164.

11. Tomlins SA, Mehra R, Rhodes DR, et al. Integrative molecular concept modeling of prostate cancer progression. *Nat Genet.* 2007;39:41–51.

12. Andriole GL, Crawford ED, Grubb RL III, et al. Mortality results from a randomized prostate-cancer screening trial. *N Engl J Med*. 2009;360:1310–1319.

13. Andriole GL, Crawford ED, Grubb RL III, et al. Prostate cancer screening in the randomized Prostate, Lung, Colorectal, and Ovarian Cancer Screening Trial: mortality results after 13 years of follow-up. *J Natl Cancer Inst*. 2012;104:125–132.

14. Schroder FH, Hugosson J, Roobol MJ, et al. Prostate-cancer mortality at 11 years of follow-up. *N Engl J Med*. 2012;366:981–990.

15. Schroder FH, Hugosson J, Roobol MJ, et al. Screening and prostate-cancer mortality in a randomized European study. *N Engl J Med*. 2009;360:1320–1328.

16. Stephenson AJ, Scardino PT, Eastham JA, et al. Preoperative nomogram predicting the 10-year probability of prostate cancer recurrence after radical prostatectomy. *J Natl Cancer Inst*. 2006;98:715–717.

17. Stephenson AJ, Scardino PT, Eastham JA, et al. Postoperative nomogram predicting the 10-year probability of prostate cancer recurrence after radical prostatectomy. *J Clin Oncol*. 2005;23:7005–7012.

18. Partin AW, Kattan MW, Subong EN, et al. Combination of prostate-specific antigen, clinical stage, and Gleason score to predict pathological stage of localized prostate cancer. A multi-institutional update. *JAMA*. 1997;277:1445–1451.

19. De Marzo AM, DeWeese TL, Platz EA, et al. Pathological and molecular mechanisms of prostate carcinogenesis: implications for diagnosis, detection, prevention, and treatment. *J Cell Biochem*. 2004;91:459–477.

20. De Marzo AM, Platz EA, Sutcliffe S, et al. Inflammation in prostate carcinogenesis. *Nat Rev Cancer*. 2007;7:256–269.

21. Nelson WG, De Marzo AM, Yegnasubramanian S. Epigenetic alterations in human prostate cancers. *Endocrinology*. 2009;150:3991–4002.

22. Bethel CR, Faith D, Li X, et al. Decreased NKX3.1 protein expression in focal prostatic atrophy, prostatic intraepithelial neoplasia, and adenocarcinoma: association with gleason score and chromosome 8p deletion. *Cancer Res*. 2006;66:10683–10690.

23. Khan MA, Partin AW. Tissue microarrays in prostate cancer research. *Rev Urol*. 2004;6:44–46.

24. Diaz JI, Mora LB, Austin PF, et al. Predictability of PSA failure in prostate cancer by computerized cytometric assessment of tumoral cell proliferation. *Urology*. 1999;53:931–938.

25. Keshgegian AA, Johnston E, Cnaan A. Bcl-2 oncoprotein positivity and high MIB-1 (Ki-67) proliferative rate are independent predictive markers for recurrence in prostate carcinoma. *Am J Clin Pathol*. 1998;110:443–449.

26. Bubendorf L, Tapia C, Gasser TC, et al. Ki67 labeling index in core needle biopsies independently predicts tumor-specific survival in prostate cancer. *Hum Pathol*. 1998;29:949–954.

27. Bettencourt MC, Bauer JJ, Sesterhenn IA, et al. Ki-67 expression is a prognostic marker of prostate cancer recurrence after radical prostatectomy. *J Urol*. 1996;156:1064–1068.

28. Cheng L, Pisansky TM, Sebo TJ, et al. Cell proliferation in prostate cancer patients with lymph node metastasis: a marker for progression. *Clin Cancer Res*. 1999;5:2820–2823.

29. Stapleton AM, Zbell P, Kattan MW, et al. Assessment of the biologic markers p53, Ki-67, and apoptotic index as predictive indicators of prostate carcinoma recurrence after surgery. *Cancer*. 1998;82:168–175.

30. Vis AN, van Rhijn BW, Noordzij MA, et al. Value of tissue markers p27(kip1), MIB-1, and CD44s for the pre-operative prediction of tumour features in screen-detected prostate cancer. *J Pathol*. 2002;197:148–154.

31. Silberman MA, Partin AW, Veltri RW, et al. Tumor angiogenesis correlates with progression after radical prostatectomy but not with pathologic stage in Gleason sum 5 to 7 adenocarcinoma of the prostate. *Cancer*. 1997;79:772–779.

32. Strohmeyer D, Rossing C, Strauss F, et al. Tumor angiogenesis is associated with progression after radical prostatectomy in pT2/pT3 prostate cancer. *Prostate*. 2000;42:26–33.

33. Strohmeyer D, Strauss F, Rossing C, et al. Expression of bFGF, VEGF and c-met and their correlation with microvessel density and progression in prostate carcinoma. *Anticancer Res*. 2004;24:1797–1804.

34. Gettman MT, Bergstralh EJ, Blute M, et al. Prediction of patient outcome in pathologic stage T2 adenocarcinoma of the prostate: lack of significance for microvessel density analysis. *Urology*. 1998;51:79–85.

35. Gettman MT, Pacelli A, Slezak J, et al. Role of microvessel density in predicting recurrence in pathologic Stage T3 prostatic adenocarcinoma. *Urology*. 1999;54:479–485.

36. Krupski T, Petroni GR, Frierson HF Jr, et al. Microvessel density, p53, retinoblastoma, and chromogranin A immunohistochemistry as predictors of disease-specific survival following radical prostatectomy for carcinoma of the prostate. *Urology*. 2000;55: 743–749.

37. Zhang YH, Kanamaru H, Oyama N, et al. Prognostic value of nuclear morphometry on needle biopsy from patients with prostate cancer: is volume-weighted mean nuclear volume superior to other morphometric parameters? *Urology*. 2000;55:377–381.

38. Zhang YH, Kanamaru H, Oyama N, et al. Comparison of nuclear morphometric results between needle biopsy and surgical specimens from patients with prostate cancer. *Urology*. 1999;54:763–766.

39. Veltri RW, Miller MC, Partin AW, et al. Ability to predict biochemical progression using Gleason score and a computer-generated quantitative nuclear grade derived from cancer cell nuclei. *Urology*. 1996;48:685–691.

40. Khan MA, Walsh PC, Miller MC, et al. Quantitative alterations in nuclear structure predict prostate carcinoma distant metastasis and death in men with biochemical recurrence after radical prostatectomy. *Cancer*. 2003;98:2583–2591.

41. Kremer CL, Klein RR, Mendelson J, et al. Expression of mTOR signaling pathway markers in prostate cancer progression. *Prostate*. 2006;66:1203–1212.

42. Sanchez D, Rosell D, Honorato B, et al. Androgen receptor mutations are associated with Gleason score in localized prostate cancer. *BJU Int*. 2006;98:1320–1325.

43. Theodorescu D, Broder SR, Boyd JC, et al. Cathepsin D and chromogranin A as predictors of long term disease specific survival after radical prostatectomy for localized carcinoma of the prostate. *Cancer*. 1997;80:2109–2119.

44. Weinstein MH, Partin AW, Veltri RW, et al. Neuroendocrine differentiation in prostate cancer: enhanced prediction of progression after radical prostatectomy. *Hum Pathol*. 1996;27:683–687.

45. McWilliam LJ, Manson C, George NJ. Neuroendocrine differentiation and prognosis in prostatic adenocarcinoma. *Br J Urol*. 1997;80:287–290.

46. Cohen RJ, Glezerson G, Haffejee Z. Neuro-endocrine cells—a new prognostic parameter in prostate cancer. *Br J Urol*. 1991;68:258–262.

47. Casella R, Bubendorf L, Sauter G, et al. Focal neuroendocrine differentiation lacks prognostic significance in prostate core needle biopsies. *J Urol*. 1998;160:406–410.

48. Shariff AH, Ather MH. Neuroendocrine differentiation in prostate cancer. *Urology*. 2006;68:2–8.

49. Nakayama M, Bennett CJ, Hicks JL, et al. Hypermethylation of the human glutathione S-transferase-pi gene (GSTP1) CpG island is present in a subset of proliferative inflammatory atrophy lesions but not in normal or hyperplastic epithelium of the prostate: a detailed study using laser-capture microdissection. *Am J Pathol*. 2003;163:923–933.

50. Brooks JD, Weinstein M, Lin X, et al. CG island methylation changes near the GSTP1 gene in prostatic intraepithelial neoplasia. *Cancer Epidemiol Biomarkers Prev*. 1998;7:531–536.

51. Bastian PJ, Yegnasubramanian S, Palapattu GS, et al. Molecular biomarker in prostate cancer: the role of CpG island hypermethylation. *Eur Urol*. 2004;46:698–708.

52. Yegnasubramanian S, Kowalski J, Gonzalgo ML, et al. Hypermethylation of CpG islands in primary and metastatic human prostate cancer. *Cancer Res*. 2004;64:1975–1986.

53. Yegnasubramanian S, Haffner MC, Zhang Y, et al. DNA hypomethylation arises later in prostate cancer progression than CpG island hypermethylation and contributes to metastatic tumor heterogeneity. *Cancer Res*. 2008;68:8954–8967.

54. Tomlins SA, Rhodes DR, Perner S, et al. Recurrent fusion of TMPRSS2 and ETS transcription factor genes in prostate cancer. *Science*. 2005;310:644–648.

55. Tomlins SA, Mehra R, Rhodes DR, et al. TMPRSS2:ETV4 gene fusions define a third molecular subtype of prostate cancer. *Cancer Res*. 2006;66:3396–3400.

56. Toubaji A, Albadine R, Meeker AK, et al. Increased gene copy number of ERG on chromosome 21 but not TMPRSS2-ERG fusion predicts outcome in prostatic adenocarcinomas. *Mod Pathol*. 2011;24:1511–1520.

57. Gopalan A, Leversha MA, Satagopan JM, et al. TMPRSS2-ERG gene fusion is not associated with outcome in patients treated by prostatectomy. *Cancer Res*. 2009;69: 1400–1406.

58. Demichelis F, Fall K, Perner S, et al. TMPRSS2:ERG gene fusion associated with lethal prostate cancer in a watchful waiting cohort. *Oncogene*. 2007;26:4596–4599.

59. Lotan TL, Toubaji A, Albadine R, et al. TMPRSS2-ERG gene fusions are infrequent in prostatic ductal adenocarcinomas. *Mod Pathol*. 2009;22:359–365.

60. Yoshimoto M, Joshua AM, Cunha IW, et al. Absence of TMPRSS2:ERG fusions and PTEN losses in prostate cancer is associated with a favorable outcome. *Mod Pathol*. 2008;21: 1451–1460.

61. FitzGerald LM, Agalliu I, Johnson K, et al. Association of TMPRSS2-ERG gene fusion with clinical characteristics and outcomes: results from a population-based study of prostate cancer. *BMC Cancer*. 2008;8:230.

62. Mao X, Shaw G, James SY, et al. Detection of TMPRSS2:ERG fusion gene in circulating prostate cancer cells. *Asian J Androl*. 2008;10:467–473.

63. Perner S, Mosquera JM, Demichelis F, et al. TMPRSS2-ERG fusion prostate cancer: an early molecular event associated with invasion. *Am J Surg Pathol*. 2007;31:882–888.

64. Saramaki OR, Harjula AE, Martikainen PM, et al. TMPRSS2:ERG fusion identifies a subgroup of prostate cancers with a favorable prognosis. *Clin Cancer Res*. 2008;14: 3395–3400.

65. Falzarano SM, Navas M, Simmerman K, et al. ERG rearrangement is present in a subset of transition zone prostatic tumors. *Mod Pathol*. 2010;23:1499–1506.

66. Netto GJ. TMPRSS2-ERG fusion as a marker of prostatic lineage in small-cell carcinoma. *Histopathology*. 2010;57:633–634.

67. Albadine R, Latour M, Toubaji A, et al. TMPRSS2-ERG gene fusion status in minute (minimal) prostatic adenocarcinoma. *Mod Pathol*. 2009;22:1415–1422.

68. Rostad K, Hellwinkel OJ, Haukaas SA, et al. TMPRSS2:ERG fusion transcripts in urine from prostate cancer patients correlate with a less favorable prognosis. *APMIS*. 2009;117: 575–582.

69. Rice KR, Chen Y, Ali A, et al. Evaluation of the ETS-related gene mRNA in urine for the detection of prostate cancer. *Clin Cancer Res*. 2010;16:1572–1576.

70. Nguyen PN, Violette P, Chan S, et al. A panel of TMPRSS2:ERG fusion transcript markers for urine-based prostate cancer detection with high specificity and sensitivity. *Eur Urol*. 2011;59:407–414.

71. Park K, Tomlins SA, Mudaliar KM, et al. Antibody-based detection of ERG rearrangement-positive prostate cancer. *Neoplasia*. 2010;12:590–598.

72. Chaux A, Albadine R, Toubaji A, et al. Immunohistochemistry for ERG expression as a surrogate for TMPRSS2-ERG fusion detection in prostatic adenocarcinomas. *Am J Surg Pathol*. 2011;35:1014–1020.

73. Wu Y, Chhipa RR, Cheng J, et al. Androgen receptor-mTOR crosstalk is regulated by testosterone availability: implication for prostate cancer cell survival. *Anticancer Res*. 2010;30:3895–3901.

74. Bismar TA, Yoshimoto M, Vollmer RT, et al. PTEN genomic deletion is an early event associated with ERG gene rearrangements in prostate cancer. *BJU Int*. 2011;107: 477–485.

75. Bubendorf L. Words of wisdom. Re: Aberrant ERG expression cooperates with loss of PTEN to promote cancer progression in the prostate. *Eur Urol*. 2009;56:882–883.

76. Han B, Mehra R, Lonigro RJ, et al. Fluorescence in situ hybridization study shows association of PTEN deletion with ERG rearrangement during prostate cancer progression. *Mod Pathol*. 2009;22:1083–1093.

77. King JC, Xu J, Wongvipat J, et al. Cooperativity of TMPRSS2-ERG with PI3-kinase pathway activation in prostate oncogenesis. *Nat Genet*. 2009;41:524–526.

78. Sarker D, Reid AH, Yap TA, et al. Targeting the PI3K/AKT pathway for the treatment of prostate cancer. *Clin Cancer Res*. 2009;15:4799–4805.

79. Squire JA. TMPRSS2-ERG and PTEN loss in prostate cancer. *Nat Genet*. 2009;41:509–510.

80. Chaux A, Peskoe SB, Gonzalez-Roibon N, et al. Loss of PTEN expression is associated with increased risk of recurrence after prostatectomy for clinically localized prostate cancer. *Mod Pathol*. 2012;25:1543–1549.

81. Lotan TL, Gurel B, Sutcliffe S, et al. PTEN protein loss by immunostaining: analytic validation and prognostic indicator for a high risk surgical cohort of prostate cancer patients. *Clin Cancer Res*. 2011;17:6563–6573.

82. Armstrong AJ, Netto GJ, Rudek MA, et al. A pharmacodynamic study of rapamycin in men with intermediate- to high-risk localized prostate cancer. *Clin Cancer Res*. 2010;16: 3057–3066.

83. Brewster SF, Oxley JD, Trivella M, et al. Preoperative p53, bcl-2, CD44 and E-cadherin immunohistochemistry as predictors of biochemical relapse after radical prostatectomy. *J Urol*. 1999;161:1238–1243.

84. Stackhouse GB, Sesterhenn IA, Bauer JJ, et al. p53 and bcl-2 immunohistochemistry in pretreatment prostate needle biopsies to predict recurrence of prostate cancer after radical prostatectomy. *J Urol*. 1999;162:2040–2045.

85. Bauer JJ, Sesterhenn IA, Mostofi FK, et al. Elevated levels of apoptosis regulator proteins p53 and bcl-2 are independent prognostic biomarkers in surgically treated clinically localized prostate cancer. *J Urol*. 1996;156:1511–1516.

86. Bauer JJ, Sesterhenn IA, Mostofi KF, et al. p53 nuclear protein expression is an independent prognostic marker in clinically localized prostate cancer patients undergoing radical prostatectomy. *Clin Cancer Res*. 1995;1:1295–1300.

87. Moul JW, Bettencourt MC, Sesterhenn IA, et al. Protein expression of p53, bcl-2, and KI-67 (MIB-1) as prognostic biomarkers in patients with surgically treated, clinically localized prostate cancer. *Surgery*. 1996;120:159,66; discussion 166–167.

88. Osman I, Drobnjak M, Fazzari M, et al. Inactivation of the p53 pathway in prostate cancer: impact on tumor progression. *Clin Cancer Res*. 1999;5:2082–2088.

89. Theodorescu D, Broder SR, Boyd JC, et al. p53, bcl-2 and retinoblastoma proteins as long-term prognostic markers in localized carcinoma of the prostate. *J Urol*. 1997;158: 131–137.

90. Kuczyk MA, Serth J, Bokemeyer C, et al. The prognostic value of p53 for long-term and recurrence-free survival following radical prostatectomy. *Eur J Cancer*. 1998;34: 679–686.

91. Markert EK, Mizuno H, Vazquez A, et al. Molecular classification of prostate cancer using curated expression signatures. *Proc Natl Acad Sci U S A*. 2011;108: 21276–21281.

92. Lacombe L, Maillette A, Meyer F, et al. Expression of p21 predicts PSA failure in locally advanced prostate cancer treated by prostatectomy. *Int J Cancer*. 2001;95:135–139.

93. Aslan G, Irer B, Tuna B, et al. Analysis of NKX3.1 expression in prostate cancer tissues and correlation with clinicopathologic features. *Pathol Res Pract*. 2006;202:93–98.

94. Gurel B, Iwata T, Koh CM, et al. Nuclear MYC protein overexpression is an early alteration in human prostate carcinogenesis. *Mod Pathol*. 2008;21:1156–1167.

95. Gurel B, Iwata T, Koh CM, et al. Molecular alterations in prostate cancer as diagnostic, prognostic, and therapeutic targets. *Adv Anat Pathol*. 2008;15:319–331.

96. Hammond ME, Fitzgibbons PL, Compton CC, et al. College of American Pathologists Conference XXXV: solid tumor prognostic factors-which, how and so what? Summary document and recommendations for implementation. Cancer Committee and Conference Participants. *Arch Pathol Lab Med*. 2000;124:958–965.

97. Lapointe J, Li C, Giacomini CP, et al. Genomic profiling reveals alternative genetic pathways of prostate tumorigenesis. *Cancer Res*. 2007;67:8504–8510.

98. Taylor BS, Schultz N, Hieronymus H, et al. Integrative genomic profiling of human prostate cancer. *Cancer Cell*. 2010;18:11–22.

99. Karnes RJ, Bergstralh EJ, Davicioni E, et al. Validation of a genomic classifier that predicts metastasis following radical prostatectomy in an at risk patient population. *J Urol*. 2013;190:2047–2053.

100. Ross AE, Feng FY, Ghadessi M, et al. A genomic classifier predicting metastatic disease progression in men with biochemical recurrence after prostatectomy. *Prostate Cancer Prostatic Dis*. 2014;17:64–69.

101. Cooperberg M, Simko J, Falzarano S, et al. Development and validation of the biopsy-based genomic prostate score (GPS) as a predictor of high grade or extracapsular prostate cancer to improve patient selection for active surveillance. *J Urol*. 2013; 189(4):e873.

102. Knezevic D, Goddard AD, Natraj N, et al. Analytical validation of the Oncotype DX prostate cancer assay—a clinical RT-PCR assay optimized for prostate needle biopsies. *BMC Genomics*. 2013;14:690.

103. Bastian PJ, Ellinger J, Wellmann A, et al. Diagnostic and prognostic information in prostate cancer with the help of a small set of hypermethylated gene loci. *Clin Cancer Res*. 2005;11:4097–4106.

104. Bastian PJ, Nakayama M, De Marzo AM, et al. GSTP1 CpG island hypermethylation as a molecular marker of prostate cancer. *Urologe A*. 2004;43:573–579.

105. Bastian PJ, Palapattu GS, Lin X, et al. Preoperative serum DNA GSTP1 CpG island hypermethylation and the risk of early prostate-specific antigen recurrence following radical prostatectomy. *Clin Cancer Res*. 2005;11:4037–4043.

106. Bussemakers MJ, van Bokhoven A, Verhaegh GW, et al. DD3: a new prostate-specific gene, highly overexpressed in prostate cancer. *Cancer Res*. 1999;59:5975–5979.

107. de Kok JB, Verhaegh GW, Roelofs RW, et al. DD3(PCA3), a very sensitive and specific marker to detect prostate tumors. *Cancer Res*. 2002;62:2695–2698.

108. Groskopf J, Aubin SM, Deras IL, et al. APTIMA PCA3 molecular urine test: development of a method to aid in the diagnosis of prostate cancer. *Clin Chem*. 2006;52: 1089–1095.

109. Deras IL, Aubin SM, Blase A, et al. PCA3: a molecular urine assay for predicting prostate biopsy outcome. *J Urol*. 2008;179:1587–1592.

110. Haese A, de la Taille A, van Poppel H, et al. Clinical utility of the PCA3 urine assay in European men scheduled for repeat biopsy. *Eur Urol*. 2008;54:1081–1088.

111. Sokoll LJ, Ellis W, Lange P, et al. A multicenter evaluation of the PCA3 molecular urine test: pre-analytical effects, analytical performance, and diagnostic accuracy. *Clin Chim Acta*. 2008;389:1–6.

112. Aubin SM, Reid J, Sarno MJ, et al. PCA3 molecular urine test for predicting repeat prostate biopsy outcome in populations at risk: validation in the placebo arm of the dutasteride REDUCE trial. *J Urol*. 2010;184:1947–1952.

113. Nakanishi H, Groskopf J, Fritsche HA, et al. PCA3 molecular urine assay correlates with prostate cancer tumor volume: implication in selecting candidates for active surveillance. *J Urol*. 2008;179:1804,9; discussion 1809–1810.

114. van Poppel H, Haese A, Graefen M, et al. The relationship between Prostate CAncer gene 3 (PCA3) and prostate cancer significance. *BJU Int*. 2012;109:360–366.

115. Aubin SM, Reid J, Sarno MJ, et al. Prostate cancer gene 3 score predicts prostate biopsy outcome in men receiving dutasteride for prevention of prostate cancer: results from the REDUCE trial. *Urology*. 2011;78:380–385.

116. Laxman B, Morris DS, Yu J, et al. A first-generation multiplex biomarker analysis of urine for the early detection of prostate cancer. *Cancer Res*. 2008;68:645–649.

117. Kantoff P. Recent progress in management of advanced prostate cancer. *Oncology (Williston Park)*. 2005;19:631–636.

118. Pizer ES, Pflug BR, Bova GS, et al. Increased fatty acid synthase as a therapeutic target in androgen-independent prostate cancer progression. *Prostate*. 2001;47:102–110.

119. Wu L, Birle DC, Tannock IF. Effects of the mammalian target of rapamycin inhibitor CCI-779 used alone or with chemotherapy on human prostate cancer cells and xenografts. *Cancer Res*. 2005;65:2825–2831.

120. Jimeno A, Carducci M. Atrasentan: a rationally designed targeted therapy for cancer. *Drugs Today (Barc)*. 2006;42:299–312.

121. Jimeno A, Carducci M. Atrasentan: a novel and rationally designed therapeutic alternative in the management of cancer. *Expert Rev Anticancer Ther*. 2005;5:419–427.

122. Aggarwal S, Singh P, Topaloglu O, et al. A dimeric peptide that binds selectively to prostate-specific membrane antigen and inhibits its enzymatic activity. *Cancer Res*. 2006;66:9171–9177.

123. Elsasser-Beile U, Wolf P, Gierschner D, et al. A new generation of monoclonal and recombinant antibodies against cell-adherent prostate specific membrane antigen for diagnostic and therapeutic targeting of prostate cancer. *Prostate*. 2006;66:1359–1370.

124. Ikegami S, Yamakami K, Ono T, et al. Targeting gene therapy for prostate cancer cells by liposomes complexed with anti-prostate-specific membrane antigen monoclonal antibody. *Hum Gene Ther*. 2006;17:997–1005.

125. Jayaprakash S, Wang X, Heston WD, et al. Design and synthesis of a PSMA inhibitor-doxorubicin conjugate for targeted prostate cancer therapy. *Chem Med Chem*. 2006;1: 299–302.

MACROS

As described in the text, the use of macros (canned text) has many advantages. Listed in the following sections are some of the macros that we most commonly use in our diagnoses. One may alter these macros to suit individual cases or one's individual preference.

BENIGN DIAGNOSES

/BPT = Benign prostate tissue.

The macro "/BPT" is used for the diagnosis of benign tissue on prostate needle biopsy.

/BPH = Benign prostatic hyperplasia.

The macro "/BPH" is only used on transurethral resections of the prostate.

/BFM = Benign fibromuscular tissue.

/SVED = Benign portion of seminal vesicle/ejaculatory duct.

/CROWDED = Prostate tissue with focus of benign crowded glands.

The macro "/CROWDED" is used for a small cluster of glands that is not sufficiently extensive to justify the diagnosis of adenosis.

/PTAT = Benign prostate tissue with partial atrophy.

/BPTAT = Benign prostate tissue with postatrophic hyperplasia.

/ADENOSIS = Benign prostate tissue with focus of adenosis. See note.

Note: This case is characterized by a fairly well-circumscribed collection of close-packed glands of different sizes. The diagnosis of adenosis rests on the nuclear and cytoplasmic similarity of the small, crowded glands to admixed larger and more recognizably benign glands. Although adenosis mimics infiltrating adenocarcinoma architecturally, it has not been shown to have any association to carcinoma.

/BPTRT = Benign prostate tissue with radiation atypia.

/CRYST = *Note:* Studies have demonstrated that the finding of crystalloids in benign glands is not associated with a higher risk of adenocarcinoma on subsequent biopsy.

DIAGNOSES WITH ATYPIA OR PROSTATIC INTRAEPITHELIAL NEOPLASIA

/ATYP = Prostate tissue with small focus of atypical glands. See note.

Note: Although these findings are atypical and suspicious for adenocarcinoma, there is insufficient cytologic and/or architectural atypia to establish a definitive diagnosis. Repeat biopsy is recommended. (See *Urology.* 1998;52:803–807 for biopsy protocol to increase the likelihood of detecting prostate cancer after an initial atypical biopsy.)

In the macro "/ATYP," one may leave off the last two sentences concerning repeat biopsy. Some pathologists may not feel comfortable recommending the repeat biopsies. We also leave off these last two sentences in this macro when the patient is very elderly or when the patient has already had multiple biopsies in the past. We modify to /ATYPHI and ATYPLOW when the findings are highly and minimally atypical, respectively.

/ATYPNN = Prostate tissue with small focus of atypical glands.

We use the macro "/ATYPNN" in cases where there is carcinoma elsewhere in the diagnosis and we merely want to describe another focus of atypical glands.

/DAPZ = *Note:* Throughout these biopsies, there are scattered foci of mildly atypical glands. It may be that this patient's "normal" prostate has an abnormal morphology consisting of clusters of small, mildly atypical glands. We have seen several patients whose prostates show similar morphology where, on repeat biopsy, there appears to be an increased risk of cancer. Repeat biopsy is recommended. (See Diffuse adenosis of the peripheral zone in prostate needle biopsy and prostatectomy specimens. *Am J Surg Pathol.* 2008;32:1360–1366.)

/PINATYP = Focus of high-grade prostatic intraepithelial neoplasia (HGPIN) with adjacent small atypical glands. See note.

Note: Adjacent to glands of HGPIN, there are a few small adjacent atypical glands. Although these small glands may represent a microscopic focus of infiltrating cancer, we cannot exclude that they represent a tangential section or outpouchings of the adjacent PIN glands. Repeat biopsy is recommended.

/PIN = High grade prostatic intraepithelial neoplasia.

/HGPIN = *Note:* The median risk recorded in the literature for cancer following the diagnosis of HGPIN on needle biopsy is 24.1%, which is not much higher than the risk reported in the literature for a repeat biopsy following a benign diagnosis. The majority of publications that have examined in the same study the risk of cancer following a needle biopsy diagnosis of HGPIN to the risk of cancer following a benign diagnosis on needle biopsy have shown no differences between the two groups. Clinical parameters do not help in stratifying which men with HGPIN are at increased risk of being diagnosed with cancer. A major factor contributing to the decreased incidence of cancer following a diagnosis of HGPIN on needle biopsy in the contemporary era relates to increased needle biopsy core sampling, which detects many associated cancers on the initial biopsy such that rebiopsy, even with good sampling, does not detect many additional cancers. It is recommended that men do not need a routine repeat needle biopsy within the first year following the diagnosis of HGPIN on extended biopsy. It may be reasonable to perform a repeat biopsy 3 years following an initial HGPIN diagnosis on needle biopsy as a result of the uncertainty as to the long-term significance of this finding. (See *J Urology*. 2006;175:820–834; *J Urology*. 2006;175:121–124.)

/EXTPIN = As a result of multifocal HGPIN on biopsy, a repeat biopsy is recommended with relative increased sampling of the areas of pin.

/DUCTPIN = *Note:* This case is characterized by crowded glands with a complex papillary architecture and cytologic atypia. The differential diagnosis is between HGPIN and ductal adenocarcinoma. The quantity and/or complexity of these glands is beyond what is typically seen in HGPIN; however, the morphologic features are insufficient for a diagnosis of ductal adenocarcinoma. Repeat biopsy is recommended with relative increased sampling of the initial atypical site.

/LGPIN = Benign prostate tissue. See note.

Note: There are foci that may represent low-grade PIN. However, we do not diagnose low-grade PIN, because its recognition is subjective and it lacks clinical relevance.

We use the macro "/LGPIN" for cases where there is a focus that stands out at low magnification as suggestive of PIN, yet it fails to satisfy the criteria for HGPIN.

/CRIB = Atypical cribriform glands suspicious for cribriform adenocarcinoma; however, HGPIN cannot be excluded with certainty.

/PINDCIS = Atypical glands surrounded by basal cells where the differential diagnosis is between HGPIN and intraductal carcinoma of the prostate. Repeat biopsy is recommended with relative increased sampling of the initial atypical site.

/NOCAAT = Due to atrophic features, a definitive diagnosis cannot be made.

/NOCAPIN = High-grade PIN cannot be excluded with certainty.

/NOCAINF = Due to the presence of inflammation, a definitive diagnosis cannot be made.

/NOCAAD = Adenosis cannot be excluded with certainty.

/NOCACRU = In part due to mechanical distortion, a definitive diagnosis cannot be made.

The macros beginning with "/NOCA . . ." can be used at the end of an atypical macro describing why a definitive cancer diagnosis was not made (i.e., /ATYP/NOCAAT).

DIAGNOSES DESCRIBING IMMUNOHISTOCHEMISTRY FOR BASAL CELLS

/COMBOCA = *Note:* The diagnosis of carcinoma is supported by the failure of immunoperoxidase staining for high molecular weight cytokeratin and p63 to demonstrate basal cells in the atypical glands. Also favoring the diagnosis of cancer is that stains for racemase (a marker preferentially expressed in prostate cancer) are positive.

/903 = *Note:* The diagnosis of carcinoma is supported by the failure of immunoperoxidase staining for high molecular weight cytokeratin to demonstrate basal cells in the atypical glands.

/P63 = *Note:* The diagnosis of carcinoma is supported by the failure of immunoperoxidase staining for p63 to demonstrate basal cells in the atypical glands.

/COMBOATP = *Note:* By itself, negative staining for high molecular weight cytokeratin and p63 in a small focus of glands, as seen in this case, is not diagnostic of cancer. The immunohistochemical stain for alpha-methylacyl-CoA racemase (P504S) is positive. However, this marker is also found positive in the majority of HGPIN and occasional benign glands and mimickers of cancer. Therefore, a positive P504S staining does not equate to prostate cancer. (See Luo et al. *Cancer Res.* 2002;62: 2220–2226.)

/NP63903 = *Note:* In a small focus, negative staining for high molecular weight cytokeratin and p63 is not of itself diagnostic of cancer.

/PP63903 = *Note:* Stains for high molecular weight cytokeratin and p63 are positive in a patchy fashion in some of the glands.

/NEG903 = *Note:* By itself, negative staining for high molecular weight cytokeratin in a small focus is not diagnostic of cancer.

/PATCHY = *Note:* Stains for high molecular weight cytokeratin are positive in a patchy fashion in some of the glands.

/NEGP63 = *Note:* By itself, negative staining for p63 in a small focus of glands, as seen in this case, is not necessarily diagnostic of adenocarcinoma.

/PP63 = *Note:* Stains for p63 are positive in a patchy fashion in some of the glands.

/RACE = *Note:* The diagnosis of prostate cancer is supported by a positive staining for alpha-methylacyl-CoA racemase, a marker that is preferentially expressed in prostate cancer. (See *Cancer Res.* 200215:2200–2206.)

/NEGRACE = *Note:* The immunohistochemical stain for alpha-methylacyl-CoA racemase (P504S) is negative. However, this marker is not positive in 100% of prostate cancer; therefore, a negative staining does not rule out prostate cancer. (See Luo et al. *Cancer Res.* 2002,62:2220–2226.)

/POSRACE = *Note:* The immunohistochemical stain for alpha-methylacyl-CoA racemase (P504S) is positive. However, this marker is also found positive in the majority of HGPIN and occasional benign glands and mimickers of cancer. Therefore, a positive P504S staining does not equate to prostate cancer. (See Luo et al. *Cancer Res.* 2002;62(8):2220–2226.)

/FPOS903 = *Note:* Some of the small atypical glands contain a patchy basal cell layer on immunohistochemistry. These glands represent either outpouchings off of HGPIN or retention of basal cells by early cancer. Other small atypical glands are negative for basal cell markers consistent with carcinoma. (See *Am J Surg Pathol.* 2002;26:115–160.)

/903NBC = *Note:* Although stains are positive for high molecular weight cytokeratin, staining is not in a basal cell distribution.

/ABERP63 = *Note:* The tumor stains aberrantly for p63. (See Aberrant diffuse expression of p63 in adenocarcinoma of the prostate on needle biopsy and radical prostatectomy: report of 21 cases. *Am J Surg Pathol.* 2008;32:461–467.)

/COMBOB9 = *Note:* Immunoperoxidase stains for high molecular weight cytokeratin and p63 demonstrate basal cells in the glands in question, whereas stains for racemase (a marker preferentially expressed in prostate cancer) are negative, supporting a benign diagnosis.

DIAGNOSES DESCRIBING TUMOR

We have separate macros for each Gleason score; for example, the macro "/336" comes out as "adenocarcinoma of the prostate Gleason score 3 + 3 = 6."

/345 = *Note:* In cases with patterns 3, 4, and 5 on needle biopsy, the Gleason score is derived by adding the most common and highest grade patterns. (See *Am J Surg Pathol.* 2005;29:1228–1242).

/PI = Perineural invasion identified in this case.

/SKEL = The tumor is seen within skeletal muscle. The presence of tumor infiltrating skeletal muscle does not necessarily indicate extraprostatic extension.

/ATROPHIC = *Note:* The tumor has atrophic features. (See *Am J Surg Pathol.* 1997;21:289–295.)

/PSEUDO = *Note:* This tumor has features of "pseudohyperplastic carcinoma." (See *Am J Surg Pathol.* 1998;22:1239–1246.)

/FOAMY = *Note:* The tumor in areas has the appearance of foamy gland carcinoma. (See *Am J Surg Pathol.* 1996;20:419–426.)

/RTCA = *Note:* The tumor in this case shows treatment effect in that there are individual cells with abundant vacuolated cytoplasm where the nuclei show smudged chromatin and absent nucleoli. Cancers that show radiation therapy effect have in some studies been associated with a better prognosis than tumors that appear unaltered by radiation. (See *Cancer.* 2008;115:673–679)

/DUCT8 = Prostatic duct adenocarcinoma. See note.

Note: The behavior of this tumor is analogous to acinar adenocarcinoma Gleason score 4 + 4 = 8.

/DCISP = Intraductal carcinoma involving the prostate. See note.

Note: "Intraductal carcinoma" is used when there is an intraductal glandular proliferation, typically highlighted with basal cell stains, that is architecturally and/or cytologically much more atypical than HGPIN. This includes either (a) solid or dense cribriform patterns or (b) loose cribriform or micropapillary patterns with either marked nuclear atypia (nuclear size 6× normal) or comedonecrosis. Whether these lesions represent cancerization of ducts and glands by invasive carcinoma or a de novo lesion arising within the ducts, from a practical standpoint, almost all cases with similar morphology have been associated with infiltrating high-grade aggressive cancer, and definitive treatment is recommended (*Mod Pathol.* 2006;19:1528–1535.)

/PINDUCT = Prostatic ductal adenocarcinoma resembling HGPIN. See note.

Note: Usual prostatic duct adenocarcinomas tumors are analogous in their behavior to acinar adenocarcinoma, Gleason score 4 + 4 = 8. However, a recent study shows that prostatic ductal adenocarcinomas resembling HGPIN appear to behave more like acinar adenocarcinoma, Gleason score 3 + 3 = 6. On hematoxylin and eosin (H&E)–stained sections, these foci resemble HGPIN. However, in these areas, the glands are too crowded, and too many atypical glands are negative for basal cell markers.

/STUMP = Prostatic stromal tumor of uncertain malignant potential. See note.

Note: This lesion has features of a prostatic stromal tumor of uncertain malignant potential (STUMP). In some cases, STUMPs may represent a focal incidental lesion of little clinical significance. However, STUMPs may also be extensive tumors that can rapidly recur, leading to urinary obstruction. There are also rare examples of dedifferentiation of STUMPs into high-grade stromal sarcoma. Also, one can have STUMPs on transurethral resection (TUR) or biopsy where there is unsampled sarcoma in the prostate. Treatment options include (a) additional sampling in an attempt to identify the extent of the lesion and to rule out a higher grade component; (b) close clinical follow-up, especially in older men where the lesion is focally present as in this case and the lesion is nonpalpable; and (c) radical prostatectomy, especially in younger men where there is a palpable lesion or a lesion is seen on imaging and the lesion is more extensive. (See Herawi M, Epstein JI. Specialized stromal tumors of the prostate: a clinicopathologic study of 50 cases. *Am J Surg Pathol.* 2006;30(6):694–704.)

/PRGIST = *Note:* Gastrointestinal stromal tumors (GISTs) may be seen on "prostate" needle biopsy specimens, representing either sampling of

GISTs confined to the rectum or less commonly of malignant rectal GISTs extending into the prostate. Even more exceptionally, GISTs may arise from soft tissue between the prostate and the rectum. Large exophytic rectal GISTs may compress the adjacent prostate and appear on imaging studies as primary prostatic masses. One should consider performing immunohistochemistry for CD117 (c-kit) to exclude a gist before diagnosing a solitary fibrous tumor (SFT), some variants of specialized prostatic stromal tumors, cellular smooth muscle tumor, or schwannoma on prostate needle biopsy. (See Herawi M, Montgomery EA, Epstein JI. Gastrointestinal stromal tumors (GIST) on prostate needle biopsy: a clinicopathologic study of 8 cases. *Am J Surg Pathol.* 2006;30:1389–1395.)

INDEX

Page numbers followed by f indicate figures; those followed by t indicate tables.

A

Acinar (usual) adenocarcinoma,
  280–282, 281f
  mimicker of PIN, 55–60, 55f
Adenocarcinoma. *See also* and the
    specific type; Carcinoma
  antiandrogen effect, 301–302f
  apoptotic body in, 98f
  architectural features, 84–93, 85t
  atrophic, 112–113f
  clear cell, urethral, 390
  crowded glands with straight bor-
    ders, 84f, 86f
  cytoplasmic features, 98–100
  distinction from urothelial carci-
    noma, 314–323, 315–317f, 321t
  edge of core, 91f
  enlarged hyperchromatic nuclei,
    96f
  glomerulations, 106f
  grading of, 202–234
    historical background, 202–204,
      203t, 204f
  grading variants of, 223–225
  high-grade, 109
  histologic features, 104–108f,
    104–109, 104t
  infiltrative pattern on needle biopsy,
    92f
  intraluminal contents in diagnosis,
    100–104, 100–104f
  mimickers of, Gleason score 2–6,
    130–146, 131t
    adenosis, 130, 132–136f, 137t,
      138–146f
    atrophy, 148–157, 148–157f

basal cell hyperplasia, 157–164,
  158–164f
colonic mucosa, 164–165, 165f
Cowper glands, 165–166, 165–166f
mesonephric remnant hyperplasia,
  166–167, 166f
nephrogenic adenoma, 167
radiation atypia, 167
seminal vesicles, 168–169f, 168–170
verumontanum mucosal gland
  hyperplasia, 170–171, 171f
mimickers of, Gleason score 7–10,
  172–173, 172t
clear cell cribriform hyperplasia,
  171–173, 172t
nonspecific granulomatous prostatitis, 173–175, 174f
paraganglia, 175, 175f
sclerosing adenosis, 176–178f,
  176–179
signet ring lymphocytes, 179, 180f
xanthoma, 179, 180f
mitotic figures, 96f
mucinous differentiations, 291–297,
  292–294f
with neuroendocrine differentiation,
  269–270, 270f
with Paneth cell-like neuroendocrine change, 270–274, 271–274f
mucinous fibroplasia, 105f
needle biopsy, 83–84
nuclear features in diagnosis, 93–98,
  94–96
perineural invasion by, 107f
pleomorphic giant cells, 98f
prostatic duct, 254–267

radiated, 305, 306f
rectum, invasion of prostate, 371, 372f
row going across core, 90f
small atypical glands, 88–90f
small glands with amphophilic cytoplasm, 87–89f, 99f
small glands with prominent
nucleoli, 93f
wrapping around a nerve, 106f
Adenosis
diffuse, mimicker of adenocarcinoma, 146–147, 147f
mimicker of adenocarcinoma, 130,
132–136f, 137t, 138–146f
Adenosquamous carcinoma, 303f
Allergic granulomatous prostatitis, 34,
35f
AMACR (alpha-methylacyl-CoA-
racemase), 123–125
Amyloid, 357, 357f
Amyloidosis, primary, 390
Anaplastic prostate cancer, 285–286
Androgen receptor status, 393
Angiosarcoma, prostatic, 350, 351f
Antiandrogen therapy, 298–303, 299t,
300–303f
Apoptotic body, 97, 98f
Atrophic adenocarcinoma, 112–113f
antiandrogen therapy, 300f
Atrophy, mimicker of adenocarcinoma,
148–157, 148–157f
Atypical diagnosis
cancer risk after, 237–238
histology, 239–249f, 239–251
interobserver reproducibility,
236–237
on needle biopsy, 236
rebiopsy techniques after, 238
terminology, 235–236
Atypical hyperplasia. See Atypical
small acinar proliferation
Atypical small acinar proliferation
(ASAP), 235
Atypical small glands, histology,
239–249f, 239–251

B

Bacillus Calmette-Guérin (BCG)
immunotherapy, 27–29, 28f, 29f

Basal cell carcinomas, 361–365,
362–364, 363t
Basal cell hyperplasia
antiandrogen therapy, 300f
mimicker of adenocarcinoma,
157–164, 158–163f, 158t
mimicker of PIN, 51–54, 52–54f, 52t
STUMP with, 338f
Basal cells, 18, 20f, 21f
identification, 108–109
Benign prostatic hyperplasia (BPH),
16, 22–23
antiandrogen therapy, 298
Biomarkers, 392–410
Biopsy
after radical prostatectomy, 307–308,
307f
clinical correlates, 1–7
needle (see Needle biopsy)
Blastomycosis, 27
Blue nevus of the prostate, 356, 356f
Bouin, 10
BPH. See Benign prostatic hyperplasia

C

Calculi and calcification (prostatic),
357–358
Carcinoid tumor, 274–276, 275f
Carcinoma. See also Adenocarcinoma;
and the specific type
acinar, 280–282, 281f
foamy gland, 110–112f
immunohistochemical adjunctive
tests for diagnosis, 119–125
large cell neuroendocrine (LCNEC),
279–280, 279–280f
mimicking benign glands, 109–116,
110–116f
small cell, 276–279, 277f
with squamous differentiation,
365–366, 365f
Cartilaginous metaplasia, 350
Castration-resistant prostate cancer,
small cell carcinoma–like clinical presentation, 285–286
CD68, 179
CDX-2, 263
Central zone histology, mimicker of
PIN, 48–49, 49f

Chondroma, 350
Chondrosarcoma, 350
CK7, 321
CK20, 321
Clear cell cribriform hyperplasia
  mimicker adenocarcinoma, 172–173, 172t
  mimicker of PIN, 49–51f, 51
Coccidiomycosis, 27
Colonic mucosa, mimicker of
  adenocarcinoma, 164–165, 165f
Colorectal adenocarcinoma, invasion
  of prostate, 371
ConfirmMDx, 404
Cowper glands, mimickers of, Gleason
  score 2–6, 165–166, 166f
Cribriform acinar adenocarcinoma,
  74–75, 75f, 75t
Cribriform pattern
  clear cell hyperplasia, 49–51, 51
  intraductal carcinoma, 70–74f
Cryotherapy, 308–310, 309f
Cryptococcosis, 27
Cytomegalovirus, 35

D
Differential display code 3 (DD3)
  (PCA3), 402–403, 403f
Diffusion-weighted images (DWI), 2
Digital rectal examination (DRE), 1
Dihydrotestosterone (DHT), 298
DRE. *See* Digital rectal examination
Ductal adenocarcinoma
  versus IDC-P, 76t
  mimicker of PIN, 60–62, 60t, 61–62f
Dynamic contrast-enhanced images
  (DCE), 2

E
Ectomesenchymoma, 370
Ectopic salivary gland tissue, in pros-
  tate, 360
Endodermal sinus tumor (yolk sac
  tumor), 370
Endometriosis, 360
Eosinophilic metaplasia, 361f
Epigenetic changes, prostate cancer,
  393–396, 394–395t
ERG-ETS gene fusions, 396, 397–398f

Extramedullary hematopoiesis, 360
Extraprostatic expression (EPE),
  prediction, 188–189

F
F18-Fluorodeoxyglucose (FDG), 2
Finasteride, 298
Fixative, for prostate needle biopsy,
  10
Fluorescence in situ hybridization
  (FISH)
  biomarkers for prostatic carcinoma,
    392
  neuroendocrine differentiation in
    prostate cancer, 286
Foamy gland carcinoma, 109, 110–112f,
  223–224, 225f
Focal/ablative therapies, 308–310
Formalin, 10

G
Ganglioneuroma, 360, 370
Gastrointestinal stromal tumor (GIST),
  347–349, 348f
GATA3, 321
GenomeDx Decipher test, 401–402
Giant cell arteritis, 360
Gleason patterns
  5, 217f, 220–223, 220–223f
  4, 213–215f, 213–220, 217–219f
  1 and 2, 208, 209f
  reporting secondary and tertiary,
    226–227
  3, 208–213, 209–213f, 218f
Gleason score
  2005 modifications, 204–206, 206t,
    207f
  change of grade over time, 231–232
  correlation between biopsy and
    radical prostatectomy grade,
    227–229, 228t
  general applications, 206–207
  interobserver reproducibility, 229
  mimickers of
    2 to 6, 130–146, 131t
    7 to 10, 171–173, 172t
  modifications: 1974 and 1977,
    203t
  needle biopsy and, 9

original system, 203t
prognostic grouping, 229–231, 230f, 231t
reporting on biopsy, 225–227
Glomerulations, 106f
Granular cell tumor, 350
Granulomatous prostatitis, systemic, 26–27, 34

H
Hair granuloma, 360
Hemangioma, 350
Hemangiopericytoma, 350
Hematopoietic tumors, 368–370, 369f
Hematoxylin and eosin–stained sections, identification of basal cells, 108–109
Herpes zoster, 35
High-intensity focused ultrasound (HIFU), 308–310
HMWCK, 120, 122f
in urothelial carcinoma, 320
Hollande, 10
Hormonal therapy, antiandrogen, 298–300, 299t, 300–303f
HOXB13, 319
Hyperchromasia, 96f, 119
Hyperthermia, 310

I
Imaging techniques, 1–2
Immunohistochemistry (IHC)
adjunctive tests, 119–125
biomarkers for prostatic carcinoma, 392
neuroendocrine differentiation in prostate cancer, 286
Infarcts (prostatic), 358, 359f
Inflammation, acute and chronic, 25–26, 26f
Inflammatory conditions, 25–37
Inflammatory myofibroblastic tumor (IMT), 344–346, 345t, 346f
Inflammatory pseudotumor, 344
International Society of Urological Pathology, modified Gleason system, 204–206, 206t, 207f. *See also* Gleason score

Intraductal carcinoma of the prostate (IDC-P), 68–78, 68f, 69t
versus ductal adenocarcinoma, 76t
versus intraductal urothelial carcinoma, 77t
Intraductal urothelial carcinoma, *versus* IDC-P, 77t
Inverted papilloma, prostatic urethra, 388–390, 389f

L
Large cell lymphoma, 368–370, 369f
Large cell neuroendocrine carcinoma (LCNEC), 279–280, 279–280f
Leiomyoma/leiomyosarcoma, 342–343, 343f
Lipofuscin, in benign prostate, 20f
Luteinizing hormone-releasing hormone (LHRH) agonist, 299
Lymphangiolipomatosis, 360
Lymphomas, 368–370, 369f

M
Macros (canned text), 185
Magnetic resonance imaging (MRI), 2, 17
Malakoplakia, 26, 27f
Malignant fibrous histiocytoma, 350
Malignant mixed germ cell tumor, 370
Malignant mixed tumor, 370
Malignant peripheral nerve sheath tumor, 350
Malignant perivascular epithelioid cell tumor (PECOMA), 371
Malignant phyllodes tumors, 340, 341f
McNeal's anatomic model, 17
MDxHealth, 404
Median bar, 22
Melanosis, 356, 356f
Melanotic lesions, 356–357
Mesenchymal tumors and tumor-like conditions, 333–354
Mesonephric remnant hyperplasia, mimicker of adenocarcinoma, 167–168, 167f
Microvessel density, 393
Microwave thermotherapy, 308–310
Mixed neuroendocrine carcinoma—acinar adenocarcinoma, 280–282, 281f

Mucinous differentiation, 291–297, 292–294f
Mucinous fibroplasia, 105f
Multiocular cyst of the prostate, 355–356
Multiparametric MRI (mpMRI), 2
Multiple endocrine neoplasia (MEN) IIB syndrome, 275
Multiplex urine assays, 403
Mycobacterial prostatitis, 27–29
Mycotic prostatitis, 27
Myofibroblastoma, 344

N
Needle biopsy
 changes after, 310
 core location, 189–191, 190t
 direct staging on, 193–195f, 193–196
 fixative, 10
 high-grade PIN, 64–67
 incidence of atypical diagnosis, 236
 intervening unstained slides, 10–11
 limited adenocarcinoma of prostate, 83–84
 macros (canned text), 185
 number of levels, 10
 number of tissue cores, 11–12
 perineural invasion, 191–193, 191t
 processing, 10–11
 quantification of amount of cancer, 185–189
 technique, 8–10
 urothelial carcinoma, 327–328, 327f
Nephrogenic adenoma, 380–388, 382–388f
 histology, 381t
 mimicker of adenocarcinoma, 168
Neuroendocrine differentiation markers, 393
Neuroendocrine (NE) cells
 differentiation, 268–290, 269t
  Paneth cell-like, 360
 histology, 18, 21
Neurofibroma, 350
Neuron-specific enolase (NSE), 268
Neurovascular bundle (NVB), prediction, 188–189
Next-generation sequencing technologies, 401–402

NKX3.1, 286, 296, 319
Nodular fasciitis of bladder, 344
Nomograms, 193
Nonepithelial prostatic spindle cell lesions, 338t
Nonspecific granulomatous prostatitis (NSGP), 29–31, 30–32f
 mimicker of adenocarcinoma, 173–175, 174–175f
Nuclear morphometry, 393

O
Oncogenes, 393, 399
Oncotype DX Prostate Cancer Assay, 402

P
Paneth cell-like change, 270–274, 271–274f, 360
Papillary cystadenocarcinoma, 370
Paracoccidiomycosis, 27
Paraganglia, mimicker of adenocarcinoma, 175–176, 176f
Paraganglioma, 390
Pathologic stage and margins, prediction, 185–187, 186t
PCA3, 403–404
Perineural invasion, needle biopsy, 191–193, 191t
Peripheral neuroectodermal tumor (PNET), 371, 371f
Peripheral zone, diffuse adenosis, 146–147, 147f
Phytotherapy, 310
PIN. *See* Prostatic intraepithelial neoplasia
PINATYP. *See* Prostatic intraepithelial neoplasia, atypical
PI3K/mTOR pathway, 393, 396, 399
Pleomorphic giant cell carcinoma, 98f, 319f
Polyarteritis nodosa, 360
Polypoid urethritis, 380, 380f
Positron emission tomography (PET), tracers, 2
Postbiopsy granulomas, 32–34, 33f
Postneedle biopsy changes, 310
Post-teflon injection granulomas, 310

Posttreatment progression, prediction, 187
Prognostic factors, 392–401
Proliferation index (ki67), 393
Proliferation markers, 307
ProMark, Metamark Genetics, Inc, 402
Prostate
  gross anatomy, 16–18
  histology, 18–22
  involvement by secondary tumors, 371–372
  miscellaneous infections, 35–36
  miscellaneous primary tumors, 370–371
  zonal anatomy, 17f
Prostate, Lung, Colorectal, and Ovarian (PLCO) Cancer Screening Trial, 6
Prostatectomy, radical
  after cancer diagnosed postatypical biopsy, 238–239
  biopsies after, 307–308, 307f
  finding of high-grade PIN, 67–68
  Gleason score and correlation with biopsy, 227–229, 228t
  needle biopsy prediction of tumor volume, 187–188
Prostate-specific acid phosphatase (PSAP), 19, 393
Prostate-specific antigen (PSA)
  age-specific references ranges, 4
  density, 3–4
  versus emerging biomarkers for detection, 392
  markers, 393
  molecular forms, 4–5
  relation to post-therapy follow-up biopsies, 5–6
  total serum, 3
  velocity (rate of change), 4
Prostate-specific membrane antigen (PSMA)
  markers, 393
  PET tracers, 2
  urothelial carcinoma, 319
Prostatic cysts, 355
Prostatic duct adenocarcinoma, 254–267, 255–259f, 264–265f
  architectural patterns, 255t

PIN-like, 260–262f
solid papillary pattern, 263, 263f
Prostatic intraepithelial neoplasia (PIN)
  androgen deprivation effects, 302
  architecturally benign glands, 40f
  atypical (PINATYP), 250–251
    mimicker of PIN, 56–60, 56–60f
  cribriform, 45–46f
  flat high-grade, 39f, 42f
  foamy, 47f
  high-grade, 38-42, 41–42f
    clinical predictors, 65
    finding at radical prostatectomy, 67–68
    finding on TURP, 67
    incidence on needle biopsy, 63–64
    number of cores sampled, 66
    overall risk of cancer, 64–65
    pathologic predictors, 65–66
    repeat biopsy, 63-68
  link to cancer, 48
  low-grade, 38, 49f
    risk of cancer on rebiopsy, 63
  with microinvasive carcinoma, 48
  micropapillary, 43–44f
  mimickers of, 11, 17
    acinar (usual) adenocarcinoma, 55–60, 55f
    basal cell hyperplasia, 51–54, 52t, 52–54f
    central zone histology, 48–49, 49f
    clear cell cribriform hyperplasia, 49–51f, 51
    ductal adenocarcinoma, 60–62, 60t, 61–62f
  mucinous secretions, 46f
Prostatic urethral polyps, 377, 378f
Prostatitis, 25–26, 26f
  granulomatous, 26–27
  mycobacterial, 27–29
  mycotic, 27
  nonspecific granulomatous, 29–31, 30–32f
  systemic granulomatous, 34
Prostein (P501S), 319, 320f
PSA. *See* Prostate-specific antigen

PSAP. *See* Prostate-specific acid phosphatase
Pseudocystic prostate carcinoma, 116, 116f
Pseudohyperplastic adenocarcinoma, 114–116, 114–116f, 225
Pseudosarcomatous fibromyxoid tumor, 344
Pseudosarcomatous myofibroblastic proliferation, 344
p63, 120–125, 122–123f
PTEN, 403–404

R
Radiation atypia, mimicker of adeno-carcinoma, 168
Radiotherapy, 303–307, 305–306f
 distinction between benign and malignant glands, 304t
Reduction by Dutasteride of Prostate Cancer Events (REDUCE) trial, 403
Renal-type clear cell carcinoma, 370
Retention cyst, 355
Rhabdoid tumor, 370
Rhabdomyosarcoma, 349–350, 350f

S
Sarcoidosis, 26
Sarcomatoid carcinoma, 366–367f, 366–368
Schwannoma, 350
Sclerosing adenosis, mimicker of adenocarcinoma, 176–179, 177–179f
Seminal vesicles, mimicker of adenocarcinoma, 168–171, 169–170f
Seminoma, 370
Sextant biopsy technique, 8
Signet ring lymphocytes, mimicker of adenocarcinoma, 180, 180f
Small cell carcinoma, 276–279, 277f
 clinical manifestations associated with, 285t
Small lymphocytic lymphoma, 368–370, 369f
Solitary fibrous tumor (SFT), 346–347, 347f

Somatic genetic alterations, prostate cancer, 393, 393f
Sperm, in prostates, 360
Squamous metaplasia, antiandrogen therapy, 300f
Stromal nodule, 22–23, 22f
Stromal sarcomas, 333–342, 340–341f
Stromal tumors of uncertain malignant potential (STUMPs), 333–342, 334–339f
Synovial sarcoma, 350, 351f

T
TMPRSS2-ERG gene, 263, 295, 396
Transition zone biopsy, 8–9
Transitional cell carcinoma. *See* Urothelial carcinoma
Transrectal ultrasound (TRUS), 1–2
Transurethral resection of the prostate (TURP)
 in BPH, 23
 diagnosis of cancer, 116–119, 117–119f, 195–197
 high-grade PIN on, 67
 sampling of, 12–13
Tubulocystic clear cell adenocarci-noma, 370
Tumor suppression genes, 393, 399
TURP. *See* Transurethral resection of the prostate

U
Urethral polyps, 377, 379–380, 379–380f
Urothelial carcinoma, 314–332, 315–317f, 321t, 322–323f
 intraductal, 323–326, 325–326f
 primary, 328–329
 secondary infiltration of prostate, 371
 seen on needle biopsy, 327–328, 327f
Urothelial metaplasia, 18, 19f
Urothelial (transitional cells), 18

V
Vacuoles, adenocarcinoma with, 223, 224f
Vascular-targeted photodynamic therapy (PDT), 308–310

Vasculitis, involving prostate, 360,
    360f
Verumontanum mucosal gland
    hyperplasia (VMGH), mimicker
    of adenocarcinoma, 171–172,
    171f

W
Wegener granulomatosis, 360

X
Xanthoma, mimicker of adenocarci-
    noma, 180, 181f